# PROSTATE CANCER
## A NEW APPROACH TO TREATMENT AND HEALING

Dr. Emilia A. Ripoll, M.D.
Mark B. Saunders

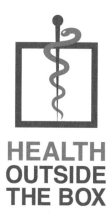

**HEALTH
OUTSIDE
THE BOX**

Emilia A. Ripoll, M.D. - Mark B. Saunders
Prostate Cancer: A New Approach To Treatment and Healing

Vital Health Press/Health Outside the Box
6899 Countryside Lane, #261
Niwot, Colorado USA
Health-OTB.com
info@health-otb.com

This 408-page book provides men who have been diagnosed with prostate can cer with the most up-to-date information about types of cancer, treatment option treatment by cancer type, success rates, complications, dealing with the emotio impact, and how to improve overall prostate health. All the information in *Prosta Cancer: A New Approach to Treatment and Healing* is presented in an easy-to- read format that is designed to make the decision-making process simple.

Cover Design by Just Designs
Inside layout & interior design by ZoeSnyder.com

To inquire about speaking engagements for Dr. Emilia A. Ripoll, M.D. and Mark E Saunders, or for bulk book purchasing information, email: mark@health-otb.com

Printed in the United States of America

# SPECIAL THANKS

*We would like to thank the following physicians for providing their stories about prostate cancer. Your perspectives added credibility, meaning, and depth.*

# TABLE OF CONTENTS

# SPECIAL SECTIONS

# GRATITUDES & DEDICATIONS

## Dr. Emilia A. Ripoll, MD

### For my family

Your patience and unconditional support have made the two years it took to complete this book easier and a lot less stressful. Thank you!

### For my patients

You continue to be my best teachers and my inspiration. Thank you for putting your trust and faith in me.

### For my patients' families

You are the silent heroes who make healing possible. Without you, recovering from prostate cancer would be a much tougher mountain to climb.

## Mark B. Saunders

### For Sophie

Your loss and your encouragement made you my shining source of inspiration and support. Thank you with all my heart.

### For Zayden

May you and all the boys of your generation grow up thinking about prostate cancer as you would smallpox — a disease that killed a lot of people a long time ago.

## Zoë Snyder

Working with Mark and Emilia on this project has proved challenging, productive, and rewarding. What I have learned as an artist and co-creator from the completion of this project has contributed to my betterment and produced a top-quality and informative book on men's health. I am grateful to both of you for your diligence, support, and heart.

# PROSTATE CANCER
## IS *NOT* A DEATH SENTENCE

> "" Everything should be made
> as simple as possible,
> but not simpler.
> — *Albert Einstein*

# Patient Story

## MARK

*Prostates are tricky. They get a bad rap for being the little gland that brings big trouble. Maybe that's because we know so little about them.*

*As a 10-year prostate cancer survivor, I have come to see my prostate as a canary in a coal mine. I think of it as a barometer for my overall health & wellness, especially the health of all the organs in my pelvis.*

*If you are "sick in the prostate," then there's a good chance something's wrong with your overall health that prevents your immune system from kickin' cancer's butt.*

*Here's a Top-5 list of what I've learned from prostate cancer in 10 years:*

*1. Listen to your intuition — especially if you don't like the message. That's the Big Kahuna talking.*

*2. Take an active role in your healing. Moving from cancer victim to cancer victor requires daily effort.*

*3. Take a 360° approach to finding the help you need. Be relentless. Explore unfamiliar territory.*

*4. Doctors can work wonders, but you're the one who has to decide which treatment option is right for YOU. It's your body, your life, your decision!*

*5. Even though a prostate cancer diagnosis feels like getting whopped upside the head by the cosmic 2 x 4, if you are willing to embrace this healing challenge, it can be the gift that allows you to peel away the old patterns that no longer serve you and embrace the man you always wanted to be.*

# INTRODUCTION

If you're reading the introduction to this book (which many people skip), you're probably not lounging on the sofa on a quiet Sunday morning with cup of coffee, wondering if today would be a good day for a bike ride.

In order to be motivated enough to open this book, one of four events recently happened:

1. You were diagnosed with prostate cancer
2. Your doctor told you that either a PSA test or a digital rectal exam (or both) found some areas of concern
3. Someone you know was just diagnosed with prostate cancer
4. Someone gave you this book because prostate cancer runs in your family

Regardless of which of these events best describes your situation, you're understandably concerned, perhaps even "freaked out." That's normal.

Since this book is about helping men gain a better understanding about prostate cancer and how to treat it, let's skip the fluffy stuff and get down to it.

## OUR GOAL

We seek to empower you to ask the right questions and make informed decisions. As advocates for prostate health and wellness, we do NOT have a stake in which types of treatment you choose, as long as they are the best one for you.

## OUR PURPOSE

We hope to provide men, their families, and their support network with the most up-to-date information about prostate cancer in an easy-to-read format.

This book is not intended as a stand-alone medical guide. Specific medical information about the health of your prostate should come from conversations with your healthcare providers. We encourage you to use this book as a point of departure for those discussions.

## THE EVOLUTION

The effectiveness of PSA blood tests is inarguable. This statement is confirmed by a 2002 study of 2,042 prostate cancer patients at the Walter Reed Army Medical Center between 1988 and 1998. In this study, the percentage of men who were initially diagnosed with metastatic prostate cancer (disease that had already spread outside the prostate) decreased from 17 percent from 1988 to 1990 to 4 percent from 1996 to 1998. The percentage of patients who, on initial evaluation, had prostate cancer that extending through the prostate capsule or into adjacent structures fell from 15 to 6 percent over the same period (1988 - 1998).

PSA blood testing is one of the primary reasons for this dramatic decrease in the number of men who have metastatic disease when they are first diagnosed.

PSA testing allows for early detection of the kind of prostate cancer that is likely to become metastatic disease. Since the early 1990s, PSA testing has saved untold lives and prevented needless suffering all over the world.

PSA testing remains a powerful tool in the battle against prostate cancer; however, it has its limitations. For example, elevated PSA numbers do not identify the culprit. Infection (prostatitis), enlarged prostate (BPH), and pelvic floor issues have raised the PSA of countless men who did NOT have prostate cancer, which led them to undergo an unnecessary prostate biopsy.

Today, we are entering a new era in prostate cancer prevention, detection, and treatment. This next generation of prostate care provides doctors and patients with new tests and tools that pick up where PSA testing leaves off.

These tests and tools help doctors find hidden cancers and identify potentially deadly cancers while they are still in their infancy — when their cure rate is highest.

These new tests also identify men with low-risk, low volume cancers who do not need the same level of treatment as men with moderate-to-high risk cancers — effectively reducing the number of unwanted complications and side effects (See **Chapter 2**).

## HOW THIS BOOK IS LAID OUT

# THIS BOOK IS DIVIDED INTO THREE SECTIONS

## THE BASICS | TOOLBOX | DIGGING DEEPER

**The Basics** distills complex medical ideas and presents the information you need to know in a simple and direct way. This "in a nutshell" approach helps you understand the key concepts, ask the right questions, and select the best possible treatment for the kind of cancer you have.

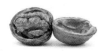

**The Toolbox** is the interactive part of this book. It is a collection of tools that allows you to tailor the information presented in each chapter to best serve your situation: assessments, checklists, worksheets, and questionnaires.

**Digging Deeper** provides you with information about topics that are new, unique, controversial, or complex. Digging Deeper provides us with the opportunity to explore these topics in greater depth.

### At the beginning of each chapter, you will find

- A Patient's Story of Surviving Prostate Cancer
- Chapter Summary
- Flow Chart
- Debunking Myths
- Vocabulary List

### At the end of the each chapter, you will find

- A Doctor's Story about Prostate Cancer
- Looking Ahead
- What's Next
- **The Toolbox**
- "Notes" page(s)

### At the end of the book, you will find

- **Digging Deeper**
- Glossary of terms
- Index
- References

We encourage you to take advantage of these features. They can make the difference between choosing the right treatment option or making a decision you regret.

Regardless of whether you are reading a paper or elec-

## HOW TO USE THIS BOOK

tronic version of this book, we do **NOT** recommend that you read the book "cover to cover."

Instead, we suggest you treat *Prostate Cancer: A New Approach to Treatment and Healing* as a reference — like an encyclopedia. Of course, there's nothing wrong with reading this book from beginning to end — it's just not required.

We recommend you read as much or as little as you like about each topic, then go the **Toolbox** at the end of each chapter and plug in your information.

Each chapter is relatively short, full of diagrams and illustrations, and can be read in 20 minutes. This easy-to-digest format gives you the essential information you need — without overwhelming you with medical acronyms and words you cannot pronounce. Each **Toolbox** section takes between 5-15 minutes to complete.

After reading each chapter and completing the **Toolbox** section, you will have a better understanding of your prostate, prostate cancer, and what your next steps are.

For example, let's say you want to know more about PSA testing. Using the Index, you locate the pages on PSA testing. The **Chapter 2 Toolbox** allows you to record your PSA info plus results from other tests.

We also suggest that you write down your questions about PSA testing in the Notes Section at the end of **Chapter 2**. This way, you are more likely to remember your questions during your next medical appointment.

PSA testing has become somewhat controversial. If you want to know more about this controversy, go to the **Digging Deeper** section (**Page 295**).

If you Google "prostate cancer," you will receive about 30 million results. At 5 minutes per result, that's about 2.3 million hours of reading. You wouldn't have time to read them all, even if you lived to be 200 — and Google probably wouldn't exist by then anyway!

## WE'VE DONE THE HEAVY LIFTING FOR YOU

Instead of reading a half dozen Google searches and feeling utterly lost, we have assembled the best-available information on the medical, surgical, psychological, and lifestyle aspects of prostate cancer — presented in a format that is free from scientific jargon and doctor speak.

As you read on, we will provide you with the ideal amount of information about the following topics:

- Innovative new tests and treatments

- The different types of prostate cancer and how to treat them

- The success and complication rates for various treatment options

- How to successfully ride the emotional roller coaster of a prostate cancer diagnosis

- How to reverse the disease process going on in your prostate (and the rest of your body), and begin the journey back to health and wellness.

## HEADS UP

Just by reading this introduction, you have embarked on a healing journey. Like all journeys, this one defies straight-line logic — one day you move ahead by leaps and bounds, only to slide backwards on the next. You'll also be thrown a couple of curve balls along the way. That's all part of this hero's journey. And yes, surviving cancer is heroic work.

## REGAINING CONTROL

In order to heal from prostate cancer, you are going to have to make some major changes. Big changes are often accompanied by serious resistance — within yourself and from others. Why? Because change messes with the status quo and our sense of control. And most men like feeling in control. (For more, see **Chapter 9.**)

Here's an illustration of how this book helps you regain control over your life.

Clinically **insignificant** prostate cancer ("hidden cancer" that is usually found during an autopsy) is a small cluster of slow-growing cells that are inactive and do **NOT** present an immediate health risk.

Around the world, men develop remarkably similar levels of clinically **insignificant** prostate cancer as they age — regardless of their race, ethnicity, economic status, genetics, lifestyle, career, country of origin ... and so on.

Most clinically **significant** prostate cancers (everything from low-risk to high-risk) are a red flag that some type of treatment is required: active surveillance, surgery, radia-

tion, or freezing the prostate to destroy the disease.
Clinically **significant** prostate cancer rates vary greatly
by race, ethnicity, economic status, genetics, country of
origin, career, current country, vocation, diet, exercise,
stress levels, and a host of other factors

## WHAT DOES THIS DIFFERENCE TELL US?

The difference in the rates for these two types of prostate cancer speaks directly to the role that lifestyle and
environmental factors play in developing **significant**
prostate cancer — factors that you have a great deal
of control over. For more information on this topic, see
**Chapter 10** and the **Chapter 10 Toolbox.**

## WHAT DOES THIS DIFFERENCE MEAN FOR MEN WITH PROSTATE CANCER?

As **Figure Intro 1.1** on **Page 10** shows, the progression
from healthy prostate cells to clinically **significant** prostate cancer is a two-way street.

The seven health factors that we discuss in **Chapter 10**
(diet, inactivity, stress, immune system, hormones, structure, and toxic substances) all have an impact on inflammation, which can make healthy prostate cells more likely
to develop prostate cancer.

| FACTORS WE ONCE THOUGHT OF AS "SET IN STONE" | FACTORS WE NOW KNOW TO BE "*FLUID*" |
|---|---|
| YOUR FAMILY HISTORY & GENETICS | • "Epigenetics" (gene modifications that do not involve genetic mutations) can change the expression of certain genes (small sections of DNA), and therefore the proteins these genes instruct the cell to produce. These changes can affect both "tumor suppressor genes" (which protect against cancer) and "oncogenes" (which promote cancer).<br>• 90% of prostate cancers are associated with "gene silencing" (a form of epigenetics that blocks the expression of DNA repair genes). Gene silencing makes it harder for the cells to repair the genetic modifications and mutations that contribute to cancer.<br>• Folate, vitamin B12, tea polyphenols, genistein, and other foods can cause "epigenetic" modifications that turn these genes back on. |
| YOUR PAST | • Physical injuries to your lower back, pelvis, or legs can affect your pelvic floor; therefore, your prostate, which in turn can lead to changes that promote prostate disease.<br>• Many physical, emotional, and sexual traumas from your youth can turn certain genes on or off, which can lead to prostate disorders including cancer. Healing physical and emotional trauma can change the expression of these genes (epigenetics). |
| EXPOSURE TO ENVIRONMENTAL TOXINS | • Many of the chemicals that are known to promote prostate cancer (carcinogenic compounds) can be measured and treated via detox protocols and eliminated from your body.<br>• You cannot control which chemicals you were exposed to before, but you can detox and limit your future environmental exposure. |
| BIOLOGICAL VS. CHRONOLOGICAL AGE | • Diet, exercise, and stress, are the three biggest contributors to how young and vibrant your body looks, functions, and feels. A healthy diet, daily exercise, and low stress levels all help prevent the initiation and promotion of cancer. |
| YOUR STRESS LEVEL | • Stress hormones are known contributors to the initiation and promotion of cancer. Identifying and changing stress patterns in your life can help you prevent the development of cancer and other diseases. |
| YOUR THOUGHTS | • Dwelling on recurring negative thoughts can increase your level of stress hormones; therefore, increasing the chance of developing all sorts of diseases, including prostate cancer. |

**Figure Intro 1.0** lists a few factors (bedrock truths) that medical science once believed were fixed and permanent, which we now know are more plastic than previously thought.

# 7 FACTORS THAT DECREASE INFLAMMATION AND REDUCE THE RISK OF PROSTATE CANCER

1. Diet      2. Inactivity      3. Stress      4. Structure
5. Immune System      6. Hormones      7. Toxic Substances

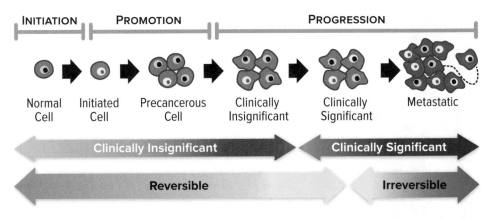

Inspired by Dr. Stephen Strum, Dr. Richard Beliveau, and Dr. Denis Gingras, **Figure Intro 1.1** visually displays how plastic the process of developing prostate cancer is. Bottom line: Prostate cancer is treatable (and reversible) if caught early enough. Regardless of when prostate cancer is detected, one of the keys to reversing cancer's progress is eliminating the "hits" healthy prostate cells receive that spark the initiation, promotion, and progression of this disease.

**OUR CORE MESSAGE**

*The core message of this book is:*
## You can heal from prostate cancer.

As the title of this book states, we are offering you a new approach to the treatment of prostate cancer. It also provides leading-edge information about how you can return your prostate to its natural state of health and wellness (provided you have "reversible" prostate cancer). Both of us have seen amazing recoveries — true stories of healing from life-threatening disease.

For example, Mark has met two men who previously had triple-digit PSA numbers and now have PSAs of less than 1.0 with no signs of the cancer that once ravaged their bodies. (One of them had a four-digit PSA number.)

This type of healing from advanced metastatic disease is rare to be sure; however, the fact remains that your body is capable of incredible healing.

In fact, **your health never leaves you** — even if you have been diagnosed with prostate cancer.

One way to conceptualize this idea of your health always being there is to think about what happens to the darkness when you walk into a room and turn on a light. Once your health (the light) shines brightly, the darkness (disease) goes away.

If you turn your health light off again, the disease will likely return. That's not magical thinking; that's called "relapse."

We recognize that not every doctor you talk to will agree with us, and that's OK. It has been our experience, however, that men who are willing to embrace the challenge of changing their lifestyle and choosing the right type of treatment for the kind of prostate cancer they have — a whole new world of possibility opens up that they never knew existed.

With these thoughts in mind, let's begin the journey of healing your prostate and returning you to your rightful state of health and wellness.

*Dr. Emilia A. Ripoll, M.D.*

*Mark B. Saunders*

# Doctor Story
## DR. SHANDRA WILSON, MD

Urology, Urologic Oncology
University of Colorado Hospital
Aurora, Colorado

*As a surgeon, my favorite prostate cancer story is about a surgery patient, of course.*

*My patient is a lovely professor from Southern Colorado. He is a kind man who sports a thick ponytail and teaches students about college chemistry. My patient and his wife are one of those graceful couples who love people and express such gratitude for everything in their lives.*

*In 2006, this 50-something Ph.D. was diagnosed with aggressive prostate cancer and needed treatment. After extensive research (as one would expect), he decided to have a nerve-sparing prostatectomy at my hospital, which brought him to me.*

*The operation was difficult because of a previous pelvic surgery. I worked and worked to peel those delicate hair-like nerves away from his cancerous prostate.*

*When my patient came for his first follow-up appointment, he and his wife brought more than $300 of books for my children (who were 2 and 3 at the time). His wife, who is also a teacher, explained that the kindest thing anyone can do for a mom is to care for her kids.*

*She was right about that. My kids and I spent hours and hours reading and re-reading those delightful books.*

*Six months later, I received a Christmas card that said he had fully recovered and everything was working great. I sent him a card back.*

*Since then, we have developed a delightful friendship. My patient even says that he is "almost glad he got cancer," because it resulted in our friendship. I would never wish cancer on anyone, but I am in awe at how such a gift can come from something as horrible as cancer.*

## LOOKING AHEAD

**CHAPTER 1:** You or your doctor is concerned about your prostate — We provide you with **Prostate 101**: where it lives, what it does, plus relevant statistics.

**CHAPTER 2:** Your doctor told you to **schedule a prostate biopsy** — We give you a **Prostate Biopsy Assessment Tool** to see if you actually need one, and what to expect if you do.

**CHAPTER 3:** You have a prostate biopsy — We explain the steps you need to take, whether you have a **negative biopsy or a positive biopsy**.

**CHAPTER 4:** You have a **positive prostate biopsy** — We provide you with a **Prostate Cancer Assessment Tool** to help you understand which kind of cancer you have.

**CHAPTER 5:** You need to select a prostate cancer treatment — We provide you with a summary of the most common types of treatment based on your **cancer risk type** (low-risk, moderate-risk, and high-risk).

**CHAPTER 6:** You have **low-risk, low-volume prostate cancer** and need to learn more about emerging treatments — We provide you with a summary of these treatments to help you understand the differences between focal, minimally invasive, alternative, whole gland, and traditional treatments.

**CHAPTER 7:** You have prostate cancer that is more advanced than low-risk, low-volume and need to know more about **whole-gland treatments** (both stand-alone traditional and combination treatments) — We provide you with a summary of these treatments.

**CHAPTER 8:** You want to know the **success and complication rates** for each type of treatment and for each cancer risk type (low-risk, moderate-risk, and high-risk) — We provide you with unbiased information to support your decision-making process.

**CHAPTER 9:** You feel **overwhelmed** by the news of a positive prostate biopsy — We give you the tools to surf this tidal wave of emotion and overcome the feeling of panic that almost always accompanies a positive biopsy report.

**CHAPTER 10:** You want to **use your cancer diagnosis as a springboard to better health** — We help you address your wellness goals with a proven plan that covers inflammation, diet, inactivity, stress, immune system, hormone optimization, structure, and removing toxic substances.

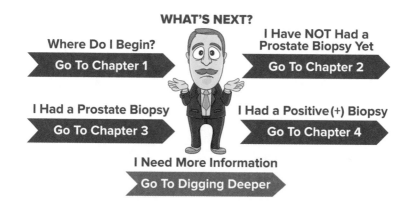

**WHAT'S NEXT?**

Where Do I Begin?
**Go To Chapter 1**

I Have NOT Had a Prostate Biopsy Yet
**Go To Chapter 2**

I Had a Prostate Biopsy
**Go To Chapter 3**

I Had a Positive (+) Biopsy
**Go To Chapter 4**

I Need More Information
**Go To Digging Deeper**

# WELCOME TO THE TOOLBOX
# INTRODUCTORY **TOOLBOX**

In the Toolbox section at the end of each chapter, you will find questionnaires, checklists, resource lists, assessment tools, and other interactive documents that are designed to help you put ideas into action.

The point of having a **Toolbox** section is to give you the opportunity to interact with the information presented in each chapter and make it personal and relevant for you and your situation.

Instead of one big Toolbox at the end of the book, we thought it would be easier to have a Toolbox section at the end of each chapter.

## EACH TOOLBOX SECTION IS DESIGNED TO HELP YOU:

- Grasp what's going on inside your prostate
- Ask the right questions
- Make the most of your medical appointments
- Connect with your support team (or create one)
- Understand what your treatment options are
- Select the right doctor
- Pick the best possible treatment plan for you, your body, and the kind of cancer you have

---

*The following pages provide you with questions to ponder and space to write down your answers. The goal of the Toolbox section is to help you better understand your condition and give you a foundation of knowledge from which you make your medical decisions. We invite you to skip ahead and look at the other Toolbox sections to gain a sense of how this section works and what's to come.*

TOOLBOX

## 7 FACTORS THAT DECREASE INFLAMMATION AND REDUCE THE RISK OF PROSTATE CANCER

1. Diet    2. Inactivity    3. Stress    4. Structure
5. Immune System    6. Hormones    7. Toxic Substances

**PLEASE ANSWER THESE 8 QUESTIONS TO GET A REALISTIC VIEW OF YOUR HEALTH**

1. How would you describe your diet? (Paleo, gluten-free, fast food ...)

2. What do you do for exercise?
(How often? How much time? How intense?)

3. How do you manage your stress?
(walking, singing, meditation...)

4. Have you had any major physical injuries that required surgery, physical therapy, osteopathic/chiropractic adjustments, acupuncture, or massage therapy? (circle one)   Yes    No
(If "Yes," please describe.)

5. Do you have an inflammatory medical condition like arthritis, diabetes, allergies, chronic infections, or other auto-immune disease? (circle one)      Yes    No

6. Are you now taking, or have you previously taken, any medications to suppress your immune system? (circle one)      Yes    No

7. Have you been evaluated for low testosterone or any other hormone deficiency? (circle one)    Yes    No

8. Have you ever been exposed to toxic materials at home, school, work, or in your community? (circle one)    Yes    No

TOOLBOX

**TOOLBOX**

# KNOW YOUR HISTORY

| | |
|---|---|
| **YOUR FAMILY HISTORY & GENETICS** | Have any men in your immediate family (blood relatives) been diagnosed with prostate cancer? If so, at what age?<br><br>Have any women in your immediate family been diagnosed with breast or cervical cancer? If so, at what age?<br><br>Do you know if anyone in your immediate family has been diagnosed with the BRCA gene or other genetic markers? |
| **YOUR PAST** | Have you had any physical injuries that affected your lower back, pelvis, or lower extremities?<br>(sports injuries, car accidents, work injuries, a fall on the ice)<br><br>What kind of treatment, if any, have you had for these injuries? Do they still bother you today?<br><br>Have you experienced intense emotional trauma?<br>Loss of a child, parent, job, significant relationship, abuse (physical, emotional, sexual), or other major trauma?<br>(circle one)<br><br>Yes          No |
| **EXPOSURE TO ENVIRONMENTAL TOXINS** | Have you been exposed to? (circle any that apply)<br>• Radiation (medical or environmental)<br>• Pesticides<br>• Herbicides<br>• Tobacco products or second-hand smoke<br>• Hormones<br>• Other toxic substances |

# KNOW MORE ABOUT YOURSELF

**YOUR CHRONOLOGICAL AGE
AND BIOLOGICAL AGE MAY BE DIFFERENT.**

1. How much energy do you have? (On a scale of 1-10, with 1 being little to none and 10 being abundant energy.)

2. How flexible are you? (On a scale of 1-10, with 1 being very inflexible and 10 being very flexible)

3. Do you exercise regularly (3 times/week or more)? (Circle one)
   Yes          No

4. Does your body hurt most of the time? (Circle one)
   Yes          No

5. Can you stand on one foot for 30 seconds without putting your other foot down? (Circle one)
   Yes          No

6. How good is your memory?
   (On a scale of 1-10, with 1 being very poor and 10 being excellent.)

**YOUR AGE (BIOLOGICAL VS CHRONOLOGICAL)**

Are you excited to see what tomorrow brings? (Circle one)
   Yes          No

Do you feel like your life is out of control? (Circle one)
   Yes          No

Do you feel like your life has purpose? (Circle one)
   Yes          No

**YOUR FUTURE**

Do you spend more time thinking about what you want or what you don't want?

What percentage of your time do you spend in worry or fear?

**YOUR THOUGHTS**

TOOLBOX

**NOTES:**

TOOLBOX

# chapter ONE
# Getting Started

" What Cancer Cannot Do —
Cancer is so limited...
It cannot cripple love,
It cannot shatter hope,
It cannot corrode faith,
It cannot destroy peace,
It cannot kill friendship,
It cannot suppress memories,
It cannot silence courage,
It cannot invade the soul,
It cannot steal eternal life,
It cannot conquer
the spirit.

— *Anonymous*

# Patient Story

## CLIFF

*I was diagnosed with Stage 1 prostate cancer at the end of 2014, right before my 50th birthday. The first urologist I saw immediately recommended a radical prostatectomy, and also mentioned that radiation treatment was another option. I initially thought, "Sure. I don't need this organ to live."*

*Then I found out about the possible side effects of the surgery, including being impotent and incontinent — for the rest of my life!*

*I did some research, and what I learned gave me permission to try other options.*

*I eliminated sugars (including alcohol), dairy, meat, gluten and soy from my diet (and added apricot seeds, cannabis oil, apple cider vinegar and blackstrap molasses), and my weight dropped from 208 to 185 in two months (23 pounds). I started addressing my stress level, going to a holistic doctor, using a far-infrared heating pad, getting monthly acupuncture treatments, and taking dried Chinese herbs and mushrooms daily.*

*My PSA dropped dramatically, but I still had this one big nagging issue: How could I be sure the cancer wasn't growing?*

*From my research, I didn't believe I needed an annual prostate biopsy, as they can have negative side-effects too.*

*I am now working with urologist who supports my choices, and I feel great! I have a goal of living to 90, and I want to celebrate the second half of my life by being healthy. If I eventually need surgery or radiation, that's fine — but I have made it a priority to not let my health get to that point.*

# chapter
## ONE
# summary

**Chapter 1** introduces you to your prostate, where it is located, what it does, as well as some important information about prostate cancer.

*If you have already been diagnosed with prostate cancer, we invite you to skip ahead to the **Chapter 4 Toolbox**, where our **Prostate Cancer Assessment Tool** shows you how to figure what kind of cancer you have (low-risk, moderate-risk, or high-risk).*

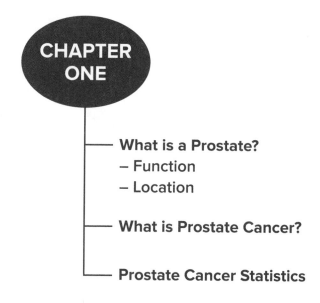

**CHAPTER ONE**

- **What is a Prostate?**
  - Function
  - Location

- **What is Prostate Cancer?**

- **Prostate Cancer Statistics**

**Figure 1.0** Illustrates the three major topics covered in Chapter 1.

**DEBUNKING MYTHS**

## No Two Cancers Are Identical

*Just as no two people are biologically the same, no two men have exactly the same kind of prostate cancer, which explains why one type of treatment may work perfectly for one man and poorly for another.*

*That's why it's so important to select a doctor who is an expert in prostate cancer and understands the pros and cons of pairing an individual who has a specific kind of prostate cancer with a particular type of treatment. This approach is the opposite of a doctor who performs the same procedure regardless of the patient or what kind of cancer he has.*

*The purpose of this book is to help you find the right treatment for the type of cancer you have. Ideally, this treatment is powerful enough to eliminate the cancer while preserving normal bowel, bladder, urinary, and erectile function. (We go into detail about selecting the right treatment plan and the right doctor in* **Chapter 5.***).*

*Also, we do NOT have a stake in any procedures, products, tests, or medications. We just want you to be well.*

---

**VOCABULARY**

See Glossary for Definitions

Bladder

Bio-individuality

BPH
(Benign Prostatic Hyperplasia)

Digital Rectal Exam (DRE)

DNA (deoxyribonucleic acid)

Gene

Gleason score

Hormones

Mutation

Pelvic Floor

Prostate Biopsy

Prostate Cancer

Prostate Zones

PSA (Prostate Specific Antigen)

PSA Testing

Rectum

Seminal Vesicles

Urethra

Urinary Retention

Urinary Sphincter

Urinary Stricture

## THE LAY OF THE LOINS

Before discussing whether a prostate biopsy is right for you (**Chapter 2**), we would like to give you a short course in prostate anatomy and physiology, clarify a few terms, and provide you with the information you need to know to become an informed patient.

## WHERE IS YOUR PROSTATE GLAND LOCATED?

Found only in men, the prostate is a walnut-shaped gland located below the bladder, behind the muscular wall of the abdomen, in front of the rectum at the bottom of the pelvis (See **Figure 1.1**). Since the prostate rests up against the rectum, the best way to access the prostate is by a digital rectal exam (DRE — See **Page 45**).

The tube that allows urine to drain from the bladder and out the penis (the urethra) passes through the middle of the prostate. One way to think of the prostate gland is that it's like a spongy golf ball with a straw running through the middle of it. Your prostate surrounds your urethra and sits in between your bladder and urinary sphincter (See **Figure 1.1**). If there's congestion or blockage in the prostate (an enlarged prostate, a prostate cancer tumor) or below it (tight urinary sphincter or scar tissue in the urethra) urine can back up, causing varying degrees of pain and urine retention.

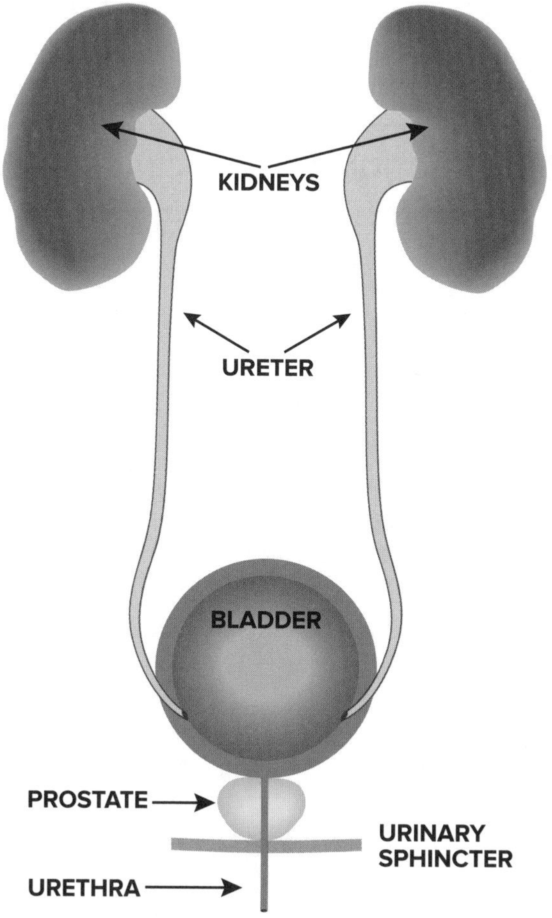

**KIDNEYS**

**URETER**

**BLADDER**

**PROSTATE**

**URINARY SPHINCTER**

**URETHRA**

Figure 1.1 This simple drawing shows the prostate gland in relationship to the rest of the urinary system.

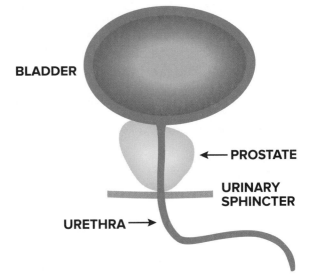

BLADDER

PROSTATE

URINARY
SPHINCTER

URETHRA

**Figure 1.2** shows a slice of the lower urinary system, with the bladder on top of the prostate and the muscular hammock of the pelvic floor/urinary sphincter below. An enlarged prostate, prostate cancer, urinary strictures (scar tissue in the urethra), or a tight urinary sphincter can cause urine to back up into the prostate, which may lead to inflammation and symptoms similar to prostate cancer.

## URINARY RESTRICTION AND BLOCKAGE

*There are four main causes of urinary restriction and blockage:*

1. *Enlarged prostate (BPH)*
2. *Tight urinary sphincter (pelvic floor dysfunction)*
3. *Urethral strictures (scar tissue in the urethra)*
4. *Prostate cancer*

*Both an enlarged prostate and prostate cancer can cause urinary restriction and blockage within the prostate. A tight pelvic floor/urinary sphincter pinches the urethra just below the prostate. Urethral strictures can occur anywhere along the urethra.*

*Regardless of what causes the blockage/restriction, if it occurs "downstream" from the prostate, urine will back up into the glands of the prostate.*

*Since the urine of most Americans has a pH of 5 (the same acidity as black coffee), a urinary restriction or blockage is like soaking your urethra and prostate in a cup of black coffee all day and night. No wonder men with urinary restriction/blockage feel a painful, itching, burning sensation in their prostates!*

WHAT DOES
YOUR
PROSTATE
GLAND DO?

## THE PROSTATE HAS TWO MAIN FUNCTIONS:

1. It secretes and stores the fluid that contains Prostate Specific Antigen (PSA), which acts like the "semen solvent" that allows individual sperm to swim on their own, instead of sperm being clumped together in groups.

2. The smooth muscles of the prostate contract during ejaculation, propelling semen down the urethra and out of the body during orgasm.

Like all the glands and organs in the pelvis, the prostate is affected by the health of the supporting structures, particularly the abdominal muscles, the lumbosacral spine, and the hammock of muscles and connective tissue that forms the pelvic floor/urinary sphincter.

ZONES OF THE
PROSTATE

The prostate is composed of three main zones: Central, Transitional, and Peripheral. (See **Figure 1.3** on **Page 26**)

**The Central Zone** surrounds the ejaculatory ducts and accounts for approximately 25 percent of the prostate volume. Only 2.5 percent of prostate cancers occur in the Central Zone; however, these cancers are usually more aggressive and invade the seminal vesicles.

**The Transitional Zone**, which surrounds the urethra in the middle of the gland, accounts for only 5 percent of total prostate volume at puberty; however, this portion of the prostate continues to grow throughout a man's life and is responsible for an enlarged prostate (BPH). Approximately, 10-20 percent of prostate cancer occurs in this zone.

**The Peripheral Zone** contains most of the "glandular" tissue in the lower half of the prostate, and surrounds the urethra as it leaves the prostate. This zone accounts for a whopping 70-80 percent of prostate cancer and is the most easily accessible by a digital rectal exam (DRE).

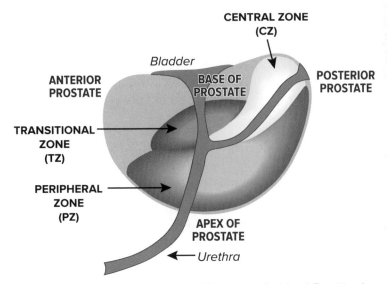

**Figure 1.3** displays the three main zones of the prostate: Peripheral, Transitional, and Central.

## WHAT CAUSES PROSTATE CANCER?

It is difficult to isolate a single cause of prostate cancer. We know that certain inherited DNA mutations (BRCA1, BRCA2, RNASEL, MLH1, MSH2) as well as mutations that occur during a man's lifetime can cause prostate cancer. Inherited DNA mutations appear to cause only 5-10 percent of prostate cancers. This means that mutations that occur after birth account for the other 90-95 percent of the prostate cancer cases.

If you look at **Figure Intro 1.1** on **Page 10**, you'll see that it takes multiple "hits" to prostate cells before cancer can find a foothold. It is important to realize that these hits come from the aspects of our lives that we can control (diet, exercise, stress management) as well as those we cannot (your family history, exposure to toxic chemicals).

### WHAT DOES THAT TELL US?

If you're a pessimist, **Figure Intro 1.1** is proof that life is out to get you. If you're an optimist, it is proof that you have a lot more control over your health in general, and your prostate health in particular, than you thought possible.

In **Chapter 10,** you will learn more about how diet, inactivity, stress, immune system, hormone levels, structure, and toxic substances impact your overall health, and the health of your prostate.

## WHAT IS PROSTATE CANCER?

*Cancer happens when cells begin to grow in an out-of-control way. Normal cells grow, divide, and die in a predictable manner. Cancer cells, on the other hand, lose the ability to self-regulate, stop communicating with other cells, replicate faster than normal cells, and simply refuse to die. In fact, under the right laboratory conditions, cancer cells can live in Petri dishes for decades.*

*This hard-to-kill quality is what allows prostate cancer to invade territory beyond the prostate gland — lymph nodes, seminal vesicles, bladder, rectum, nearby bones, and eventually the entire body.*

*For more information on the longevity of prostate cancer cells, see the* **Chapter 1** Digging Deeper *section.*

*It is generally accepted that cancer is caused by changes (mutation or modification) in a cell's DNA (genetic code) that occurs while the cell is dividing and replicating. Once a mutation/modification occurs (assuming it doesn't kill the cell), it is passed on to all future copies of that cell.*

*Prostate Cancer can be seen as the result of microscopic changes to a small section of a cell's DNA (genes) that increase the rate at which cells divide and replicate. Theoretically, turning these genes off — or turning on other genes that slow down the rate of cell division and replication — could stop prostate cancer from spreading.*

*Mutations/modifications can also control a cell's ability to repair itself. "Gene silencing" prevents a cell's microscopic mechanics from repairing the cell's DNA. When this happens, a cell can be overrun by invading molecules from nearby cancer cells.*

*Obviously, a lot of research is going on in these areas.*

**NOTE**

*In the United States, approximately 15 percent of men will be diagnosed with prostate cancer during their lifetime. That information says nothing about which 1-in-7 men will develop prostate cancer. More importantly, it ignores who the other six are and why they were spared from this disease (or at least a diagnosis).*

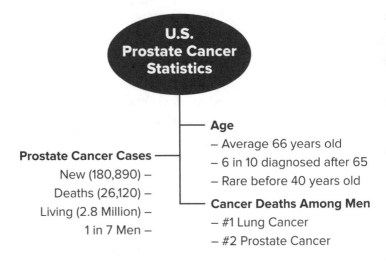

**Figure 1.4** When reviewing the 2016 prostate cancer statistics from the American Cancer Society, keep in mind how much these numbers have fallen since the 1990s.

## PROSTATE CANCER STATISTICS

Here are the American Cancer Society's prostate cancer estimates for 2016. (All of these numbers are better than the 2015 numbers):

- New cases of prostate cancer (all ages): 180,890 (down from 220,800 in 2015). Approximately 1 in 7 men in the United States will be diagnosed during his lifetime.
- Prostate cancer has the highest incidence rate of all cancers in the United States: 131.5/100,000 men.
- Death from prostate cancer (all ages): 26,120 (down from 27,545 in 2015). Between 2008-2012, approximately 21 out of 100,000 men in living in the United States died of prostate cancer.
- Prostate cancer is the second leading cause of cancer death in American men; lung cancer is # 1. About 1 man in 38 will die of prostate cancer (2.6%).
- Prostate cancer occurs mainly in older men. About 6 out of 10 cases are diagnosed in men aged 65 or older, and it is rare before age 40. The average age at the time of diagnosis is 66.
- Race is a factor: African American men are almost twice as likely to develop prostate cancer than white American men — and more than twice as likely to die from prostate cancer.
- The probability of a man developing prostate cancer (and dying from prostate cancer) increases with age.

- Between 2005-2011, the 5-year prostate cancer survival rate for all-stages was 99%. The rate was more than 99% for cancer still inside the prostate; however, for cancer that had spread throughout the body (metastatic disease), the 5-year survival rated dropped to 28%.

Thanks to PSA testing, early detection, and better care, fewer men are dying of prostate cancer. For example, between 2008-2012, 21.4 out of 100,000 U.S. men died from prostate cancer, compared to 39.2 per 100,000 men in 1992, just before PSA testing became widespread. That's a **83 percent improvement!**

In addition to the statistics about new prostate cancer cases and deaths, statistics are available for each risk factor, type of prostate cancer treatment, and the complications of those treatments.

## BIO-INDIVIDUALITY AND PROSTATE CANCER

*The term bio-individuality means that no two people are biologically the same (even identical twins). So it shouldn't come as a surprise that there is no one-pill-cures-all treatment for prostate cancer. If such a treatment existed, there would*

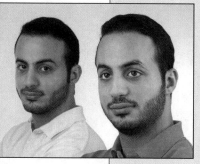

*be no need for a urologist to make a cancer diagnosis — a computer could do that.*

*Bio-individuality isn't just an interesting idea; it is leading-edge cancer research. Dr. Steven Rosenberg, M.D. of the National Cancer Institute and his colleagues have developed a new form of immunotherapy (enhancing the body's immune system) that targets the specific mutations (changes in a cell's DNA) of a particular person's cancer.*

*This form of cancer therapy creates a completely individualized form of treatment that kills 100 percent of the cancer cells and leaves all the other cells (cells that lack a specific mutation) alone. (For more information about Dr. Rosenberg's work, please visit: https://ccr.cancer.gov/Surgery-Branch/steven-a-rosenberg.) Dr. Rosenberg's therapy goes right to the heart of the question behind all prostate cancer research: How can we destroy all the cancer while sparing the healthy tissue around it?*

*The answer to that question is what keeps urologists up at night.*

# Doctor Story
## DR. ELIZABETH CEILLEY, MD

Radiation Oncology

Banner Health

Loveland, Colorado

*No matter how sophisticated the technology, or how precise the treatment plan, a patient's experience is shaped predominately by their interactions with their medical team.*

*My colleagues like to tease radiation oncologists like me about our love of "fancy toys." So as expected, I was thrilled that our center was among the first to acquire a new TrueBeam STx Linear Accelerator. Our center was already known for its warm environment and caring staff. Now we were going to be a state-of-the art radiation oncology center.*

*The first patient to be treated on the new machine was A.A., a gentleman who had previously had a prostatectomy. His PSA was now rising and radiation therapy was recommended. Our hospital wanted to publicize our new technology, and A.A. was the perfect first patient, because the technical aspect of his treatment was greatly improved by the True Beam Linear Accelerator.*

*However, A.A. was less than excited about being the first patient on the new machine. "I don't buy new cars for a reason," he said. He was also a bit bothered by all the attention surrounding his treatment. I ended up asking another patient to be interviewed for an article in a local magazine about our new linear accelerator.*

*A.A.'s seven weeks of radiation treatment went well. In follow-up, he was doing great, and his PSA was undetectable. Later, I suggested that someone on our PR staff should interview A.A. about his experience.*

*When A.A. was asked for an interview, he said "Yes," and then added, "It was not that machine that made my treatment successful... it was the PEOPLE."*

## LOOKING AHEAD

**CHAPTER 1:** You or your doctor is concerned about your prostate — We provide you with **Prostate 101**: where it lives, what it does, plus relevant statistics.

**CHAPTER 2:** Your doctor told you to **schedule a prostate biopsy** — We give you a **Prostate Biopsy Assessment Tool** to see if you actually need one, and what to expect if you do.

**CHAPTER 3:** You have a prostate biopsy — We explain the steps you need to take, whether you have a **negative biopsy or a positive biopsy**.

**CHAPTER 4:** You have a **positive prostate biopsy** — We provide you with a **Prostate Cancer Assessment Tool** to help you understand which kind of cancer you have.

**CHAPTER 5:** You need to select a prostate cancer treatment — We provide you with a summary of the most common types of treatment based on your **cancer risk type** (low-risk, moderate-risk, and high-risk).

**CHAPTER 6:** You have **low-risk, low-volume prostate cancer** and need to learn more about emerging treatments — We provide you with a summary of these treatments to help you understand the differences between focal, minimally invasive, alternative, whole gland, and traditional treatments.

**CHAPTER 7:** You have prostate cancer that is more advanced than low-risk, low-volume and need to know more about **whole-gland treatments** (both stand-alone traditional and combination treatments) — We provide you with a summary of these treatments.

**CHAPTER 8:** You want to know the **success and complication rates** for each type of treatment and for each cancer risk type (low-risk, moderate-risk, and high-risk) — We provide you with unbiased information to support your decision-making process.

**CHAPTER 9:** You feel **overwhelmed** by the news of a positive prostate biopsy — We give you the tools to surf this tidal wave of emotion and overcome the feeling of panic that almost always accompanies a positive biopsy report.

**CHAPTER 10:** You want to **use your cancer diagnosis as a springboard to better health** — We help you address your wellness goals with a proven plan that covers inflammation, diet, inactivity, stress, immune system, hormone optimization, structure, and removing toxic substances.

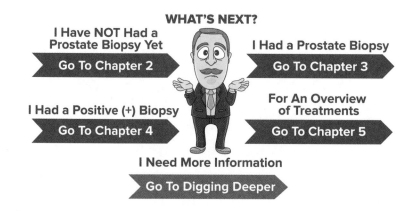

**WHAT'S NEXT?**

**I Have NOT Had a Prostate Biopsy Yet**
Go To Chapter 2

**I Had a Prostate Biopsy**
Go To Chapter 3

**I Had a Positive (+) Biopsy**
Go To Chapter 4

**For An Overview of Treatments**
Go To Chapter 5

**I Need More Information**
Go To Digging Deeper

# WELCOME TO THE TOOLBOX
# CHAPTER 1 **TOOLBOX**

*Chapter 1 is designed to provide you with a little "Prostate 101" and a few prostate cancer statistics. We begin presenting you with worksheets, checklists, assessment tools, and other resources in the Chapter 2 Toolbox. In the meantime, please use the notes section below to jot down any thoughts or questions you may have.*

**NOTES:**

# Do You Need A Prostate Biopsy?

" It's very frightening when you're told you have any form of the C-word, but because of early detection, they caught it before it had hardly begun. I'm completely cured, and will go on to have a wonderful, fruitful life. I'll never die of prostate cancer.

— *Mandy Patinkin, actor*

# Patient Story

## JOEL

*Here's the one thing I want to share with other men like me: If prostate cancer runs in your family, it's very important to get tested — even if you're still young. Just because you're 36 (like I was) doesn't mean you have to wait to get tested. I am glad I pushed it, because they wouldn't have discovered the cancer until it was more advanced.*

*Five years ago, I went to the doctor to find out about my prostate, because both my dad and my uncle had prostate cancer. I was only 36 years old, and my doctor said I was too young. He said to wait until I was 39.*

*When I turned 39, my doctor suggested that we wait until I was 40. I told him: 'No, I want run the tests now.' Thank God I did. We caught the cancer very early: Only 1 out of the 24 needles had a small amount of low-risk cancer.*

*I went to my oldest brother and told him, 'Bro, you should get tested too.' He did, and his biopsy was positive also. He just had CyberKnife treatment, and he's doing fine.*

*I've been on active surveillance for a year and a half, and I go in for my second MRI next month to see if the cancer is growing. And even if it is, I know I'll get the right treatment.*

*The second thing I want to share is always get a second opinion — that's what I did.*

*The first doctors I saw scared the shit out of me. They wanted to cut out my prostate. They said, "Might as well take it out and get it over with." I'm like, wait a minute, I'm only 40 years old. I don't want to wear Pampers for the rest of my life and not be able to have sex.*

*My uncle lives in Roswell, New Mexico. So he didn't have the same options I do, and 60 percent of his prostate had cancer. He had surgery, and now he leaks when he plays golf, and he still cannot get an erection even though he takes Cialis every day — and he's only 52!*

# chapter TWO summary

As with all medical decisions, you want to make an informed one about having a prostate biopsy.

**Chapter 2** walks you through the test results, images, and information that doctors use when evaluating whether or not a man needs to have a prostate biopsy.

**The Prostate Biopsy Assessment Tool** in the **Chapter 2 Toolbox** gives you a clear and concise way to use these results, images, and information to better understand why you do (or do not) need a prostate biopsy.

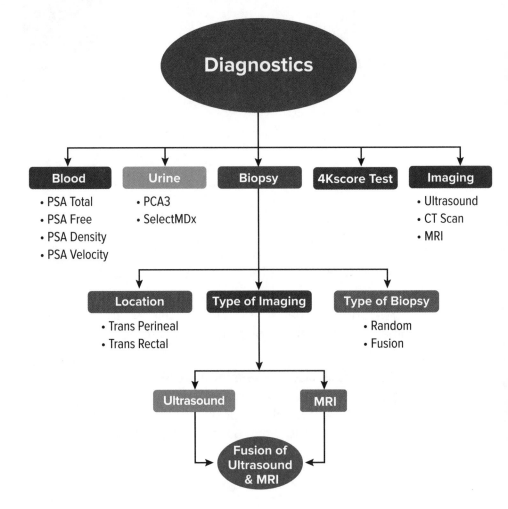

The first row of **Figure 2.0** displays the four main sources of information that doctors use to determine whether or not you need a prostate biopsy. The 4Kscore Test is a hybrid blood test plus an algorithm. The **Prostate Biopsy Assessment Tool** in the **Chapter 2 Toolbox** will help you put this information to use.

## Do Prostate Biopsies Spread Cancer?

*The short answer is NO.*

*After millions of prostate biopsies over many decades, the overwhelming clinical evidence shows nothing to support the idea that prostate cancer spreads along needle tracks after a prostate biopsy.*

*As Dr. Larry Bans, M.D. of the Cancer Treatment Centers of America puts it, "The risk of 'seeding,' or 'tracking,' or 'spreading' cancer with prostate needle biopsies, if there is a risk at all, has to be exceedingly rare and low."*

*Currently, prostate biopsies are a necessary part of making an accurate cancer diagnosis. In the near future, however, MRI and other forms of imaging may become so sensitive that biopsies become a thing of the past — or only require a few needles to make the correct diagnosis (instead of today's 12-24 needles).*

**VOCABULARY**

See Glossary for Definitions

- 4Kscore Test
- AUA Score
- Benign Prostatic Hyperplasia (BPH)
- Biopsy
- CAT Scan
- ConfirmMDx
- Digital Rectal Exam (DRE)
- Doppler
- Erectile Dysfunction (ED)
- Imaging
- Lab Tests
- Magnetic Resonance Imaging (MRI)
- MRI-fusion biopsy
- Medical History
- Needle Cores
- PCA3 Test
- Pelvic Floor
- Prostate Biopsy
- Prostatitis
- PSA (Prostate Specific Antigen)
- PSA Density
- PSA Free
- PSA Test
- PSA Total
- PSA Velocity
- SelectMDx
- TRUS (standard) Biopsy
- TURP (surgery to relieve BPH)
- Ultrasound
- Urinary Frequency
- Urinary Urgency

## WHY HAVE A PROSTATE BIOPSY?

*Simply stated: There are three main reasons to have a prostate biopsy :*

1. *Determine if you have prostate cancer*
2. *If you have cancer, find out which type and how much*
3. *If cancer is present, how life threatening is it?*

**NOTE**

*Many patients ask, "Why should I have a prostate biopsy? Don't all men develop prostate cancer eventually?" Yes and no. If men live long enough, 1-in-7 will develop some form of clinically significant prostate cancer. Most of these cancers will be low-risk low-volume cancer, which can be treated (at least initially) with active surveillance.*

**PUTTING ALL THE PIECES TOGETHER**

There is no simple equation or computer algorithm that tells doctors exactly who needs to have a prostate biopsy — and who does not. However, the following four sources of information, plus your doctor's experience, can help identify patients who may have prostate cancer:

1. Medical history
2. Physical exam
3. Lab tests
4. Imaging

To see how these four sources of information define the health of your prostate, we invite you to use the **Prostate Biopsy Assessment Tool** in the **Chapter 2 Toolbox**.

These four sources also help rule out conditions such as prostatitis, BPH, and pelvic floor problems, which can all lead to an unnecessary prostate biopsy. (See "The Great Mimickers" on **Page 40**.)

**SIGNS THAT YOU MIGHT NEED A PROSTATE BIOPSY**

When that familiar, easy feeling of going to the bathroom is replaced by any of the following, it's a good indicator that something is wrong:

- Pain during urination
- Needing to urinate frequently (more than every hour)
- Needing to go NOW!
- Straining to urinate
- Waking up to urinate multiple times at night
- Incomplete emptying of your bladder

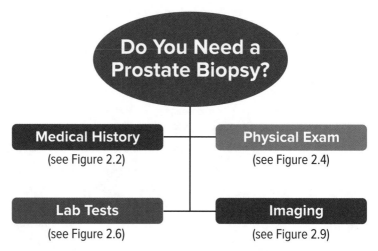

**Figure 2.1** contains the four sources of information that doctors frequently use to decide whether they think a prostate biopsy is the logical next step.

## BEFORE YOU HAVE A BIOPSY

*If your doctor has already scheduled your prostate biopsy — but has NOT discussed the results from the four sources of information listed in* **Figure 2.1** *— we recommend that you make another appointment so you are crystal clear about why your doctor thinks you need a prostate biopsy.*

*Why question your doctor's expert opinion? The invention of PSA testing has given rise to a dramatic increase in the number of prostate biopsies performed every year — more than half a million of which are unnecessary. Why expose yourself to unwanted complications from a diagnostic procedure that you don't actually need? (see* **Page 59***)*

*Sometimes it helps to have a second opinion to answer your questions and address your concerns — and to make sure that a prostate biopsy is the best course of action.*

## THE GREAT MIMICKERS

*It is important to rule out prostate cancer mimickers like BPH and prostatitis before you have a prostate biopsy; however, a prostate biopsy is worth the limited risk of complications to dismiss the possibility of advanced prostate cancer.*

### THERE ARE TWO COMMON CONDITIONS THAT MIMIC PROSTATE CANCER:

1. **Enlarged Prostate** *or* **BPH**
   *(Benign Prostatic Hyperplasia)*
2. **Prostatitis** *(pain, itching, swelling, of the prostate and/or nearby tissue)*

*Both of these conditions can cause symptoms similar to those of advanced prostate cancer. All three raise your PSA levels. (Early prostate cancer rarely has symptoms.)*

**BPH** *is a non-cancerous growth of the prostate that occurs in most men as they age. Approximately half of American men over 50 have some symptoms related to BPH.*

**Prostatitis** *(prostate inflammation or infection) is often called, "a headache in the pelvis." More than two million American men visit their doctor every year with prostatitis.*

*There are four kinds of prostatitis, but 95 percent of cases fall into the "Chronic Nonbacterial" category, which means the symptoms have been going on for months (sometimes years) and they aren't being caused by a detectable bacterial infection.*

*Both an enlarged prostate and prostatitis can cause symptoms that are similar to advanced prostate cancer:*

- *Low flow (weak urinary stream)*
- *Having to push to drain your bladder*
- *Urinary urgency (gotta go NOW!)*
- *Urinary frequency (the need to go every hour)*
- *Waking up to pee in the middle of the night (nocturia)*
- *Painful urination (dysuria)*
- *Itching, burning, or pain in the prostate area*

## 1. MEDICAL HISTORY

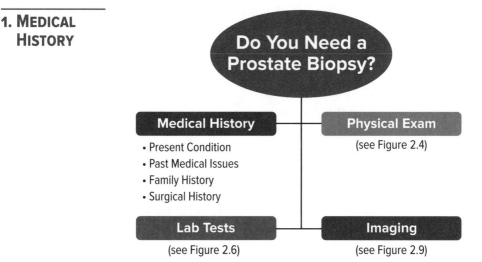

Figure 2.2 details why providing your doctor with a complete medical history is an important step in the, "Do I need a biopsy?" Process.

### PRESENT CONDITION

Men with early stage prostate cancer rarely have urinary symptoms. If you are having urinary symptoms like the ones listed on **Page 40**, there is a very high probability that the cause is BPH, prostatitis, or advanced prostate cancer.

Fortunately, BPH and prostatitis are the most common causes of urinary symptoms. For example, if your urinary problems have steadily increased for a few years, an enlarged prostate is the likely cause.

Likewise, prostatitis can create the urgent need to go to the bathroom RIGHT NOW or feeling like you have to go every-hour-on-the-hour. Prostatitis can also create pain and itching that wanders up and down the urethra or extends up into the bladder.

If you're having urination issues, we encourage you take the American Urological Association (AUA) questionnaire (See **Page 63** in the **Chapter 2 Toolbox**), and go over it with your doctor.

Unfortunately, by the time prostate cancer has advanced far enough to cause urinary symptoms, 95 percent of those men have prostate cancer outside their prostate (metastatic disease). Prostate cancer is much easier to treat when it is still inside the prostate (local disease).

According to the American Cancer Society, the 10-year survival rate for treating **all stages** of prostate cancer is 99 percent, which includes the survival rates for cancers that have spread outside the prostate but are still within the pelvis ("regional" metastatic disease).

The 10-year survival rate for treating prostate cancer that has spread to distant lymph nodes, organs, and bones throughout the body ("distant"metastatic disease), sadly, is only 28 percent.

That's why it is so important rule out distant metastatic prostate cancer. Please let your doctor know if you've ever had any of the following:

- BPH
- Prostatitis
- Urinary Tract Infections (UTIs)
- Urinary strictures (scarring inside the urethra that prevents the normal flow of urine)
- A serious car accident (or other injury) that caused significant trauma to your lower back, pelvis, hips, or lower extremities?
- Other major medical diseases such as diabetes, heart disease, stroke, autoimmune disorders, COPD, asthma, other cancers ... to name just a few.

Although these six points are only a partial list (a full list would take pages), your **past medical issues** provide your healthcare team with important clues about what's causing your prostate problems: cancer or other "easier to treat" conditions.

Also, tell your doctor about all the medications you are currently taking and all the medications you've been prescribed in the past year. This information is essential to creating a comprehensive prostate snapshot.

Bottom line: Talk to your healthcare providers. Give them all the information they need about your past and present conditions, injuries, and medications, which will help them determine whether you are a good candidate for a prostate biopsy.

## FAMILY HISTORY

Prostate cancer runs in families.

A man who has a father or brother who developed prostate cancer is two times more likely to develop this disease. The chances go up if prostate cancer was detected before the age 55, or if three or more family members develop prostate cancer. The risk of developing prostate cancer is slightly higher if a brother had the disease than if a father did.

Also, men from families in which the women have had breast or ovarian cancer are at a higher risk of developing prostate cancer.

## SURGICAL HISTORY

Previous surgeries affect the outcomes of future prostate cancer treatments. For example, if you have had a TURP (TransUrethral Resection of the Prostate) for an enlarged prostate, you may be at a higher risk for incontinence, which could affect your choice of treatment.

Your surgical history is also important because even the most successful surgeries leave scar tissue behind that can make a second surgery more difficult.

Surgeries (or injuries) to other areas of your body can also impact the health of your prostate. For example, a surgery that has a long-term affect on how you walk, run, stand, or sit can eventually impact the health of your pelvic floor (also called your "urinary sphincter").

Essentially, anything that has a negative effect on the overall health of your pelvis will probably cause problems for your prostate, too. If you've had any surgeries, it's important to tell your doctor about them.

## LABORATORY (LAB) TESTS

Blood tests like PSA (free and total), comparisons like PSA velocity and PSA density, and urine tests such as PCA3 and SelectMDx can help identify men who are more likely to have prostate cancer. Also, SelectMDx and 4Kscore Test can identify men who have a higher risk of developing aggressive (high-risk) prostate cancer.

These tests support a doctor's decision to recommend that a patient have a prostate biopsy or to wait for a period of time (usually between three months and a year) to repeat the tests.

| Risk Factors | Information | Comments |
|---|---|---|
| Age | • Median age of diagnosis is 66.<br>• 6 in 10 men are diagnosed after 65.<br>• African American should start screening after age 40. | Your health history and family health history of longevity are important factors. |
| Race (Incidence Rates per 100,000) | • African American 203.5<br>• White American 121.9<br>• Hispanic American 106.9<br>• Asian American 68.9<br>• Pacific Island American 68.9<br>• Native American/Alaskan 63.9 | Race can help doctors decide who should have a biopsy and at what age. African American men and native Hawaiian men do not have the same cancer risk, even if they are the same age and have the same test results. |
| Present Illness | • Includes suspicious signs/symptoms of advanced prostate cancer.<br>• Previous results of lab tests, imaging, and diagnostic tests are important baseline information. | Severity, duration, and timing of symptoms help rule out conditions that can mimic prostate cancer (BPH & prostatitis). |
| Past Medical | Identify other medical conditions that could increase complication rates and/or limit your survival. | These medical conditions include diabetes, heart disease, stroke, neurogenic bladder, lumbar disc disease, other cancers, and so on. |
| Urologic | • Previous urologic surgeries<br>• History of urethral strictures<br>• Presence of prostatitis or BPH<br>• History or presence of stones in the kidneys, bladder, or prostate | Certain urologic conditions should be addressed before prostate cancer treatment, as they may limit the type of treatment or hamper recovery from treatment. |
| Surgical | • Previous abdominal or pelvic surgeries can affect your structure or create scar tissue that limits proposed treatment(s).<br>• Previous orthopedic surgeries can affect function of the urinary sphincter and bladder. | Previous surgeries, spinal injuries, or orthopedic injuries may increase prostate cancer treatment complication rates and may limit future treatment choices. |
| Family | Your prostate cancer risk is 2-5 times higher if your father and/or brother has prostate cancer before age 65. | Your prostate cancer risk also rises if your mother and/or sister have had breast or cervical cancer. |
| Social (Habits) | Smoking, chronic/binge drinking, recreational drug use, or prescription drug abuse may affect your general health, liver function, and immune system. | You need to be honest with all your healthcare providers about your vices/addictions; otherwise, there could be severe complications from treatment. |

**Figure 2.3** displays the prostate cancer risk factors that can affect your choice to have a prostate biopsy.

## 2. PHYSICAL EXAM

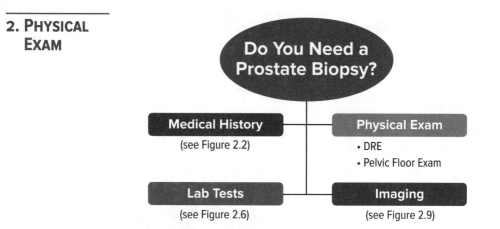

**Figure 2.4** lists the two physical exams that you should receive during your evaluation for a prostate biopsy: digital rectal exam (DRE) and pelvic floor exam. These tests can be done simultaneously.

### WHAT IS A DIGITAL RECTAL EXAM (DRE)?

A DRE is a physical exam where your doctor inserts a lubricated, gloved finger (digit) into your rectum and checks for any prostate irregularities that can be felt through the wall of the rectum. These irregularities include:

- Asymmetry (the two sides of your prostate should feel the same)
- Size (big, little, average)
- Texture (soft, hard, or both in different places)
- Lumps and bumps that could indicate cancer

A DRE can also help identify or rule out prostate cancer mimickers like prostatitis, enlarged prostate, and problems caused by lopsided tension on your urinary sphincter (pelvic floor dysfunction). Always wait 48 hours between a DRE and PSA test.

### WHAT IS THE DIFFERENCE BETWEEN A DRE AND A PELVIC FLOOR EXAMINATION?

Most doctors perform a digital rectal exam of the prostate and a pelvic floor examination at the same time. A DRE gives doctors all the prostate information listed above; a pelvic floor exam allows doctors to feel for areas of rigid and flaccid muscles. Tight, loose, or uneven muscular tone in the pelvic floor/urinary sphincter indicates a high probability of a structural component to your prostate problems.

| | If/Then | Comments |
|---|---|---|
| **DRE** *(Normal)* | **If PSA 2-4:** 15% risk of positive biopsy<br>**If PSA 4-10:** 25% risk of positive biopsy<br>**If PSA >10:** 50% risk of positive biopsy | • Highly subjective<br>• Operator dependent |
| **DRE** *(Abnormal)* | **If PSA 2-4:** 20% risk of positive biopsy<br>**If PSA 4-10:** 45% risk of positive biopsy<br>**If PSA >10:** 75% risk of positive biopsy | • Urologist is generally more accurate than a single blood test |

**Figure 2.5** illustrates the connection between digital rectal exams (DRE), PSA, and the risk of having a positive prostate biopsy.

## 3. LAB TESTS

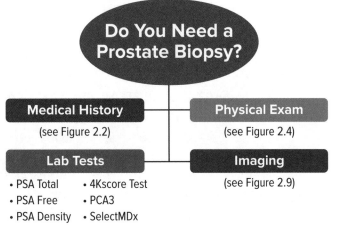

**Figure 2.6** lists the lab tests that are most likely to indicate the presence of prostate cancer; therefore, suggesting that a prostate biopsy is the next logical step.

The easiest way to classify **Lab Tests** is look at which body fluid is being tested:

### BLOOD

- **PSA (free & total):** The lower the PSA total number and the higher the PSA free number, the better.
- **PSA Density:** Includes prostate size and PSA total: the bigger the prostate, the higher the PSA total.
- **PSA Velocity:** How your total PSA numbers change (increase or decrease) over time.
- **Hormone Levels:** (recommended) Total testosterone, free testosterone, total estrogen, and testosterone/estrogen ratio.
- **4Kscore Test:** Combines 4 blood biomarkers with age, DRE result, and biopsy results (if any) to assess the probability of finding aggressive prostate cancer.

| Lab Test: Blood | |
|---|---|
| **Information** | **Comments** |
| **PSA Total** — **Normal Ranges for Adult Men**<br>• 0.0-2.5 in 40-49 year olds.<br>• 2.6-3.5 in 50-59 year olds.<br>• 3.6-4.5 in 60-69 year olds.<br>• 4.6-6.5 in 70-79 year olds. | • **Increased by:** BPH, infection, inflammation, ejaculation, prostatic massage, riding bicycles, DRE, TRUS, prostate biopsy, and cystoscopy.<br>• **Decreased by:** certain herbs, medications, and products that contain estrogen.<br>• PSA can vary by 3.6% from day to day<br>• Still the best first alert system |
| **PSA Free**<br>• PSA free is an unbound form of PSA released by BPH cells<br>• Helpful when PSA is between 4-10<br>• If PSA free > 25%, the likely culprit for an elevated PSA is an enlarged prostate (BPH). | • If free PSA is between **0-10%**: there is a 56% chance prostate cancer<br>• **10-15%**: there is a 28% chance prostate cancer<br>• **15-20%**: there is a 20% chance prostate cancer<br>• **20-25%**: there is a 16% chance prostate cancer<br>• **>25%**: there is an 8% chance prostate cancer |
| **PSA Density**<br>• PSA density is a ratio of PSA to prostate size (See **Page 54**).<br>• Calculated by dividing PSA total by the volume of prostate, calculated by ultrasound or MRI<br>• You need TRUS or MRI to determine density (DRE not reliable) | • PSA Density of less than 0.07 is likely to be caused by BPH<br>• 0.07-0.15: Uncertain<br>• PSA Density of greater than 0.15 is suspicious for prostate cancer |
| **PSA Velocity**<br>• Measures the rate of change in your PSA total over time<br>• Requires 3 PSA tests within a 2-year period | • A PSA velocity increase of 0.75 ng/ml per year, or an increase of more than 20% per year is suspicious for prostate cancer.<br>• You need to rule out: BPH, infection, inflammation, ejaculation, prostatic massage, riding bicycles, DRE, TRUS, biopsy, & cystoscopy. |
| **4Kscore Test**<br>• 4 kallikrein levels: PSA total, PSA free, PSA intact, and hK2<br>• Also takes age, DRE, and prior biopsy results into account<br>• Algorithm calculates risk of aggressive prostate cancer | • Tests like PSA and PCA3 are used to assess a man's risk of having prostate cancer; whereas the 4Kscore Test identifies a man's risk of having *aggressive* (high-risk) prostate cancer<br>• A reliable indicator that accurately identifies aggressive prostate cancer |

**Figure 2.7** explains the various values to watch for with blood tests. Please see the **Prostate Biopsy Assessment Tool** in the **Chapter 2 Toolbox (Page 56)** to include your own information.

### URINE

- **PCA3:** This test reveals a gene that highly expressed in prostate cancer cells. Unlike PSA, PCA3 is NOT affected by an enlarged prostate (BPH) or inflammation (prostatitis). A positive PCA3 test is a strong indicator of prostate cancer.

- **SelectMDx:** This test helps identify men who have a higher risk of developing aggressive prostate cancer. It also accurately predicts whether a biopsy will find low-grade or high-grade cancer.

| Lab Test: Urine | | |
|---|---|---|
| **PCA 3** | • Non-invasive urine-based, molecular test.<br>• Uses the first part of the urine stream after a DRE & prostate massage.<br>• Measures Prostate Cancer Antigen 3 (PCA3): a gene only present in the prostate and highly expressed in prostate cancer. | • PCA3 is unchanged by BPH, infection, inflammation, ejaculation, prostatic massage, riding bicycles, DRE, or previous prostate biopsies.<br>• If positive, IDs patients who need a prostate biopsy, despite previous negative biopsies.<br>• A high PCA3 score indicates an increased likelihood of a positive biopsy.<br>• A low PCA3 score indicates a decreased likelihood of a positive biopsy. |
| **SelectMDx** | • Non-invasive urine-based, molecular test.<br>• Uses first part of the urine stream after DRE and prostate massage<br>• Measures the expression of DLX1 and HOXC6 genes. Both are associated with an increased probability for high grade prostate cancer (Gleason Score ≥ 7) | • Helps identify men with a higher risk for aggressive prostate cancer.<br>• Accurately predicts the likelihood of finding low-grade & high-grade cancer in a biopsy<br>• Helps determine which patients need a follow-up biopsy right away.<br>• Reduces the need for unnecessary biopsies & other costly tests for men who have a low risk for having prostate cancer. |

Figure 2.8 lists the two main state-of-the-art urine tests that doctors use to evaluate whether a man should have a prostate biopsy or wait for another round of tests. See **Page 57** to include your own information.

**4. IMAGING**

The following imaging studies give your medical team more information about your prostate:

1. Doppler Ultrasound (also measures blood flow)
2. CAT scan
3. MRI
4. MRIS (MRI plus spectroscopy that includes info about cellular activity and metabolism)
5. MRI Fusion (merges an MRI with an ultrasound image to create a 3-D view of the prostate)

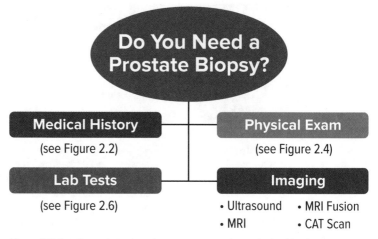

**Do You Need a Prostate Biopsy?**

**Medical History**
(see Figure 2.2)

**Physical Exam**
(see Figure 2.4)

**Lab Tests**
(see Figure 2.6)

**Imaging**
- Ultrasound
- MRI
- MRI Fusion
- CAT Scan

**Figure 2.9** lists the main images doctors use to evaluate the health of your prostate.

Both MRI and a CAT scans are used throughout the country in prostate imaging. Image quality and modalities vary from region to region.

How do you know how to choose between having an MRI or a CAT scan of your prostate? That's a tough call. We recommend you talk to your doctor(s) and local prostate cancer support groups and find out which imaging facility in your area provides the best results.

Imaging technology has come a long way in the last decade, but it has not evolved to the point where your doctor can tell whether or not you have cancer or how aggressive that cancer is.

For that, you still need a biopsy.

The **Prostate Biopsy Assessment Tool** in the **Chapter 2 Toolbox** gives you a way to look at the information from your various tests and images like a doctor would.

Obviously, a bunch of numbers on a page cannot replace the one-on-one interactions you have with your doctor; however, understanding why a prostate biopsy is (or is not) your logical next step is important.

Understanding leads to knowledge, and knowledge gives you the tools you need to make informed decisions about having a biopsy and your health in general.

We encourage you to take advantage of this opportunity, because if you have prostate cancer, it's far better to know *now* than *later*.

## TYPES OF BIOPSIES

| Biopsies | Rectal | Perineal |
|---|---|---|
| The Numbers | • Rectal Bleeding: 50%<br>• Infection Rates: 15.5%<br>• Positive Biopsy Rate: 48%<br>• Perineal swelling: 3%<br>• Less painful | • Rectal Bleeding: 3.4%<br>• Infection Rate: 3.4%<br>• Positive Biopsy Rate: 44%<br>• Perineal swelling: 14%<br>• More painful |

Figure 2.10 lists the pros and cons of rectal and perineal prostate biopsies. Urinary tract symptoms, pain/difficulty urinating, and urinary retention rates are the same for both kinds of biopsies; however, rectal bleeding, infection, perineal swelling rates, and post-procedure pain are not. Unless there is a compelling medical reason not to, we recommend that you go with the type of biopsy your urologist performs regularly. Frequency is the key here: The more frequently your doctor performs a particular type of biopsy, the better he/she is at doing that procedure.

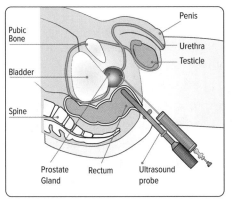

### Rectal Prostate Biopsy

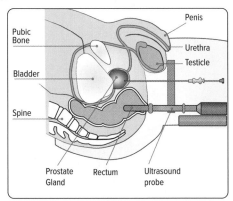

### Perineal Prostate Biopsy

Figure 2.11 (courtesy of the Irish Cancer Society) displays the difference between the two kinds of prostate biopsies: Rectal and Perineal.

### A WORD ABOUT MRI-FUSION PROSTATE BIOPSIES

*The combination of an MRI with an ultrasound image significantly improves the accuracy of a prostate biopsy, and decreases the number of biopsies needed to determine if prostate cancer is present. An MRI fusion biopsy is 70-75% accurate in diagnosing existing prostate cancer versus 30-35% for a TRUS/random biopsy. MRI fusion technology is a significant step in decreasing unnecessary biopsies, and cuts down on the number of core samples obtained during a biopsy; therefore, minimizing complications. (Higher accuracy leads to fewer biopsies; fewer biopsy needles lead to fewer complications).*

## ADVANTAGES AND DISADVANTAGES OF THE THREE MOST COMMON TYPES OF PROSTATE BIOPSIES

| | Advantages | Disadvantages |
|---|---|---|
| **TRUS / Random** | • TRUS is relatively inexpensive.<br>• The ultrasound determines the size and shape of the prostate, suggest areas of cancer, calcifications, and blood flow.<br>• Most urologists use ultrasound equipment in their office.<br>• All urologists train with TRUS.<br>• TRUS is an evenly spaced "random" needle biopsy that uses a total of 12-24 needles, depending on the size of the prostate. | • TRUS does not detect all cancer areas.<br>• TRUS is considered random in most cases.<br>• Quality of the ultrasound equipment is crucial in the improved detection of suspicious areas.<br>• Doppler can be helpful in identifying more suspicious areas.<br>• The risk of infection and trauma to rectal wall goes up with the number of biopsies.<br>• TRUS can miss up to 70% of cancers. |
| **MRI / Guided** | • Very high resolution of suspicious areas.<br>• Decreased number of needles, minimizing trauma to rectal wall; thus, reducing the risk of infection.<br>• Important for creating a baseline for future MRI monitoring.<br>• Helpful in active surveillance patients.<br>• Helpful in staging as it can detect extracapsular extension and seminal vesicle involvement.<br>• Can detect lymph node involvement and/or bone involvement. | • Expensive procedure.<br>• Claustrophobic patients may need medication to manage anxiety.<br>• Quality of the MRI technology varies<br>• Few physicians are properly trained in the use of this technology. |
| **MRI-Fusion** | • Increased detection of high-risk prostate cancer.<br>• Decreased detection of low-risk prostate cancer.<br>• Radiologists experienced in reading and interpreting MRI images are essential in mapping the abnormal areas. | • Fusion images are susceptible to a patient's movement resulting in imprecise segmentation of the gland outline and decreased accuracy<br>• Doctors must learn to read MRI images.<br>• Additional time is required for the image segmentation and matching processes. |

**Figure 2.12** outlines the advantages and disadvantages of the different types of prostate biopsies. See the **Chapter 2** Toolbox to include your own information.

For more information about prostate biopsy complications, see **Page 322** in the **Chapter 2 Digging Deeper** section.

# Doctor Story
## DR. KURT STROM, MD

Urology,
Banner Health
Loveland, Colorado

*As a medical student, I remember the chairman of Rush University Medical Center proclaiming that sometime in the near future there would be a pill that cures prostate cancer. While that "magic pill" still eludes us, I marvel at how far prostate cancer treatment of has come during my brief career.*

*Back in 2007, as a resident performing open radical prostatectomies, I watched skilled surgeons lose copious amounts of blood. Halfway through my training, our hospital bought a DaVinci S surgical robot, and I witnessed seasoned urologists struggle to become skilled robotic surgeons.*

*Despite the cost of the robot (millions of dollars), the blood loss was minimal, patients went home the next day and back to work within a week. These improvements in care were hugely important to my patients and their families — parts of the healthcare equation that economists cannot assign a dollar value.*

*In May 2012, the United States Preventative Services Task Force (USPSTF) stated that PSA screening for prostate cancer was inappropriately overused. Doctors could do little but watch as prostate cancer treatment rates fell dramatically. It was a conspiracy against men.*

*Despite how wrongheaded this decision was, it challenged urologists to rethink how to better treat men with prostate cancer — and men who may develop it.*

*For example, we have stopped treating non-lethal low-risk prostate cancer, because the unwanted complications of treatment often outweigh the benefits. It's changes like this that keep me hopeful that prostate cancer treatment is moving in the right direction.*

## LOOKING AHEAD

**CHAPTER 1:** You or your doctor is concerned about your prostate — We provide you with **Prostate 101**: where it lives, what it does, plus relevant statistics.

**CHAPTER 2:** Your doctor told you to **schedule a prostate biopsy** — We give you a **Prostate Biopsy Assessment Tool** to see if you actually need one, and what to expect if you do.

**CHAPTER 3:** You have a prostate biopsy — We explain the steps you need to take, whether you have a **negative biopsy or a positive biopsy**.

**CHAPTER 4:** You have a **positive prostate biopsy** — We provide you with a **Prostate Cancer Assessment Tool** to help you understand which kind of cancer you have.

**CHAPTER 5:** You need to select a prostate cancer treatment — We provide you with a summary of the most common types of treatment based on your **cancer risk type** (low-risk, moderate-risk, and high-risk).

**CHAPTER 6:** You have **low-risk, low-volume prostate cancer** and need to learn more about emerging treatments — We provide you with a summary of these treatments to help you understand the differences between focal, minimally invasive, alternative, whole gland, and traditional treatments.

**CHAPTER 7:** You have prostate cancer that is more advanced than low-risk, low-volume and need to know more about **whole-gland treatments** (both stand-alone traditional and combination treatments) — We provide you with a summary of these treatments.

**CHAPTER 8:** You want to know the **success and complication rates** for each type of treatment and for each cancer risk type (low-risk, moderate-risk, and high-risk) — We provide you with unbiased information to support your decision-making process.

**CHAPTER 9:** You feel **overwhelmed** by the news of a positive prostate biopsy — We give you the tools to surf this tidal wave of emotion and overcome the feeling of panic that almost always accompanies a positive biopsy report.

**CHAPTER 10:** You want to **use your cancer diagnosis as a springboard to better health** — We help you address your wellness goals with a proven plan that covers inflammation, diet, inactivity, stress, immune system, hormone optimization, structure, and removing toxic substances.

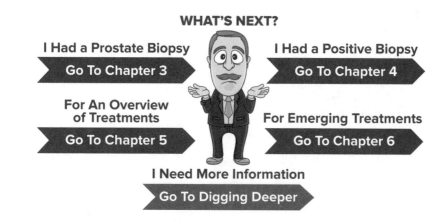

**WHAT'S NEXT?**

**I Had a Prostate Biopsy**
Go To Chapter 3

**I Had a Positive Biopsy**
Go To Chapter 4

**For An Overview of Treatments**
Go To Chapter 5

**For Emerging Treatments**
Go To Chapter 6

**I Need More Information**
Go To Digging Deeper

# WELCOME TO THE TOOLBOX
# CHAPTER 2 **TOOLBOX**

**THIS TOOLBOX SECTION INCLUDES THE FOLLOWING TOOLS AND RESOURCES TO HELP YOU MAKE AN INFORMED DECISION ABOUT HAVING A PROSTATE BIOPSY:**

- PSA Density Calculator
- Prostate Cancer Risk Factors
- Prostate Biopsy Assessment Tool
- Frequently Asked Questions
- How to Prepare for an Outpatient Prostate Biopsy Procedure
- Post-biopsy Instructions
- A Word about Blood Thinners
- AUA Score

## *PSA Density Calculator*

| | HOW TO CALCULATE | YOUR DATA |
|---|---|---|
| **Prostate Volume** | • The easiest way to calculate your Prostate Volume is with a trans-rectal ultrasound image that measures the length, width, and height of the prostate (prostate volume).<br>• Once you have these numbers, multiply them together (L x W x H), then multiply that number by 0.52 | **You have to know your Prostate Volume to calculate your PSA Density.** |
| **PSA Density** | • Calculate your Prostate Volume with either a trans-rectal ultrasound, MRI, or CT scan.<br>• Divide your PSA Total number by your total Prostate Volume to find the PSA Density.<br>• For example, if you have a PSA Total of 4.0 ng/ml and a prostate volume of 30 ml, divide 4.0 by 30.<br><br>$$4.0 \div 30 = 0.15$$ | • Less than 0.07 = likely BPH<br>• 0.07-0.15 = uncertain<br>• More than 0.15 = suspicious for prostate cancer |

**TOOLBOX**

*The information that you provide in the "Your Data" column on the next three pages gives you and your doctors a clear indication about whether a prostate biopsy is the next logical step in evaluating the health of your prostate.*

# Prostate Cancer Risk Factors

| | INFORMATION | COMMENTS | YOUR DATA |
|---|---|---|---|
| **AGE** | • If older than 75, no need for screening.<br>• If you have a family history of cancer or are African American, start screening at age 40. | • Not an exact science.<br>• Your health history is very important.<br>• History of longevity in your family is also important. | **Your Age** |
| **RACE** *(Incidence Rate per 100,000)* | • African American 203.5<br>• White American 121.9<br>• Hispanic American 106.9<br>• Asian American 68.9<br>• Pacific Island American 68.9<br>• Native American/Alaskan 63.9 | Knowing your racial identity can help determine when you should have your first prostate biopsy. | **Ethnicity** |
| **MEDICAL HISTORY** | Do you have any medical conditions that could limit your 5-year survival? | Do you have any medical conditions that could increase complications rates of prostate cancer treatments? | **Medical History** |
| **FAMILY HISTORY** | If you are under 65 years old and either your father, brother, or both have had prostate cancer, you have a 2-5 times higher risk of developing the disease. | If your mother and/or sister had breast or cervical cancer, that also increases your chances of having prostate cancer. | **Cancer History** |
| **If Digital Rectal Exam is Normal** | • If PSA 2-4, 15% probability of positive biopsy<br>• If PSA 4-10, 25% probability of positive biopsy<br>• PSA >10, 50% probability of positive biopsy | • Highly subjective<br>• Operator-dependent<br>• DREs performed by urologists are generally more accurate | **PSA w/ Normal DRE** |
| **If Digital Rectal Exam is Abnormal** | • PSA 2-4, 20% probability of positive biopsy<br>• PSA 4-10, 45% probability of positive biopsy<br>• PSA >10, 75% probability of positive biopsy | • Highly subjective<br>• Operator-dependent<br>• DREs performed by urologists are generally more accurate | **PSA w/ Abnormal DRE** |

---

# Prostate Biopsy Assessment Tool

TOOLBOX

| | INFORMATION | COMMENTS | YOUR DATA |
|---|---|---|---|
| **PSA Total** | **Normal PSA Total Range**<br>• 0.0-2.5 in 40-49 year olds<br>• 2.6-3.5 in 50-59 year olds<br>• 3.6-4.5 in 60-69 year olds<br>• 4.6-6.5 in 70-79 year olds<br>• Still the best first alert system | • Increased by: BPH, infection, inflammation, ejaculation, prostatic massage, riding bicycles, DRE, TRUS, prostate biopsy, and cystoscopy.<br>• Decreased by: certain herbs, medications such as 5 alpha reductase inhibitors, and products that contain estrogen.<br>• PSA can vary by 3.6% from day to day | **Total PSA?** |
| **PSA Free** | • PSA free is an unbound form of PSA released by BPH cells<br>• Helpful when PSA free is between 4-10<br>• If PSA free is greater than 25%, the likely culprit for an elevated PSA is an enlarged prostate (BPH). | • If PSA free is between 0-10%, there is a 56% chance of prostate cancer<br>• 10-15%, there is a 28% chance of prostate cancer<br>• 15-20%, there is a 20% chance of prostate cancer<br>• 20-25%, there is a 16% chance of prostate cancer<br>• More than 25% there is an 8% chance of prostate cancer | **Free PSA?** |
| **PSA Density** | • PSA density is a ratio of PSA to prostate size.<br>• It is calculated by dividing PSA total by the volume of prostate (calculated by ultrasound or MRI)<br>• You need TRUS or MRI to determine density (DRE not reliable) | • A PSA density of less than 0.07 is likely to be caused by BPH<br>• 0.07-0.15: Uncertain<br>• Greater than 0.15: Suspicious for prostate cancer | **PSA Density?**<br>*(See Page 54)* |
| **PSA Velocity** | Requires 3 PSA tests in a 2-year period | • A PSA velocity increase of 0.75 ng/ml per year, or an increase of more than 20% per year is suspicious for prostate cancer.<br>• You need to rule out: BPH, infection, inflammation, ejaculation, prostatic massage, riding bicycles, DRE, TRUS/BX, and cystoscopy. | **PSA Velocity?** |

# Prostate Biopsy Assessment Tool Cont.

| | INFORMATION | COMMENTS | YOUR DATA |
|---|---|---|---|
| **4Kscore Test** | • 4 kallikrein levels: PSA total, PSA free, PSA intact and hK2<br>• Includes age, DRE, and prior biopsy status<br>• Algorithm calculates risk of aggressive prostate cancer | • Highly sensitive test that is a clear indicator of aggressive prostate cancer<br>• The only blood test that accurately identifies risk for aggressive prostate cancer | **4Kscore Test** |
| **PCA3** | • Non-invasive urine-based molecular test<br>• Uses first part of the urine stream after DRE and prostate massage<br>• If you have a positive PCA-3 test and a negative biopsy, a 2nd biopsy is encouraged because of the high likelihood of having prostate cancer. | PCA-3 is not changed by BPH, infection, inflammation, ejaculation, prostatic massage, riding bicycles, DRE, TRUS/BX, or cystoscopy. | **PCA3 Score** |
| **SelectMDx** | • Non-invasive urine-based molecular test<br>• Uses first part of the urine stream after DRE and prostate massage<br>• Measures the expression of DLX1 and HOXC6 genes. Both are associated with an increased probability for high-grade prostate cancer (Gleason Score ≥ 7) | • Helps ID men with a higher risk for aggressive prostate cancer<br>• Can accurately predict the likelihood of finding low-grade & high-grade cancer in a biopsy<br>• Helps determine which patients need a follow-up biopsy sooner<br>• Reduces the need for unnecessary biopsies & other costly tests for men who have a low risk of having prostate cancer | **SelectMDx** |

TOOLBOX

# Frequently Asked Questions about Transrectal Ultrasound-Guided Needle Biopsy of Prostate (TRUS biopsy)

**TOP 6 QUESTIONS THAT PATIENTS ASK ABOUT PROSTATE BIOPSIES:**
1. Why should I have a prostate biopsy?
2. What do I need to do before I have a biopsy?
3. What are the possible complications of a prostate biopsy?
4. Will it hurt?
5. What if my prostate biopsy comes back positive?
6. Why do I need a biopsy if MRI imaging suggests I have prostate cancer?

## 1. Why should I have a prostate biopsy?

When doctors recommend that their patients have a prostate biopsy, they are attempting to do two things:

1. Rule out the presence of prostate cancer
2. If prostate cancer is present, determine type, stage, Gleason Score, and the extent of the cancer.

The earlier you catch prostate cancer, the easier it is to cure. If prostate cancer is present, it's better to know sooner than later.

## 2. What do I need to do before I have a biopsy?
The logistics of a prostate biopsy are fairly straightforward:

**BEFORE THE PROCEDURE**
- You will be asked to use an enema at home a couple of hours before the procedure.
- You will given some oral antibiotics to take as a precaution against infection from the procedure. (Some doctors prefer to give patients an antibiotic injection prior to a biopsy.)

**DURING THE PROCEDURE**
- The procedure is usually done in your doctor's office.
- It usually takes 20-30 minutes.
- Unless you require anti-anxiety medication, you can drive yourself home.
- A lubricated ultrasound probe is inserted into your

*TOOLBOX*

rectum. This probe also doubles as the guide for the biopsy needles.

- Between 12-24 needles will be used to extract a small amount of tissue from your prostate, which will be analyzed and evaluated by a pathologist (a doctor who specializes in tissue analysis).

**AFTER THE PROCEDURE**

- You will be given additional antibiotics.
- It takes about a week to get the results back.
- It is normal to pee and ejaculate blood for up to two weeks. The blood will be bright red to begin with and then fade to brown before it goes a way completely.
- If you have persistent pain or inflammation in your prostate (like you have a tennis ball between your legs), fever, flu-like symptoms, muscle aches, or your body starts to shake uncontrollably, go to the nearest emergency room or urgent care center. These are all symptoms of sepsis (a systemic blood infection), a rare but potentially fatal complication of a prostate biopsy.

**3. What are the possible complications of a prostate biopsy?**

All surgical procedures, including prostate biopsies, carry some risk of complications:

- Infection — which can be fatal in a very low percentage of cases (1 to 3 men per 1,000)
- Prostatitis (itching, scratching, and pain in the prostate and/or urethra)
- Difficulty urinating
- Urinary frequency (the urge to pee frequently)
- Urinary Urgency (gotta go RIGHT NOW!)
- Temporary erectile dysfunction (ED)
- Blood in your urine
- Blood in your semen
- Lingering pain

These complications, which usually go away on their own, often increase in number and severity with repeated biopsies.

### 4. Will it hurt?

When we explain the above information to most men, they nod their heads "yes" at all the right moments, but when we ask them if they have any questions, the first one they ask is, "Will it hurt?"

When the injection of a local anesthetic is done correctly, which happens 99% of the time, the pain of a prostate biopsy is low (1 or 2 out of 10, with 10 being the worst pain you've ever felt). If the anesthetic injection is done incorrectly, a prostate biopsy feels like what it is — a bunch of needles being shot through the wall of your rectum and into your prostate (8 out of 10 pain).

Hint: Ask the doctor to make sure that you are "totally numb" before the first biopsy needle goes in.

### 5. What if your prostate biopsy comes back positive?

One of the chief points of this book is to help men (and their loved ones) understand all the factors that go into (or should go into) the decision to have a prostate biopsy.

If your prostate biopsy finds any amount of prostate cancer, we recommend you read **Chapters 4-10** of this book.

### 6. Why do I need a biopsy if MRI imaging suggests I have prostate cancer?

Imaging technology has come a long way in the last decade. That said, MRI technology has not advanced to the point where it can tell you whether or not you have cancer, or more importantly, how aggressive that cancer is. Doctors still need a "tissue diagnosis" to do that.

## Preparation for an Outpatient Prostate Biopsy

*The following information expands upon our answers to the previous six questions. We include this information because our experience tells us that different people need to hear the same information presented in different ways before they "get it."*

This procedure is usually done in your urologist's office and involves firing and retracting several needles (12 to 24) into the prostate to retrieve small samples of tissue. A real-time ultrasound image is used to guide the needles, and the procedure usually takes between 20 to 30 minutes, depending upon the number of needles.

**Standard suggestions include:**

- Consume only clear liquids the day of the procedure.
- Use a Fleets enema, which can be purchased at any drugstore, the morning of the procedure to clear any stool from the rectum. **This is very important!**
- You will probably receive 2 prescriptions, as well as some anti-anxiety medication just before the biopsy.
- Come to the procedure with your bladder at least partially full of urine (at least one hour without urinating).
- You can go home after the biopsy.
- Continue to take the antibiotics until all the pills are gone.
- Continue to take your regular medications (except blood thinners) that you are taking under the direction of your doctor(s).

**Common biopsy complications include:**

- Bleeding from the rectum
- Blood in your urine and semen — a common and disconcerting problem that usually only lasts 2-3 weeks.
- Mild burning, pain, or increased need to urinate — these symptoms are not a concern unless they persist for more than 24 hours.

If you develop fever, chills, muscle aches, flu-like symptoms, the pain increases, or you cannot urinate —

**let your doctor know immediately!**

## Post Trans Rectal Ultrasound and Prostate Biopsy Instructions

It is extremely important that you finish your antibiotics. Also, increase your fluid intake for the first two days after the biopsy to decrease formation of blood clots in your urine. Usually, your urine will clear itself of blood clots after the first few times you pee. Blood spotting in your urine may occur for up to two weeks after the biopsy.

Your rectum or the base of your penis may hurt for a couple of days. That's normal.

Staying off your feet until the morning after your biopsy is a good idea. Limit your activity, particularly heavy lifting, for 48 hours or until the bleeding stops. Avoid cycling for one week.

**IT IS IMPORTANT TO CONTACT YOUR DOCTOR IMMEDIATELY (OR GO TO YOUR LOCAL EMERGENCY ROOM) IF ANY OF THE FOLLOWING SYMPTOMS OCCUR:**

- Sharp pain or intense burning while urinating
- Chills
- Fever
- Muscle aches
- Excessive blood clots or lots of blood in your urine or stool
- Difficulty or inability to urinate
- Overall weakness or feeling like you're going to faint

## A Word or Two about Blood Thinners

Talk to your doctor(s) about ALL the medications you are taking: prescription, over-the-counter, and nutritional supplements.

We recommend that you bring all the bottles and containers to show your doctor(s) — **BEFORE YOU HAVE A PROSTATE BIOPSY.**

If you don't want to carry all those bottles with you to your next appointment, write down a complete list of all the pills, powders, potions, and lotions you use.

The reason we want you to show your doctor(s) the medications and supplements you take is because some of them may contain blood-thinning compounds.

Avoiding blood thinners is one of the most important things you can do to ensure that you have a successful prostate biopsy.

Again, talk to your doctor(s). They will be happy to clarify what's OK for you to take before your biopsy, and more importantly, what you should NOT take!

TOOLBOX

ur **AUA score gives you and your doctors a way to quantify your**
inary symptoms. If you haven't filled out an **AUA** score recently,
ke a minute to do so, and share the results with your doctors.

## AUA Symptom score (AUASS)

| Circle One Number on Each Line | Not at All | Less Than 1 Time in 5 | Less Than Half the Time | About Half The Time | More Than Half The Time | Almost Always |
|---|---|---|---|---|---|---|
| ver the past month, how often have you had the eling of not completely emptying your bladder ter you finished urinating? | 0 | 1 | 2 | 3 | 4 | 5 |
| ver the past month, how often have you had to rinate again less than 2 hours after you finished rinating? | 0 | 1 | 2 | 3 | 4 | 5 |
| ver the past month, how often have you found at you stopped and started again several times hen you urinated? | 0 | 1 | 2 | 3 | 4 | 5 |
| ver the past month, how often have you found it ard to hold your urine? | 0 | 1 | 2 | 3 | 4 | 5 |
| ver the past month, how often have you had a eak urine stream? | 0 | 1 | 2 | 3 | 4 | 5 |
| ver the past month, how often have you had to ush or strain to begin urination? | 0 | 1 | 2 | 3 | 4 | 5 |
| | None | 1 Time | 2 Times | 3 Times | 4 Times | 5 or More Times |
| ver the past month, how many times per night d you most typically get up to urinate from the ne you went to bed at night until the time you t up in the morning? | 0 | 1 | 2 | 3 | 4 | 5 |

d the score for each number above and write the total in the space to the right  _____

MPTOM SCORE: 1-7 (Mild)  8-19 (Moderate)  20-35 (Severe)

## Quality of Life (QOL)

| Circle One Number on Each Line | Delighted | Pleased | Mostly Satisfied | Mixed | Mostly Dis-satisfied | Unhappy | Terrible |
|---|---|---|---|---|---|---|---|
| w would you feel if you had to live th your urinary condition the way it is w, no better, no worse, for the rest of ur life? | 0 | 1 | 2 | 3 | 4 | 5 | 6 |

TOOLBOX

**NOTES:**

TOOLBOX

# Biopsy Results: What to Do?

> You can be a victim of cancer,
> or a survivor of cancer.
> It's a mindset.
>
> — *Dave Pelzer, author and*
> *childhood abuse survivor*

# Patient Story
## STEPHEN

*What have I learned from my prostate cancer experience?*
*Trust the science, but also trust your heart. Gather information, but listen to your intuition.*

*At 64, I was a healthy soon-to-be-retired public school administrator who was looking forward to becoming a full-time recreational cyclist. Prostate cancer was a shock.*

*For some reason, I thought I ought to have a physical. Nothing was wrong, it had just been a while. The blood work showed an elevated PSA, so my physician suggested the urologist downstairs, who'd likely order a prostate biopsy. Somewhere, I'd heard about too many unnecessary prostate biopsies; it was enough to make me hesitate.*

*My wife suggested another urologist, so I made an appointment. My new urologist thoroughly explained all the tests, and did recommend a prostate biopsy when other tests suggested that was the right step. The biopsy was positive for cancer.*

*You could say that I only delayed the process by not following my first doctor's advice ... but that would be missing the point.*

*I have always sought a balanced approach between science and the forces that science can't explain. The most important events of my life have taught me to pay attention to seemingly random events and decisions because of how easily they turn into "circumstances" of major significance.*

*If I reverse engineer my cancer experience, the most important parts are (1) an early diagnosis and (2) being referred for CyberKnife treatment. The science, the physics and the medicine did the trick. But I had to get there. I don't know if the urologist I chose NOT to see would have made that recommendation; however, I do know that all the other treatment options were invasive and had significant side effects. It had to be CyberKnife, so I could heal and go on with my life relatively unscathed.*

# chapter
## THREE
# summary

**Chapter 3** helps you understand the information from a prostate biopsy. We also introduce you to the most common types of prostate cancer.

Our goal is to help you become a well-informed patient so you can have better conversations with your doctor(s).

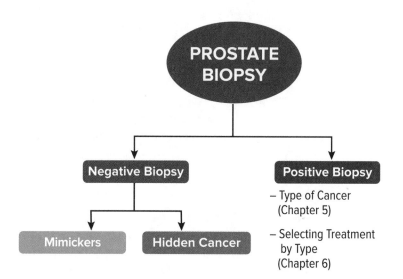

The third tier of **Figure 3.0** illustrates why a prostate cancer biopsy may not be a simple on/off, yes/no kind of procedure. Thanks to several new "epigenetic" and "genomic" tests, we can now separate prostate cancer from other conditions that have similar symptoms (mimickers), detect "hidden" prostate cancer (and detect it sooner) — as well as accurately determine how aggressive the cancer is once it's found.

**DEBUNKING MYTHS**

# DOES A NEGATIVE PROSTATE BIOPSY MEAN YOU DO NOT HAVE PROSTATE CANCER? NOT ALWAYS ...

*Of the 1.2 million prostate biopsies performed in the United States every year, over 700,000 (68%) are negative. Twenty-five percent of those 700,000 contain cancer (175,000).*

*Most of what a prostate biopsy tells you is whether the hollow-core needles that collected samples from your prostate DID or DID NOT contain any cancer.*

*Is it possible that these needles missed a tiny tumor of prostate cancer? Absolutely! Traditional prostate biopsies only sample 1% of the total prostate volume.*

*If you have any of the following, there is good reason to repeat a negative prostate biopsy, as any of these results could indicate the presence of prostate cancer:*

- *Elevated PSA total*
- *Low PSA free*
- *Rising PSA velocity*
- *Rising PSA density*
- *Higher 4KScore Test result*
- *Abnormal PCA3 or SelectMDx score*
- *Positive ConfirmMDx test*

*The "false negative" scenario mentioned above is exactly why 3D MRI-fusion prostate biopsies are such a welcomed improvement over conventional random TRUS biopsies.*

*MRI-fusion biopsies catch 70-75% of prostate cancer on the first biopsy, while conventional TRUS biopsies only catch 30-35% of prostate cancer on the first biopsy.*

*Pairing an MRI picture of the prostate with a real-time ultrasound image also allows doctors to search suspicious areas and find hidden tumors that may have been missed on previous negative biopsies.*

*In addition, MRI-fusion biopsies are 2-3 times more sensitive in detecting "clinically significant" prostate cancer and twice as accurate as standard TRUS biopsies in determining the extent of the cancer.*

*Combining MRI-fusion technology with other tests like ConfirmMDx, SelectMDx, 4Kscore Test, and PCA3 gives doctors an increased chance of uncovering hidden and aggressive cancers.*

## VOCABULARY

See Glossary for Definitions

4Kscore Test

Bone Scan

ConfirmMDx

Decipher

DRE (Digital Rectal Exam)

Epigenetic Testing

Extracapsular Extension (ECE)

False Negative

Genomic Testing

Gleason Score

Lymph Node

Methylation

MRI

MRI-Fusion Prostate Biopsy

Oncotype DX

Partin Tables

PCA3 Test (urine)

Prostatic Interstitial Neoplasia (PIN)

Perineural Invasion (PNI)

Prolaris

Prostate Biopsy

PSA (Prostate Specific Antigen)

PSA Density

PSA Free

PSA Test

PSA Total

PSA Velocity

SelectMDx

Seminal Vesicle Involvement

TRUS Prostate Biopsy

Ultrasound

## A NEW ERA IN PROSTATE CANCER DIAGNOSIS AND TREATMENT

*Prostate cancer diagnosis and treatment are swiftly moving beyond Gleason Scores, PSA, Cancer Stages, and Partin Tables.*

*Today, blood biomarker tests like the 4Kscore Test, non-invasive urine-based molecular tests such as PCA3 and SelectMDx, epigenetic tests such as ConfirmMDx, image analysis tools like ProMark, and genomic tests such as Oncotype DX provide doctors with the tools to detect prostate cancer earlier and with greater accuracy than ever before.*

*These innovations allow patients to avoid unnecessary biopsies, while improving doctors ability to locate and identify existing cancers. This improved accuracy helps doctors avoid overtreating insignificant cancers and undertreating cancers that have the potential to spread outside the prostate — even though these cancers may initially appear to be low-risk.*

*As a patient, you want to know the true nature of your cancer, so you can find the best treatment for the kind of cancer you have.*

*Bottom line: We want all men who have "clinically significant" prostate cancer to get the best possible treatment. This is especially true for men with moderate- and high-risk disease. We also do NOT want to see men with "clinically insignificant" or "low-risk, low-volume" disease get over-treated and suffer lifelong quality-of-life complications from their treatment.*

**WHAT A
BIOPSY
LOOKS LIKE**

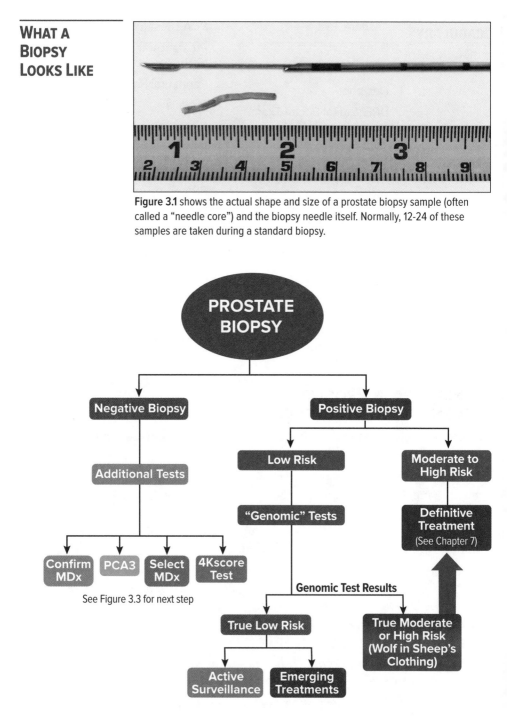

**Figure 3.1** shows the actual shape and size of a prostate biopsy sample (often called a "needle core") and the biopsy needle itself. Normally, 12-24 of these samples are taken during a standard biopsy.

**Figure 3.2** illustrates the cascade of "next steps" if your prostate biopsy is negative or positive.

## WHAT TO DO WITH YOUR BIOPSY RESULTS

If your prostate biopsy is negative, one of three things is likely:

1. You do not have cancer
2. The cancer is undetected
3. You have BPH and/or prostatitis.

If your biopsy is positive, then you need to make some choices about treatment options based on the kind of cancer you have. (We encourage you to look at the list of "12 Factors that Define Prostate Cancer" on **Page 75**).

Let's take a closer look at these two scenarios.

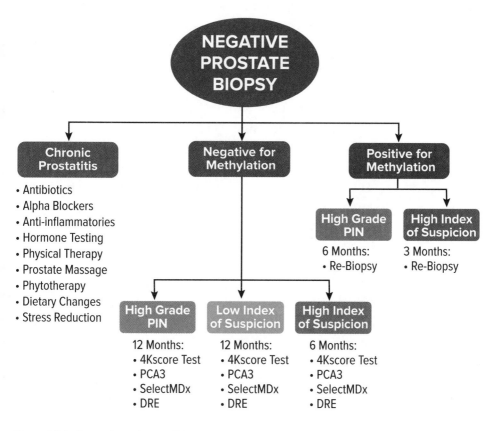

Figure 3.3 further explores the **possible scenarios** for a negative prostate biopsy and additional next steps. **(This figure outlines some of your options. Not every test listed is appropriate.)** "Index of Suspicion" means how likely you are to have cancer: A low index of suspicion means a low probability of having prostate cancer, and a high index of suspicion means you have a high probability of having cancer. See **Page 72** for information on "Methylation."

## NEGATIVE BIOPSY (NO CANCER)

### WHAT YOU NEED TO KNOW ABOUT METHYLATION

*A new generation of "epigenetic" tests are able to evaluate prostate biopsy tissue samples for the presence or absence of "methylation." A positive methylation test suggests the presence of prostate cancer. A negative methylation test suggests the absence of prostate cancer. For more information about epigenetic tests, go to* **Chapter 3 Digging Deeper.**

A negative biopsy means that your prostate biopsy showed no signs of cancer — which is great news!

Before you pop the champagne, however, we offer a few words of caution. Don't get us wrong, having a negative biopsy is a wonderful thing, it just does not completely rule out the presence of cancer.

If you've had a negative biopsy, we recommend that you talk with your doctor about where you fit in **Figure 3.3**:

**1.** No Cancer (most likely BPH or prostatitis)

**2.** Negative for methylation

**3.** Positive for methylation

This conversation with your doctor will be tempered by whether your doctor thinks you have a "low index of suspicion" (meaning you probably do NOT have prostate cancer — or if you do, it's a very low-grade cancer) or a "high index of suspicion," (meaning you probably DO have cancer, but it has not been detected yet.)

We see having a negative biopsy with a negative methylation test and a low index of suspicion as an opportunity to learn how you can modify your lifestyle to improve your health and prevent prostate cancer (See **Chapter 10**).

On the other hand, we see a negative biopsy with a positive methylation test and a high index of suspicion as a likely "false negative" biopsy (a biopsy that does not detect cancer, even though cancer is present).

A high index of suspicion usually prompts your doctor to recommend another round of tests (blood, urine, and DRE) and an additional prostate biopsy in 3-6 months.

Also, relatively new blood tests such as the 4Kscore Test, urine tests like SelectMDx, and biopsy-based tests like ConfirmMDx can help reveal the presence of hidden cancers that may be lurking in a "false negative" biopsy.

These innovative tests are so important because traditional TRUS prostate biopsies only detect 30-35 percent of clinically significant prostate cancers on the first biopsy. MRI-Fusion biopsies detect 70-75 percent of clinically significant prostate cancer on the first biopsy — which cuts down on the need for multiple biopsies (and the complications they create). However, MRI-Fusion biopsies still miss 25-30 percent of cancers on the first try.

If you need to repeat a biopsy, we highly recommend that you ask your doctor if MRI-fusion prostate biopsy technology is available in your area — or just Google "MRI fusion prostate biopsy" + your area or nearest city.

**POSITIVE
BIOPSY**

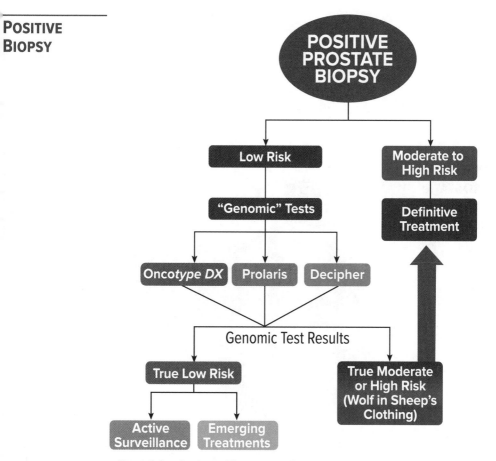

**Figure 3.4** outlines possible next steps for a prostate biopsy that reveals low-risk or moderate-to-high-risk prostate cancer.

If any of the tissue samples taken during your prostate biopsy are positive for cancer, then you have some form of prostate cancer.

If that is the case, the next step is to answer these three questions:

1.  **What type of cancer is it?**
2.  **How much cancer was discovered?**
3.  **What is the risk of this cancer developing into life-threatening (metastatic) disease?**

With the answers to these three questions, you're off to a good start toward selecting the right type of prostate cancer treatment based on the kind of cancer you have. As you can see on the next page, additional information allows you to better understand your condition and select the best treatment option.

Thanks to new genomic tests like Decipher, Onco*type* DX, and Prolaris, automated image recognition testing like ProMark, and urine/DRE tests like PCA-3 and Select MDx, doctors can now answer question #3 above with much greater certainty.

## TYPES OF PROSTATE CANCER

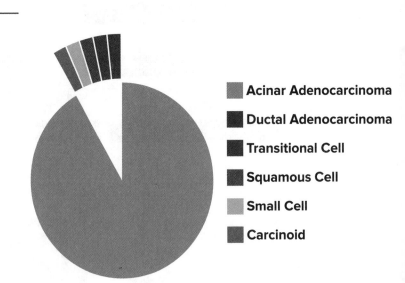

- Acinar Adenocarcinoma
- Ductal Adenocarcinoma
- Transitional Cell
- Squamous Cell
- Small Cell
- Carcinoid

**Figure 3.5** Since the vast majority (95 percent) of prostate cancer is Acinar Adeno-carcinoma, it's easy to lose sight of the fact that there are the five other types of prostate cancer, each of which requires a different treatment protocol (See **Page 332**).

## 95% OF PROSTATE CANCER IS ACINAR ADENOCARCINOMA

*Throughout this book, when we talk about "prostate cancer," we are really talking about "Acinar Adenocarcinoma." Actually, there are 5 other kinds of prostate cancer (See **Figure 3.5**). Each of these cancers is unique, requires its own treatment protocol, and represents about 1% of all prostate cancers. For more information about the different types of prostate cancer, see the **Chapter 3** Digging Deeper section.*

**12 FACTORS THAT DEFINE PROSTATE CANCER**

To answer the three questions on the previous page (and expand on them), pathologists, urologists, and other doctors look at the following 12 factors:

1. Gleason Score: How aggressive your cancer appears under a microscope
2. PSA Total: Your highest level
3. Clinical Stage: How your cancer was discovered
4. Number of Positive Biopsy Samples
5. Highest Percentage of Cancer Detected
6. Bilateral Positive Biopsy Samples (Did positive samples come from both sides of the prostate? If "yes," how many from each side?)
7. Location of Positive Biopsy Cores
8. Perineural Invasion (Has the cancer invaded the nerves that travel through the prostate? Yes/No)
9. Extracapsular Extension (Does the cancer extend into or beyond the prostate membrane? Yes/No)
10. Seminal Vesicle Involvement (Yes/No)
11. Positive Lymph Nodes (Yes/No)
12. Positive Bone Scan (Yes/No)

By evaluating these 12 factors, doctors can categorize your cancer and give you a better explanation of:

- How much cancer is there
- Where the cancer is located
- What's the risk of it spreading outside your prostate
- Whether or not the cancer has already spread outside your prostate
- And a lot more

| CANCER TYPE | LOW-RISK | MODERATE-RISK | HIGH-RISK |
|---|---|---|---|
| "CAT NAME" | KITTY CAT | BOBCAT | MOUNTAIN LION |
| Treatments | Observation or Single Treatment | Single or Dual Treatment | Dual Treatment + Hormones |
| Gleason Score | 3+3 = 6 | 3+4 or 4+3 = 7 | 8-10 |
| PSA | Less than 10 | 10-20 | More than 20 |
| Cancer Stage | T1 or T2A | T2B | T2C |

**Figure 3.6** shows the three traditional cancer markers (Gleason Score, PSA, and Cancer Stage) for clinically significant prostate cancer (low-risk, moderate-risk, and high-risk) and Dr. Ripoll's "Cat Names."

## UNDERSTANDING CANCER THROUGH ANALOGIES

Over the years, Dr. Ripoll found that certain patients simply could not take in any more "medical information" after they received a prostate cancer diagnosis. So she gave the three main risk types of local prostate cancer (cancer that is still confined inside the prostate) "cat names." This way of talking about cancer was easier and more intuitive for some patients because it bypassed using a lot of numbers and medical terminology.

The cat names (shown below) are Dr. Ripoll's way of taking the emotional charge off a diagnosis and helping her patients find a little breathing room.

It's a lot harder to freak out about being labeled a "Kitty Cat" than it is to be told you have Gleason 3 + 3, T1C, PSA: 2.5, 5% in 1 of 18 core samples, low-risk, low-volume prostate cancer. The cat analogies cut through all the abbreviations, acronyms, and mumbo jumbo.

- Clinically Insignificant Prostate Cancer: **Kitten**
- Low-risk Prostate Cancer: **Kitty Cat**
- Moderate-risk Prostate Cancer: **Bobcat**
- High-risk Prostate Cancer: **Mountain Lion**

Dr. Ripoll's cat names are useful analogies for lots of men, but they don't work for everyone. If you don't like cats (or even if you do), we invite you to come up your own names for different kinds of cancer.

So far, we've heard "The pit bull to poodle spectrum"; "Papa bear, momma bear, baby bear"; and "Birds, rabbits, and turtles."

We invite you to you come up with your own names for different classifications of prostate cancer. We would like to hear about the names you create, because your analogies might work perfectly for someone else.

Bottom line: Use whatever analogy helps you deal with your prostate cancer diagnosis.

**NOTE**

*With or without analogies, receiving a prostate cancer diagnosis almost always feels overwhelming. We wrote* **Chapter 9:** *Coping with a Prostate Cancer Diagnosis specifically to help men and their families deal with the emotional upheaval of finding out you have cancer.*

*We highly recommend this chapter to anyone who has been diagnosed with prostate cancer. It contains a simple 5-point plan to help you rebound from the psychologically and emotional shock of a prostate cancer diagnosis.*

*Also, we encourage you to read* **Chapter 10: Using Your Diagnosis as a Springboard to Better Health.** *No matter what kind of prostate cancer you have (low risk to high risk, low volume to high volume), the tools that we offer in* **Chapter 10** *can help you heal your prostate — by healing the body it lives in.*

| NEGATIVE BIOPSY | |
| --- | --- |
| **What does it do?** | **How does it do it?** |
| ConfirmMDx | • Helps identify men who have prostate cancer that was undetected by a biopsy (false negative biopsy). False negative biopsies occur in about 25% of negative biopsies.<br>• Points to specific areas of the prostate that are likely to contain cancer.<br>• Decreases the number of unnecessary biopsies.<br>• Used only with patients who have had negative biopsies. | • Detects areas within a prostate biopsy sample that contain higher concentrations of "methylation." (A molecular process that can shut down tumor-suppressors genes.)<br>• Methylation may be present even though the prostate cells look normal under a microscope.<br>• The confirmation of a methylation halo (also called a "field effect") points to the area(s) most likely to harbor hidden cancer. |

Mentioned by name in **Figure 3.2** and indirectly in **Figure 3.3** (positive and negative for "methylation"), **Figure 3.7** provides a brief outline of what the **ConfirmMDx** test does and how it works.

| POSITIVE BIOPSY | |
| --- | --- |
| The following three tests are examples of genomic tests. What are genomic tests? In the case of prostate cancer, these tests that are designed for men who have had a positive prostate biopsy. The tests measure the expression of certain DNA strands (called "genes") that are associated with aggressive prostate cancer — or the RNA strands that these genes create. For example, Onco*type* DX measures the expression of 17 such genes, Prolaris measures the expression of 46 genes, and Decipher measures 22 RNA biomarkers.<br><br>All three of these tests provide you with a score (a number) that explains how likely your prostate cancer is to grow rapidly and spread outside your prostate — where it is much harder to treat. | |
| **What does it do?** | **How does it do it?** |
| Oncotype DX | • A test for men who have recently been diagnosed with early-stage, low-risk prostate cancer.<br>• Onco*type* DX uses the prostate biopsy sample to confirm that the cancer is true low-risk cancer – and not a more aggressive form of prostate cancer that is masquerading as low-risk cancer.<br>• Gives patients a "Genomic Prostate Score" (GPS) that accurately predicts how aggressive a prostate cancer tumor is.<br>• Adds valuable information that goes beyond Gleason Score and PSA. | • Onco*type* DX is a biopsy-based test that measures the level of expression of 17 aggressive prostate cancer genes.<br>• It is performed on positive tissue samples from a recent biopsy. The result is an individualized number called a "Genomic Prostate Score" (GPS).<br>• Using these 17 prostate cancer genes, the GPS predicts how likely a man's prostate cancer is going to spread beyond his prostate.<br>• This test can use tissue samples from a prostate biopsies or a radical prostatectomy (surgery). |

## POSITIVE BIOPSY continued

| | What does it do? | How does it do it? |
|---|---|---|
| **Prolaris** | • As with Onco*type* DX, Prolaris is a tissue-based molecular test that provides men with a result that calculates how aggressive their prostate cancer is. Prolaris works in conjunction with traditional clinical prostate tests like Gleason Score and PSA.<br>• Helps identify low- to moderate-risk patients. This information identifies good candidates for active surveillance versus candidates for definitive treatment.<br>• Prolaris can test both specimens from a prostate biopsy or a radical prostatectomy (surgery). | • It is a 46-gene test designed to gauge the aggressiveness of prostate cancer in individual patients. It measures the expression of genes that govern how quickly cells divide and make new cells.<br>• Measures the expression of genes involved in cancer tumor proliferation to predict whether a man's cancer will eventually spread outside his prostate. |
| **Decipher (after surgery)** | • Analyzes a small tissue sample that is routinely taken during surgery and archived by the pathology laboratory.<br>• Provides an independent assessment of tumor aggressiveness and predicts the probability of prostate cancer spreading to other parts of the body after surgery (metastasis).<br>• Provides Information independent from Gleason Score or PSA. | • Measures the expression of 22 RNA biomarkers involved in biological pathways that are associated with aggressive prostate cancer<br>• Uses the expression of these biomarkers to calculate the probability of clinical metastasis within 5 years after surgery, and within 3 years of a rising PSA after surgery.<br>• Has been validated by over 2,000 patients in clinical studies at top U.S. cancer centers. |

### Genomic Testing in a Nutshell

Some insurance companies cover one test but not the other two. Some doctors prefer one test over the others. If you have had a positive prostate biopsy, we recommend that you use whichever test your health insurance covers and your doctor recommends.

**Figure 3.8** provides an outline of the three most common genomic tests: Onco*type* DX, Prolaris, and Decipher. These tests are given to men who have had a positive prostate biopsy to determine how aggressive their cancer is. Two of these tests, Onco*type* DX and Prolaris, can be used on positive prostate biopsy samples to identify aggressive prostate cancer that is masquerading as low-risk cancer. All three of these tests can be performed on prostate tissue samples after the prostate has been surgically removed. The results of all three tests can help men decide on the most appropriate next step in their treatment plan.

*For more information about epigenetic and genomic tests, see the* **Chapter 3 Digging Deeper** *section.*

# Doctor Story
## DR. CHERI KING N.D.

Naturopathic Medicine
Boulder Natural
Health
Boulder, Colorado

*One year after my curmudgeonly 75-year-old father had been success-fully treated with radiation and Lupron for his Gleason 8 prostate cancer, his PSA jumped to a whopping 48.*

*He took this as a death sentence and started getting his affairs in order and giving his things away. We retested, hoping the high PSA was a mistake and not metastasis. It was neither. His PSA was indeed that high, but thankfully, there was also no detectable tumor. His urologist, an integrative physician, emphasized the need to stimulate and support his immune system to destroy individual cancer cells floating around in his body before they could invade tissue and create a tumor. She called these cancer cells "floaters."*

*As a naturopathic physician, I knew there were countless things that we could do to detoxify and stimulate the immune system. If he could only change some of the bad habits he'd fallen into, I knew he would cele-brate quite a few more birthdays.*

*Over the next few months, I worked closely with his urologist. Even though he balked several times, I dragged him in for his Vitamin C IVs, made him take his anti-cancer supplements, and even checked him into an integrative medicine clinic for two weeks of intensive treatments. At the end of those treatments, his PSA was normal and not one test gave any indication of floaters.*

*Today, my dad continues to follow naturopathic protocols and is on the same trajectory in life as any healthy man his age: traveling, enjoying his family and his leisure time.*

*Maybe he's a little less of a curmudgeon these days, but now he wants his stuff back!*

## LOOKING AHEAD

**CHAPTER 1:** You or your doctor is concerned about your prostate — We provide you with **Prostate 101**: where it lives, what it does, plus relevant statistics.

**CHAPTER 2:** Your doctor told you to **schedule a prostate biopsy** — We give you a **Prostate Biopsy Assessment Tool** to see if you actually need one, and what to expect if you do.

**CHAPTER 3:** You have a prostate biopsy — We explain the steps you need to take, whether you have a **negative biopsy or a positive biopsy**.

**CHAPTER 4:** You have a **positive prostate biopsy** — We provide you with a **Prostate Cancer Assessment Tool** to help you understand which kind of cancer you have.

**CHAPTER 5:** You need to select a prostate cancer treatment — We provide you with a summary of the most common types of treatment based on your **cancer risk type** (low-risk, moderate-risk, and high-risk).

**CHAPTER 6:** You have **low-risk, low-volume prostate cancer** and need to learn more about emerging treatments — We provide you with a summary of these treatments to help you understand the differences between focal, minimally invasive, alternative, whole gland, and traditional treatments.

**CHAPTER 7:** You have prostate cancer that is more advanced than low-risk, low-volume and need to know more about **whole-gland treatments** (both stand-alone traditional and combination treatments) — We provide you with a summary of these treatments.

**CHAPTER 8:** You want to know the **success and complication rates** for each type of treatment and for each cancer risk type (low-risk, moderate-risk, and high-risk) — We provide you with unbiased information to support your decision-making process.

**CHAPTER 9:** You feel **overwhelmed** by the news of a positive prostate biopsy — We give you the tools to surf this tidal wave of emotion and overcome the feeling of panic that almost always accompanies a positive biopsy report.

**CHAPTER 10:** You want to **use your cancer diagnosis as a springboard to better health** — We help you address your wellness goals with a proven plan that covers inflammation, diet, inactivity, stress, immune system, hormone optimization, structure, and removing toxic substances.

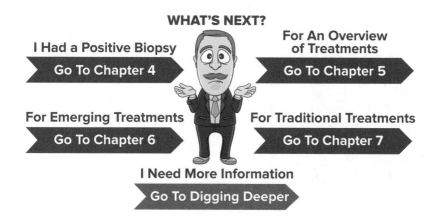

**WHAT'S NEXT?**

**I Had a Positive Biopsy**
Go To Chapter 4

**For An Overview of Treatments**
Go To Chapter 5

**For Emerging Treatments**
Go To Chapter 6

**For Traditional Treatments**
Go To Chapter 7

**I Need More Information**
Go To Digging Deeper

# WELCOME TO THE TOOLBOX
# CHAPTER 3 **TOOLBOX**

**THIS TOOLBOX SECTION INCLUDES THE FOLLOWING TOOLS AND RESOURCES TO HELP YOU UNDERSTAND THE RESULTS OF YOUR PROSTATE BIOPSY:**

- Call List of Important People
- Prostate Cancer Resources List

## *Call List*

|  | NAME | NUMBER |
|---|---|---|
| FAMILY |  |  |
| FRIENDS |  |  |
| COUNSELOR/ THERAPIST |  |  |
| RELIGIOUS ADVISOR |  |  |
| PRIMARY DOCTOR |  |  |
| UROLOGIST |  |  |
| SECOND OPINION |  |  |
| THIRD OPINION |  |  |
| NUTRITIONIST |  |  |
| SUPPORT GROUP |  |  |
| INSURANCE BENEFITS |  |  |
| WORK BENEFITS |  |  |
| FINANCIAL ADVISOR |  |  |

TOOLBOX

# Prostate Cancer Resources

We include this alphabetical list as a resource for additional information. Unfortunately, we cannot guarantee that any of these resources will be helpful in your search for leading-edge information about prostate health, prostate cancer, its treatment, or a community to support you in your search; however, we have generally found these resources to be helpful.

## CANCER TREATMENT CENTERS OF AMERICA
http://www.cancercenter.com/prostate-cancer

## CANCER COMPASS PROSTATE CANCER DISCUSSIONS
www.cancercompass.com/message-board/cancers/prostate-cancer/1,0,119,2.htm

## CANCER HOPE NETWORK                    1-877-467-3638
www.cancerhopenetwork.org
Matches cancer patients one-on-one with someone
who has recovered from a similar experience.

## DAILY STRENGTH PROSTATE CANCER SUPPORT GROUP
www.dailystrength.org/c/Prostate-Cancer/support-group

## IMERMAN ANGELS                         1-877-274-5529
www.imermanangels.org
Imerman Angels partners a person fighting cancer with someone
who has beaten the same type of cancer.

## MALE CARE
www.malecare.org

## MALECARE: MODERATED EMAIL DISCUSSION LISTS
health.groups.yahoo.com/group/prostatecancerunder50
health.groups.yahoo.com/group/prostatecancerandgaymen
health.groups.yahoo.com/group/advancedprostatecancer

## NATIONAL CANCER INSTITUTE LIFELINE
http://www.cancer.gov/cancertopics/disparities/lifelines/prostatecancer

## OUT WITH CANCER: ONLINE LGBT COMMUNITY
http://www.outwithcancer.org

## PROSTATE CANCER FOUNDATION
http://www.pcf.org

## PROSTATE CANCER FOUNDATION — SUPPORT GROUPS
http://www.pcf.org/site/c.leJRIROrEpH/b.5856543/k.6599/Finding_a_Support_Group.htm

## PROSTATE CANCER RESEARCH INSTITUTE
www.pcri.org

## PROSTATE CANCER: VOLUME, DIMENSION & DENSITY
http://www.mskcc.org/nomograms/prostate/volume

## PROSTATE CONDITIONS EDUCATION COUNCIL
https://prostateconditions.org

## PROSTATE HEALTH EDUCATION NETWORK
http://www.prostatehealthed.org

## PSA DOUBLING TIME
http://www.mskcc.org/nomograms/prostate/psa-doubling-time

## THE SCOTT HAMILTON CARES INITIATIVE    1-866-520-3197
## 4TH ANGEL PROGRAM
http://www.4thangel.org

Free, national service that provides a one-to-one supportive relationship (phone or email) to cancer patients and their caregivers.

## US TOO PROSTATE CANCER SUPPORT GROUP
http://www.ustoo.org

## US TOO INSPIRE ONLINE COMMUNITY
www.inspire.com/inspire/group/us-too-prostate-cancer

## YANA - YOU ARE NOT ALONE
## NOW PROSTATE CANCER SUPPORT SITE
www.yananow.org

## ZERO: THE END OF PROSTATE CANCER
https://zerocancer.org

TOOLBOX

**NOTES:**

**NOTES:**

TOOLBOX

# What Kind of Cancer Do You Have?

> " We have two options medically and emotionally: give up or fight like hell.
>
> — *Lance Armstrong, cancer survivor*

# Patient Story

## JOHN

*If I could go back in time and talk to the person I was a couple of years ago, here's what I'd say:*

1. *Take the time to do the research you need to make a good decision — one you won't regret. I took 6 months.*

2. *Don't overreact to everything that doctors tell you. A lot of them are in the business of removing your prostate, and that's exactly what they'll tell you to do.*

3. *Doctors, tests, scans ... none of this is a perfect science. You want minimum invasion and maximum results.*

4. *Become aware of what's going on with your body. Know your medical history and your family history.*

5. *Learn about all your different treatment options and which ones are the best for your condition. I sought out the experts in the field and asked all kinds of questions.*

6. *Choose the right doctors who perform the right type of treatment for you. I selected the best doctors who used the most sophisticated technology and knew exactly what my treatment plan was before they started.*

*Also, be aware that this is NOT a simple decision: A lot of different factors go into it:*

- *Cancer Stage*
- *Gleason Score*
- *Prostate Size*
- *Rate of Progression*
- *PSA: free, density, velocity*

*I had CyberKnife treatment, and the last one was one year to the day of writing this story. My PSA continues to drop. It was once as high as 17, and now it's 3.6.*

*My doctors told me what to expect, and I am getting the results they said I would. It's just a matter of the slow death of my prostate.*

*I still feel a certain amount of dread about PSA tests. That's normal. It's just something you learn to live with.*

# chapter
## FOUR
## summary

**Chapter 4** gives you the tools and information you need in order to figure out which kind of prostate cancer you have: low-risk, moderate-risk, high-risk, or metastatic disease.

Obviously, this chapter cannot replace your doctor. However, if you have a copy of your prostate biopsy pathology report, **Chapter 4** and the **Prostate Cancer Assessment Tool** in the **Chapter 4 Toolbox** can help you gain a better understanding of the kind of cancer you have.

This information is also important for the rest of the book, particularly **Chapter 8,** where we look at treatment success and complication rates by treatment type and cancer category.

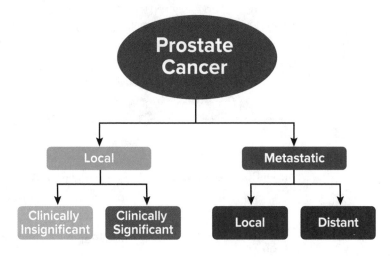

Figure 4.0 provides an overview for what **Chapter 4** and the **Prostate Cancer Assessment Tool** in the **Chapter 4 Toolbox** are attempting to do — help you determine what kind of cancer you have.

**DEBUNKING MYTHS**

## PIN VS. PNI: A DYSLEXIC'S NIGHTMARE

*PIN (Prostatic Intraepithelial Neoplasia) is a kind of inflammation that causes the appearance of certain prostate cells to change.*

*It isn't true cancer; however, PIN is present in 85 percent of all prostate cancer cases.*

*Because PIN can be detected years before the appearance of prostate cancer, it acts as a warning signal that your prostate health is heading in the wrong direction. If your prostate had a dashboard, the presence of PIN would be a yellow "check prostate" light.*

*PIN doesn't cause a rise in PSA and is undetectable in blood tests. Currently, the only way to detect PIN is by a medical procedure — usually a prostate biopsy or a TURP.*

*PNI (Perineural Invasion) happens when cancer cells surround nerve fibers inside the prostate or travel along these fibers as a pathway of escape from the prostate.*

*When PNI is discovered during a biopsy, it means there's a higher chance that the cancer has spread outside the prostate — and that's a big deal because prostate cancer is much easier to treat when it is confined to the prostate.*

*PNI usually bumps your cancer risk category to the next level. For example, if your cancer would otherwise be classified as moderate-risk, PNI will moves it to the high-risk category.*

*Does PNI always mean that cancer has spread outside the prostate? No, but it's a good indicator that the prostate cancer exodus has begun.*

---

**VOCABULARY**

See Glossary for Definitions

Bilateral Positive Biopsies

Clinical Stage

Extracapsular Extension

Gleason Score

Local Disease

Lymph Node

Metastatic Disease

Pathology Report

(PIN) Prostatic Intraepithelial Neoplasia

(PNI) Perineural Invasion

PSA

Seminal Vesicles

TURP (Transurethral Resection of the Prostate)

## WHAT KIND OF PROSTATE CANCER DO YOU HAVE?

Answering that question is the point of this chapter. Clearly, your best source for this information is your doctor; however, what if you can't get in to see your doctor for a week? Or what if you've already spoken with your doctor after your biopsy, and you still have questions?

That's why we created an easy-to-use **Prostate Cancer Assessment Tool** in the **Chapter 4 Toolbox**. This tool is designed to help you decipher your prostate biopsy pathology report, plus the numbers from other important tests.

The rest of this chapter focuses on the 12 factors that go into the **Prostate Cancer Assessment Tool.** Our goal is to provide you with clear, easy-to-understand answers to the three questions we asked in **Chapter 3**:

1. **What type of cancer is it?**
2. **How much cancer?**
3. **What is the risk of this cancer developing into life-threatening disease?**

**TO ANSWER THESE QUESTIONS, DOCTORS OF ALL STRIPES LOOK AT THE FOLLOWING 12 FACTORS:**

1.  GLEASON SCORE: How aggressive your cancer appears under the microscope
2.  PSA TOTAL: Your highest level
3.  CLINICAL STAGE: How your cancer was discovered
4.  NUMBER OF POSITIVE BIOPSIES
5.  HIGHEST PERCENT OF CANCER DETECTED
6.  BILATERAL POSITIVE BIOPSY SAMPLES
7.  LOCATION OF POSITIVE BIOPSY CORES
8.  PERINEURAL INVASION (Yes/No)
9.  EXTRACAPSULAR EXTENSION (Yes/No)
10. SEMINAL VESICLE INVOLVEMENT (Yes/No)
11. POSITIVE LYMPH NODES (Yes/No)
12. POSITIVE BONE SCAN (Yes/No)

## STAGING FACTORS

1. GLEASON SCORE
2. PSA
3. CANCER STAGE

## 1. GLEASON SCORE

Gleason Score is the most important of the three staging factors (Gleason score, PSA, and cancer stage). Why? Because it is the most accurate predictor of how aggressive your cancer is; therefore, how likely it is to spread outside your prostate.

Gleason score describes the microscopic appearance of your cancer. The scale of Gleason numbers goes from 1 to 5. The higher the Gleason score (pattern), the more aggressive the cancer is — and the more distorted and crazy-looking the cells are.

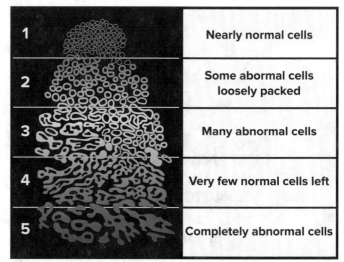

| | |
|---|---|
| 1 | Nearly normal cells |
| 2 | Some aformal cells loosely packed |
| 3 | Many abnormal cells |
| 4 | Very few normal cells left |
| 5 | Completely abnormal cells |

**Figure 4.1** is the standard Gleason Score illustration. As your Gleason number goes up from 1 to 5, so does the aggressiveness of your prostate cancer.

Low Gleason scores (1 & 2) are uncommon and difficult to distinguish from normal prostate cells. The most common Gleason prostate cancer score is 3, which is considered a low-risk of spreading outside the prostate. Scores of 4 or 5 are considered a higher risk of escaping the prostate and invading the nearby tissue.

**Your Gleason Score is defined by two numbers added together to create one sum.**

A Gleason Score equation looks like this:  **3 + 4 = 7**

The first number (3 in the example above) refers to the most common pattern (grade) of cancer cells found in the prostate biopsy. The second number refers to the second most common pattern of cancer found in the biopsy sample (4 in example above). The sum of the two numbers (7) is the number doctors use describe the cancer: "Gleason 7" in this example.

If more than two cell patterns are present, more data is needed to establish a definitive Gleason score.

Also, it is important to note that a "Gleason 3 + 4" is much less aggressive than a "Gleason 4 + 3," even though they both equal 7.

## 2. PSA

As discussed in **Chapter 2**, PSA (Prostate Specific Antigen) is a critical marker for prostate health. There are several different PSA blood tests that are useful when evaluating the possibility of having prostate cancer:

- PSA total
- PSA free
- PSA velocity
- PSA density

For the purpose of identifying the kind of prostate cancer you have, doctors use your highest PSA total. Other culprits like prostatitis, BPH, and a tight urinary sphincter can cause you to have a higher PSA, which alters the accuracy of this factor in the prostate cancer equation.

| TWO SYSTEMS OF CANCER STAGING | | | |
|---|---|---|---|
| **STAGE** | **DEFINITION** | **STAGE** | **DEFINITION** |
| STAGE I (A) | Cannot be felt | T1 | Not palpable |
| STAGE II (B) | Elevated PSA Confined to prostate | T2 | Confined within the prostate |
| STAGE III (C) | Outside the capsule | T3 | Extends through capsule |
| STAGE IV (D) | Spread to lymph nodes | T4 | Invades adjacent structures |

**Figure 4.2** gives you a simple comparison between the two most common systems of staging prostate cancer. As you can see, both systems are roughly equivalent.

## 3. CANCER STAGE

Your cancer stage (The letter "T" followed by number) explains how the cancer was discovered.

There are four main categories ranging from T1 to T4 and three subcategories for T1 and T2. The bigger the number, the more advanced the cancer is.

For example, T1 cancers are small tumors that are only found during a transurethral resection of the prostate (TURP) or prostate biopsy and not felt during a rectal exam. T2 cancers can be felt during a DRE and are confined within the prostate. T3 cancers are aggressive and may have spread outside your prostate (local extension). T4 cancers have already spread outside the prostate and tumors are present in the surrounding tissues.

**T1:** Your doctor does not feel anything unusual during a DRE or notice anything out of the ordinary in a transrectal ultrasound or MRI.

**T1a:** The cancer is found while performing a TURP to relieve the symptoms of Benign Prostatic Hyperplasia (BPH). This incidental discovery of cancer during a TURP occurs in no more than 5 percent of the prostate tissue removed during the procedure.

**T1b:** Similar to T1a, except *more* than 5 percent of the tissue removed contains prostate cancer.

**T1c:** Cancer is discovered by a needle biopsy after an elevated Total PSA blood test.

**T2:** Your doctor feels something unusual (a lump or bump) during a DRE or sees the cancer on a transrectal ultrasound or MRI, but the cancer is still confined within the prostate.

**T2a:** The cancer is only detected on one half (or less) of one side of your prostate (left or right) — and it is NOT present on both sides.

**T2b:** The cancer is detected in more than half of one side of your prostate (left or right) — and it is NOT present on both sides of the prostate.

**T2c:** The cancer is detected on both sides.

**T3:** The cancer has spread outside your prostate and may/may not have spread to your seminal vesicles.

**T3a:** The cancer has spread outside the prostate but not to the seminal vesicles.

**T3b:** The cancer has spread to the seminal vesicles.

**T4:** The cancer has grown into the tissues next to your prostate including the urinary sphincter (muscle that helps control urination), the rectum, the bladder, and/or the wall of the pelvis.

**OTHER STAGING FACTORS**

## 4. NUMBER OF POSITIVE BIOPSY SAMPLES

You don't have to be a urologist to figure out that the more prostate cancer you have, the more prostate biopsy needles are likely come back positive. If you have a lot of prostate cancer (high volume), it will probably be found in several biopsy needle cores.

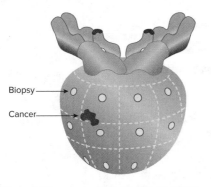

Likewise, if you have a small amount of prostate cancer (low volume), it may only show up in one prostate biopsy needle core — or not at all.

The number of positive biopsy core samples (1 out of 12, 3 out of 16...) gives doctors a better idea about the extent of the cancer in your prostate.

**Figure 4.3** (courtesy of MDxHealth) illustrates how difficult it is for a prostate biopsy needle to strike a small prostate cancer tumor. A standard 12-needle biopsy only samples 1% of the total prostate volume.

*Figure 4.3 illustrates how a 12-needle prostate biopsy may only sample 1 percent of the total prostate volume, leaving lots of room for small prostate cancer tumors to hide. Finding "hidden" cancer tumors that would otherwise indicate a (false) negative biopsy, is why epigenetic testing like ConfirmMDx is so important.*

**NOTE**

*Before a biopsy, the 4Kscore Test helps identify men who are at greater risk of having aggressive prostate cancer. After a positive biopsy, genomic tests like Prolaris, Decypher, and Oncotype DX help men determine if they have high-risk cancer.*

## WHAT CAN THE PERCENTAGE OF PROSTATE CANCER TELL YOU?

A biopsy needle core that contains 10 percent prostate cancer tells a different story about the health of your prostate than one that contains 50 percent cancer.

The 10-percent (or less) needle core means that either the needle "nicked" a prostate cancer tumor (which could be large or small) or went directly through a small tumor (see **Figure 4.4**). It's hard to tell.

On the other hand, the 50-percent needle indicates the presence of a large prostate tumor, which means the patient has high-volume disease. This kind of volume rules out certain types of treatment (see **Chapter 5**).

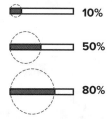

Figure 4.4 displays the difference between a 10% positive biopsy core sample, a 50% positive core, and an 80% positive core. When you see this difference visually, it's easier to comprehend the significance of these numbers.

## 5. HIGHEST PERCENTAGE OF CANCER DETECTED

The percent of a positive prostate biopsy core sample is another way of estimating the size/amount of your cancer.

There are two ways to measure the percent of cancer in a prostate biopsy:

  A. The percent of cancer detected in a single prostate biopsy core sample.

  B. The percent of cancer detected in all the core samples.

Scientific studies support the idea that A and B closely mirror each other. The data shows NO appreciable difference between A & B in quantifying the amount of cancer.

The advantage of method B is that it's so easy: 4 out of 12 needle core samples (30%) contained prostate cancer.

After decades of analyzing surgically removed prostate glands, doctors can accurately predict the total amount (volume) of prostate cancer and how aggressive the cancer is/will become based on the percentage of positive prostate cancer biopsy needles.

## 6. BILATERAL POSITIVE BIOPSIES

If you have prostate cancer on both sides of your prostate (what doctors call "multi-focal disease"), it is safe to assume that your entire prostate contains cancer. This finding rules out "focal treatments" that treat only small areas of your prostate. A bilateral positive biopsy puts you in the "whole-gland treatment only" category.

## 7. LOCATION OF POSITIVE BIOPSY NEEDLE CORES

The location of a prostate cancer tumor is an important element in deciding the right type of treatment. For example, if a tumor near the capsule of the prostate begins to grow rapidly, it doesn't have far to go before it extends into, or grows through, the capsule of the prostate. This is extra capsular extension (Factor #9).

Also, the location of a prostate cancer tumor can affect treatment results. For example, a tumor in the apex of the prostate is more likely to have "positive surgical margins," meaning the surgeon is more likely to leave behind some cancer after a prostatectomy. (See **Figure 4.5**).

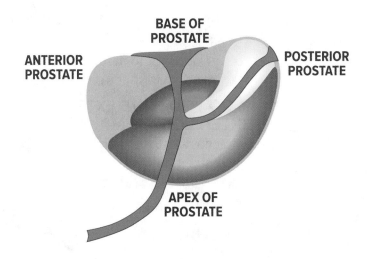

Figure 4.5 illustrates the location of the four regions of the prostate: anterior, posterior, apex, and base.

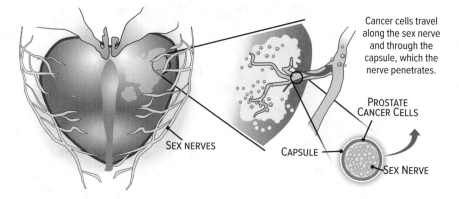

Cancer cells travel
along the sex nerve
and through the
capsule, which the
nerve penetrates.

PROSTATE
CANCER CELLS

SEX NERVES

CAPSULE

SEX NERVE

**Figure 4.6** (courtesy of ProstRcision) displays how Perineural Invasion (PNI) surrounds nerve fibers and uses them as pathways to spread outside the prostate. Once outside the prostate, these cells take up residence in nearby tissues. If these cells reach the circulatory system (blood and lymph vessels), they can travel all over the body.

## 8. IS THERE EVIDENCE OF PERINEURAL INVASION?

Perineural Invasion (PNI) is one of the ways that prostate cancer gets outside the prostate gland and spreads throughout the body. Think of the nerves traveling through the prostate like the Prostate Cancer Autobahn.

Once cancer cells invade the nerves traveling through the prostate (See **Figure 4.6**), it is easier for them to get outside the prostate and spread throughout the body.

If you have PNI, your cancer risk category moves up a notch — low-risk to moderate-risk, moderate-risk to high-risk, which limits your treatment options (See **Chapter 5).**

**LOCAL METASTASIS**

## 9. DO YOU HAVE EXTRACAPSULAR EXTENSION?

Extracapsular Extension (ECE) is a form of high-risk, local, advanced prostate cancer that occurs when the cancer extends into, or goes through, the prostate capsule. ECE

A prostate gland is like an orange: The rind is the capsule, and the meat of the orange is the prostate. The dark cloud in **Figure 4.7** illustrates a prostate tumor that has grown into the prostate capsule (extracapsular extension) and is about to spread outside the prostate (become locally invasive).

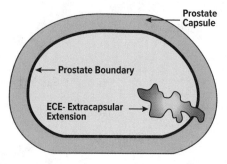

Prostate
Capsule

Prostate Boundary

ECE- Extracapsular
Extension

is usually detected by MRI or transrectal ultrasound.

If you have ECE, your treatment options change because of what doctors call "positive margins," which means the edges of your prostate gland (the margins), are positive for prostate cancer. In some cases, prostate cancer is a hair's width from the edge of the prostate; in others, it has already broken through the capsule.

Once ECE occurs, surgically removing the prostate is no longer a complete form of treatment. In 60 percent of ECE cases, even the best prostate cancer surgeons in world leave some cancer behind.

## 10. HAS THE CANCER SPREAD TO YOUR SEMINAL VESICLES? (SEMINAL VESICLE INVOLVEMENT)?

As with Extra Capsular Extension (above), if the cancer has spread to your seminal vesicles, it reduces your treatment options and increases the number, types, and combinations of treatments required to kill all the cancer and create a cure.

**DISTANT METASTASIS**

## 11. HAS THE CANCER SPREAD TO NEARBY LYMPH NODES?

The further the cancer spreads from your prostate, the harder it is to destroy. The success rates for the combination of treatments required to eradicate this kind of cancer are much lower than for the same cancer when it is still contained inside to your prostate. If cancer invades your lymph nodes, cancer cells now have access to the entire body through the circulatory system.

## 12. HAVE YOU HAD A POSITIVE BONE SCAN?

Prostate cancer prefers to invade bones the same way termites love to burrow into wood, especially the big bones of the pelvis, hips, upper legs, and lower spine. Once cancer has spread to your bones, your treatment plan shifts from killing the cancer to managing it.

A positive bone scan often backs up your doctor's suspicion that you may have "distant metastatic disease," which means that prostate cancer that has spread throughout your body.

**PROSTATE
CANCER
ASSESSMENT
TOOL**

These 12 factors form the **Prostate Cancer Assessment Tool** in the **Chapter 4 Toolbox**. We recommend that you turn to **Page 104** and write in all the information you have. If you need additional information from your prostate biopsy report or other tests, please contact your doctor's office.

Don't stress if you haven't had certain tests (or don't have the results). No problem. What's important here is for you to begin to familiarize yourself with your cancer numbers and how they affect your treatment options.

The information from the **Prostate Cancer Assessment Tool** will help you have more in-depth discussions with your doctors, which ought to help you find the best type of treatment for the kind of cancer you have.

So let's get started.

Also, see the **Chapter 4 Digging Deeper** section for more information on prostate cancer calculators and how MRI-fusion biopsies can help detect prostate cancer and put the 12 prostate cancer factors mentioned in **Chapter 4** to use.

# Doctor Story
## DR. LEE MCNEELY, MD

Radiation Oncology

Anova Cancer Center

Lone Tree, Colorado

*My patient, Jerry, is a healthy, physically active man in a vibrant relationship with his wife. The day he arrived for his initial radiation therapy consultation, however, he looked anything but his robust self.*

*We talked about prostate cancer specifics like Gleason score, PSA, tumor extent on biopsy — all indicating he had a very good prognosis for complete recovery.*

*As doctors, we naturally assume that this kind of news would be a welcomed relief. The look on Jerry's face, however, told a different story.*

*I noticed a change in Jerry as the conversation shifted to treatment options, which can be confusing with all the different types of radiation treatment available — seeds, external beam, combination protocols (both with and without hormonal therapy), and so on.*

*The more I talked about treatment options, the more relaxed Jerry became; it was as if someone had lifted a weight from his shoulders. "You mean I don't have to have surgery? Doc, I just don't want to be cut on 'down there.'"*

*Suddenly, he was a new man.*

*The more medicine advances, the more tools we have that empower patients to make healthy choices about their care and their lives. Some patients feel burdened by the responsibility of making the "right choice." For those patients, know that doctors struggle with that challenge every day.*

*Today, Jerry is alive and well after his seed implantation (Brachytherapy). He recovered quickly from the irritating urinary symptoms. In follow-up visits, he thanked me every time for helping him make the right choice. And my reply was always the same, "You did that, Jerry. Not me."*

## LOOKING AHEAD

**CHAPTER 1:** You or your doctor is concerned about your prostate — We provide you with **Prostate 101**: where it lives, what it does, plus relevant statistics.

**CHAPTER 2:** Your doctor told you to **schedule a prostate biopsy** — We give you a **Prostate Biopsy Assessment Tool** to see if you actually need one, and what to expect if you do.

**CHAPTER 3:** You have a prostate biopsy — We explain the steps you need to take, whether you have a **negative biopsy or a positive biopsy**.

**CHAPTER 4:** You have a **positive prostate biopsy** — We provide you with a **Prostate Cancer Assessment Tool** to help you understand which kind of cancer you have.

**CHAPTER 5:** You need to select a prostate cancer treatment — We provide you with a summary of the most common types of treatment based on your **cancer risk type** (low-risk, moderate-risk, and high-risk).

**CHAPTER 6:** You have **low-risk, low-volume prostate cancer** and need to learn more about emerging treatments — We provide you with a summary of these treatments to help you understand the differences between focal, minimally invasive, alternative, whole gland, and traditional treatments.

**CHAPTER 7:** You have prostate cancer that is more advanced than low-risk, low-volume and need to know more about **whole-gland treatments** (both stand-alone traditional and combination treatments) — We provide you with a summary of these treatments.

**CHAPTER 8:** You want to know the **success and complication rates** for each type of treatment and for each cancer risk type (low-risk, moderate-risk, and high-risk) — We provide you with unbiased information to support your decision-making process.

**CHAPTER 9:** You feel **overwhelmed** by the news of a positive prostate biopsy — We give you the tools to surf this tidal wave of emotion and overcome the feeling of panic that almost always accompanies a positive biopsy report.

**CHAPTER 10:** You want to **use your cancer diagnosis as a springboard to better health** — We help you address your wellness goals with a proven plan that covers inflammation, diet, inactivity, stress, immune system, hormone optimization, structure, and removing toxic substances.

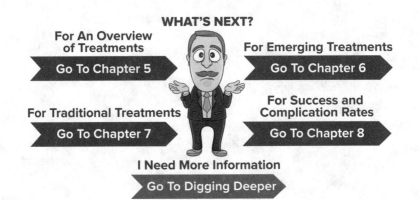

**WHAT'S NEXT?**

**For An Overview of Treatments**
Go To Chapter 5

**For Emerging Treatments**
Go To Chapter 6

**For Traditional Treatments**
Go To Chapter 7

**For Success and Complication Rates**
Go To Chapter 8

**I Need More Information**
Go To Digging Deeper

# WELCOME TO THE TOOLBOX
## CHAPTER 4 **TOOLBOX**

## THIS TOOLBOX SECTION INCLUDES THE FOLLOWING TOOLS AND RESOURCES TO HELP YOU UNDERSTAND WHAT TYPE OF PROSTATE CANCER YOU HAVE:

- Prostate Cancer Assessment Tool
- Prostate Cancer Grade
- Gleason Score
- Prostate Cancer Stage
- Lymph Node Involvement Numbers
- Metastatic Disease Evaluation

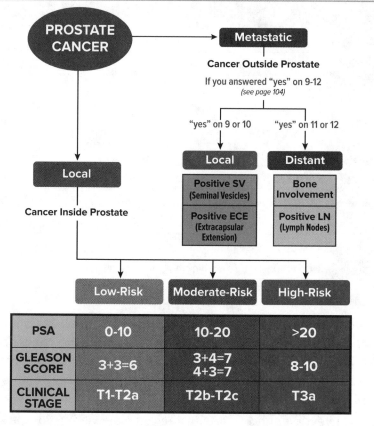

**Figure 4.0 Toolbox** provides a different way of looking at the information in the **Prostate Cancer Assessment Tool**. This figure uses the same information, but presents it as a flow chart. The goal of **Figure 4.0 Toolbox** and the **Prostate Cancer Assessment Tool** is to categorize your cancer as low-risk, moderate-risk, or high-risk. With that information, you can go to **Chapter 5** and start previewing treatment options based on the kind of cancer you have. Also, if you have "distant" metastatic disease (right side of the figure), chances are very high that you have "local" metastatic disease as well.

## *PROSTATE CANCER ASSESSMENT TOOL*

**The information you need and where to get it:**

1. Highest PSA total (Blood test — primary care doctor or urologist)
2. Clinical stage (Digital Rectal Exam — urologist)
3. Gleason Score, number of biopsies/percent of biopsies, Perineural Invasion, Extra Capsular Extension (Pathology Report — urologist)
4. Extracapsular Extension, Seminal Vesicle involvement, positive Lymph Nodes, and Bone Lesions (Imaging Studies such as CT scan, PET scan, or MRI — radiologist or urologist)
5. Bone involvement (Bone scan — radiologist)

| | CLINICAL DATA | YOUR RESULTS |
|---|---|---|
| **TRADITIONAL INFORMATION** | Gleason score (X + Y = your score) | **1.** |
| | PSA total (at its highest level) | **2.** |
| | Clinical stage (T1, T2, T3) | **3.** |
| **OTHER MODIFIERS** *(These modifiers may bump you up into a higher category)* | Number of positive biopsies (1, 2, ...) | **4** |
| | Percent of cancer in the biopsy (from 1 – 100%) | **5.** |
| | Bilateral positive biopsies (yes or no) | **6.** |
| | Location of positive biopsies (apex, base, anterior ...) | **7.** |
| | Do you have perineural invasion? (yes or no) | **8.** |
| **LOCAL METASTASIS** | Do you have extra capsular extension? (yes or no) | **9.** |
| | Do you have seminal vesicle involvement? (yes or no) | **10.** |
| **DISTANT METASTASIS** | Do you have positive lymph nodes? (yes or no) | **11.** |
| | Do you have a positive bone scan? (yes or no) | **12.** |

The Prostate Cancer Assessment Tool allows you to look at your cancer the way your doctor(s) would. The goal is to categorize the cancer as low-risk, moderate-risk, or high-risk. Once you understand which risk category best describes your cancer, then you can start evaluating treatment options to find the one that is the "best fit."

This "tool," however, cannot pinpoint the kind of cancer you have, nor can it determine the exact type of treatment that would be right for you. **Any of these 12 pieces of information** could dramatically shift your cancer diagnosis, which would alter your treatment options (more on that in **Chapter 5**).

TOOLBOX

# How Prostate Cancer is Categorized

The grade ("G") of the cancer tells you the degree of difference between cancerous tissue and normal tissue. Technically, the prostate cancer "grade" is a separate evaluation from the prostate cancer "stage"; however, both grade and stage use some of the same information to arrive at their numbers. There are 4 different grades of prostate cancer.

## Circle or highlight the one that best matches your condition.

**1.** GX:     Cannot assess grade.

**2.** G1:     The tumor closely resembles normal tissue (Gleason 2–4)

**3.** G2:     The tumor somewhat resembles normal tissue (Gleason 5–6)

**4.** G3–4:   The tumor barely resembles normal tissue or not at all (Gleason 7–10)

Today, pathologists (doctors who specialize in evaluating tissue samples) rarely assign a tumor with a Gleason pattern of less than 3, particularly in biopsy tissue. A more contemporary consideration of Gleason pattern is one of the following four choices:

## Circle or highlight the number that best matches the information from your prostate biopsy:

**1. Gleason 3+3 = 6** (low-grade cancer)

**2. Gleason 3+4 = 7 / 3+5 = 8** (mostly low grade with some high grade)

**3. Gleason 4+3 = 7 / 5+3 = 8** (mostly high grade with some low grade)

**4. Gleason 4+4 / 4+5 / 5+4 / 5+5** (all high grade)

**The presence of Gleason 5 cancer is a serious red flag!** If any Gleason pattern 5 is present, it is always included in the final score (Gleason 5+4, instead of Gleason 9).

TOOLBOX

## Cancer Stage (the "T" numbers)

There are four basic prostate cancer stages: T1, T2, T3, and T4, with several sub-stages that are given as letters (a, b, c ... ). TX and T0 are used by doctors to say that they cannot detect any cancer.

A variation of this cancer staging system (T0 - T4) is also used for all cancers, not just prostate cancer.

## Please circle or highlight the T number that best matches your cancer stage:

**TX:** Doctors cannot evaluate the primary tumor.

**T0:** There is no evidence of tumor.

**T1:** Prostate cancer is present, but it is not detectable clinically or with imaging.

**T1a:** Prostate cancer was found incidentally in less than 5 percent of prostate tissue resected (for example, to relieve BPH).

**T1b:** Prostate cancer was incidentally found in more than 5 percent of prostate tissue resected.

**T1c:** Prostate cancer was found in a needle biopsy performed after an elevated PSA.

**T2:** A prostate cancer tumor can be felt on examination, but has not spread outside the prostate.

**T2a:** The cancer is in half or less than half of one of the prostate gland's two lobes.

**T2b:** The cancer is in more than half of one lobe, but not both.

**T2c:** The cancer is in both lobes but within the prostatic capsule. ("T2c" implies a tumor is palpable in both lobes of the prostate. Tumors that are found to be bilateral on biopsy only and are not palpable bilaterally should not be staged as T2c.)

**T3:** The cancer has spread through the prostatic capsule. (If it is only part-way through, it is still T2.)

**T3a:** The cancer has spread through the capsule on one or both sides.

**T3b:** The cancer has invaded one or both seminal vesicles.

**T4:** The cancer has invaded other nearby structures.

TOOLBOX

# The evaluation of the regional lymph nodes (the 'N' numbers)

Lymph node involvement numbers are straight forward (yes, no, can't tell).

## Please highlight the Lymph Node number that best matches your condition:

**NX:**  Cannot evaluate the regional lymph nodes

**N0:**  There has been no spread to the regional lymph nodes

**N1:**  There has been spread to the regional lymph nodes

# Evaluation of distant metastasis (the 'M' numbers)

The evaluation of metastatic disease (cancer that has spread outside the prostate) is more complicated than the N numbers above, but not as complex as a prostate cancer stage (T numbers).

## Please highlight the Distant Metastasis number that best matches your condition:

**MX:**  Distant metastasis cannot be evaluated.

**M0:**  There are no distant metastases.

**M1:**  There are distant metastases.

**M1a:** The cancer has spread to lymph nodes beyond those close to the prostate.

**M1b:** The cancer has spread to bone.

**M1c:** The cancer has spread to other sites (regardless of bone involvement).

TOOLBOX

**NOTES:**

TOOLBOX

# Treatment By Type

> " If the only tool you have is a hammer, everything looks like a nail.
>
> — *Abraham Maslow*

# Patient Story

## BOB

*The beginning of a long and tough process began with my annual check-up back in 2012, when my doctor showed me pretty big jump in my PSA from the previous year.*

*Next came a prostate biopsy and MRI. The biopsy revealed that a small part of one sample that contained cancer; thankfully, the MRI showed low probability of the cancer extending beyond the prostate gland, which was good news. What followed was a lot of conversations about what all this information meant and what my treatment options were.*

*Ten years ago, my prostate would have been surgically removed, which is the "safe" but most aggressive form of treatment. In some places, this is still the treatment of choice. After discussing the side effects, my doctor told me there was no way she would recommend this procedure at this time. She felt that I was a good candidate for Active Surveillance (a PSA tests every six months and an MRI once a year), which is what I elected to do.*

*Things went smoothly until the summer of 2014 when my doctor ordered an MRI with contrast that theoretically identifies areas of concern that can later be pinpointed for biopsy. Mine showed a number of hot spots, so I had another biopsy. Thankfully, this biopsy was negative.*

*As of this writing (summer of 2015), I am now due for another MRI and set of lab work, and I'm not overly concerned, which speaks volumes about how I have settled into a relative comfort zone with this disease. I will have to monitor it for the rest of my life, but I think it is unlikely that prostate cancer will kill me.*

*More likely, raising two adopted teen-age girls as a single dad is going to do me in. And there is no treatment for that... except time.*

# chapter
## FIVE
# summary

Using the **Prostate Cancer Assessment Tool** in the **Chapter 4 Toolbox**, you learned how to combine your prostate biopsy information with the results of other tests to determine the kind of prostate cancer you have.

**Chapter 5** uses this information and directs you to the types of prostate cancer treatments that are the best match for you and the kind of cancer you have.

Knowledge is power. You cannot make an informed decision about your treatment options without accurate information.

The goal of this chapter is to help you learn more about each type of treatment and narrow the field of treatment options.

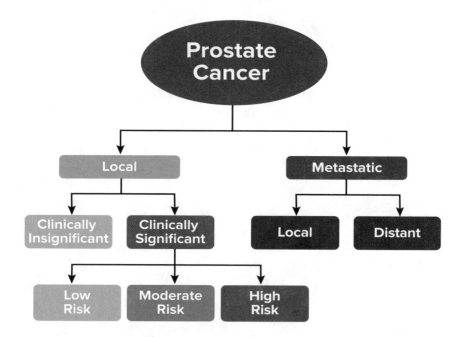

**Figure 5.0** displays the different kinds of prostate cancer. More than 90 percent of prostate cancer diagnosed today is "clinically significant but not metastatic."

## VOCABULARY

See Glossary for Definitions

Active Surveillance

Bobcat Prostate Cancer

Brachytherapy

Cancer Stage

Clinically Insignificant Prostate Cancer

Combination Therapy

Cryosurgeon

Cryotherapy

CyberKnife

Digital Rectal Exam (DRE)

External Beam Radiation

Gleason Score

Goldilocks Treatment

HIFU (High Frequency Ultrasound)

High-risk Prostate Cancer

Hormone Therapy

Kitten Prostate Cancer

Kitty Cat Prostate Cancer

Local Prostate Cancer

Low-risk Prostate Cancer

Metastatic Disease

Moderate-risk Prostate Cancer

Mountain Lion Prostate Cancer

Needle Core

Oncologist

Partin Tables

Perineural Invasion (PNI)

Prostate Biopsy

Proton Beam Radiation

PSA

PSA Testing

Radiation Oncologist

Radical Prostatectomy

Trifecta

Urologist

Watchful Waiting

**DEBUNKING MYTHS**

## THE PROSTATE CANCER CHALLENGE: NOT ALL TREATMENT TYPES ARE A MATCH FOR THE KIND OF CANCER YOU HAVE

*The first goal of any prostate cancer specialist is to determine if the patient has an aggressive or non-aggressive form of cancer.*

*The second goal is to pair the ideal type of treatment with the precise kind of prostate cancer a man has. This ideal treatment neither overtreats nor undertreats the cancer — or the man who has it.*

### What Does The Ideal Prostate Cancer Treatment Look Like?

- *Allows for the complete elimination of the cancer*
- *No complications during (or after) the procedure*
- *Complete and rapid recovery of urinary, bowl, and sexual function*
- *Balances cancer control with quality of life*
- *The patient lives a long and healthy life and eventually dies of something other than prostate cancer.*

*If you haven't already, we recommend you go through the* **Prostate Cancer Assessment Tool** *in the* **Chapter 4 Toolbox,** *to figure out which type of prostate cancer you have.*

*Partin Tables combine your PSA total, Gleason score, and clinical stage to estimate the aggressiveness of your prostate cancer. These five tables are 95 percent accurate and designed to help predict how likely the cancer is to:*

**NOTE**

1. *Remain inside the prostate (organ-confined)*
2. *Penetrate the capsule of the prostate (extracapsular extension)*
3. *Spread to the seminal vesicles (seminal vesicles involved)*
4. *Spread to local lymph nodes (lymph nodes involved)*

*Please use the link to the official Johns Hopkins University Partin Table Calculator in the* **Chapter 5 Toolbox** *to learn more about the kind of cancer you have.*

**CHOICE**

We are huge proponents of choice.

When it comes to prostate cancer treatment, every man should feel like he has some measure of choice — even if there is only a minor difference between choices.

As your advocates, we want you to make the best possible decision about your prostate cancer treatment based on the information available. We don't have a stake in which type of treatment you choose. Our only concern is helping you find the right treatment for you.

The purpose of **Chapter 5** is to help you find the "Goldilocks Treatment": treatment that kills all the cancer, yet maintains healthy bowel, bladder, urinary, and erectile function. Your doctor may refer to this type of treatment as the "Trifecta": it kills the cancer, while the maintaining normal urinary, erectile, and bowel function — and the patient eventually dies of something else.

If you have moderate-risk (Bobcat) prostate cancer, you won't find a powerful enough treatment by looking at options for clinically insignificant (Kitten) cancer. Likewise, if you have low-risk (Kitty Cat) cancer, many high-risk (Mountain Lion) treatment options would be overkill — like using a sledgehammer as a flyswatter.

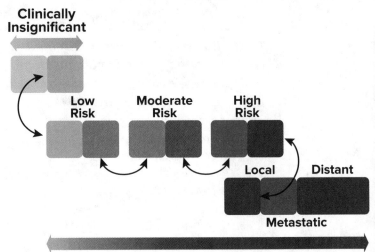

The arrows in **Figure 5.1** shows the overlap between different kinds of prostate cancer and their treatment. For example, the low end of moderate-risk (low volume) cancer can be treated in a similar way as the high end of low-risk (moderate-to-high volume) prostate cancer.

| FACTORS THAT INFLUENCE CANCER TREATMENT | Treatment Categories |
|---|---|
| **LOW-RISK (LOW-VOLUME)** | |
| **STAGE:** T1-T2a <br> **GLEASON SCORE:** 6 or less <br> **PSA:** 10 or less <br> **POS. (+) BIOPSY:** Less than 34% | **Active Surveillance** |
| **LOW-RISK (MODERATE-TO-HIGH VOLUME)** | |
| **STAGE:** T1-T2a <br> **GLEASON SCORE:** 6 or less <br> **PSA:** 10 or less <br> **POS. (+) BIOPSY** More than 34% | **Single Treatment** |
| **MODERATE-RISK (LOW-VOLUME)** | |
| **STAGE:** T2b-T2c <br> **GLEASON SCORE:** 7 (3+4) <br> **PSA:** 10-20 <br> **POS. (+) BIOPSY** Less than 34% | **Single Treatment** |
| **MODERATE-RISK (MODERATE-TO-HIGH VOLUME)** | |
| **STAGE:** T2b-T2c <br> **GLEASON SCORE:** 7 (3+4) or (4+3) <br> **PSA:** 10-20 <br> **POS. (+) BIOPSY** More than 34% | **DUAL Treatment** |
| **HIGH-RISK** | |
| **STAGE:** T3-T4 <br> **GLEASON SCORE:** 8 or more <br> **PSA:** More than 20 | **Dual Treatment + Hormones** |

**Figure 5.2** previews the five prostate cancer risk categories discussed in this chapter. This chapter outlines the range of treatment options for each type of cancer with the goal of finding a healthy balance between overall effectiveness and post-treatment quality of life.

**NOTE**

*Cancer categories were created to allow doctors to communicate meaningful information among themselves and with their patients. These categories help doctors ensure that they are not overtreating or undertreating their patients.*

*Undertreating prostate cancer would be foolish, and overtreating prostate cancer can cause complications that are worse than living with the disease.*

## CLINICALLY INSIGNIFICANT PROSTATE CANCER

Clinically insignificant prostate cancer is defined as low-grade, low-risk, low-volume disease that is unlikely to spread or pose a threat to a man's health.

Clinically insignificant prostate cancer is difficult to detect and normally only discovered during an autopsy — not a prostate biopsy. The question is what to do about it once it is discovered.

In the past, the tendency was to overtreat this inconsequential cancer and the men who had it. Doctors felt morally obligated to treat the cancer when they found it.

Today, most doctors agree that this category of prostate cancer does not require treatment outside of active surveillance (lifestyle modifications). These modifications often serve as a springboard to a healthier and happier life. For more information on lifestyle modifications, see **Chapter 10**.

### RECOMMENDED TREATMENT OPTION FOR CLINICALLY INSIGNIFICANT PROSTATE CANCER

Active surveillance, including:

- Lifestyle modifications (diet, exercise, stress management, and others)
- PSA testing & Digital Rectal Exam (every 6 months)

## LOW-RISK, LOW-VOLUME PROSTATE CANCER

| LOW-RISK/LOW-VOLUME PROSTATE CANCER | |
|---|---|
| Cancer Stage | T1C - T2A |
| Gleason Score | 3+3 = 6 or less |
| PSA | Less than 10 |
| # of positive core samples | Less than 3 |
| % Cancer in Biopsy | Less than 34% |

Figure 5.3 displays the basic information for low-risk, low-volume prostate cancer. "Low volume" is defined as less than 34% of cancer in a positive prostate biopsy (either a single core sample or entire biopsy). Low-volume patients are ideal candidates for active surveillance or emerging treatments. If the "% of Cancer in Biopsy" is more than 34%, the volume goes from "low" to "moderate-to-high."

As Dr. Ripoll's analogy implies, "kitty cat" is early-stage, low-risk local prostate cancer that has a statistically low probability of becoming metastatic disease. As cancers go, this category is considered non-aggressive.

Typically, these low-risk, low-volume clinically significant patients do well with either active surveillance or emerging treatments such as focal cryotherapy, brachytherapy, and HIFU. (See **Chapter 6** for information about these types of treatment.)

The good thing about a low-risk, low-volume prostate cancer diagnosis is knowing that you are going to be cured. For some men with this kind of cancer, the biggest challenge is making up their minds about which type of treatment to choose.

Even with the world's most compassionate doctor who provides the latest clinical information seasoned with sage advice, some men find making life-altering decisions like choosing between focal cryotherapy and brachytherapy beyond agonizing.

Understandably, there's a lot of anxiety about selecting the "right" treatment. Every patient wants the "Goldilocks" treatment — the one that's *just* right. Fortunately, with low-risk, low-volume prostate cancer, all the major treatment options are very successful. (For the success and complication rates of several types of treatment, please see **Chapter 8**.)

## SUCCESSFUL TREATMENT OPTIONS FOR LOW-RISK, LOW-VOLUME PROSTATE CANCER

- Active Surveillance (For more information on Active surveillance, see the **Chapter 5 Digging Deeper**)
- Electroporation (IRE)
- Freezing: Focal Cryotherapy
- Focal Hyperthermia
- Photodynamic Therapy (PDT)
- Radiation (External): Proton therapy, External Beam Radiation Therapy (EBRT), CyberKnife, and Intensity Modulated Radiation Therapy (IMRT)
- Radiation (Internal): Focal or whole gland
- Brachytherapy

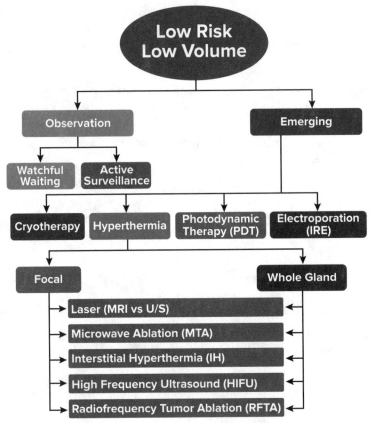

**Figure 5.4** displays the successful treatment options for low-risk, low-volume prostate cancer that we discuss in **Chapter 5.** For a more in-depth discussion of cryotherapy and brachytherapy, see **Chapter 6.**

## LOW-RISK, MODERATE-TO-HIGH VOLUME PROSTATE CANCER

| LOW-RISK/MODERATE-TO-HIGH VOLUME PROSTATE CANCER | |
|---|---|
| Cancer Stage | T1 - T2A |
| Gleason Score | 3+3 = 6 |
| PSA | Less than 10 |
| No. of Pos. Core Samples | More than 3 |
| % Cancer in Total Biopsy | Greater than 34% |

**Figure 5.5** displays the cancer information for low-risk, moderate-to-high volume cancer. Moderate-to-high volume disease is defined as more than 34% of cancer in any positive biopsy needle core. The number of positive core samples (more than 3) is also greater than low-volume disease (less than 3). Low-risk, moderate-to-high volume patients are ideal candidates for emerging treatments as well as traditional ones.

The principal difference between low-risk, low-volume and low-risk, moderate-to-high volume prostate cancer is the amount of cancer present. It's worth noting that 34 percent is the cut-off point between low-volume and moderate-volume prostate cancer. If there is more than 34 percent cancer in a total prostate biopsy (or any single prostate biopsy core sample), the cancer is considered "moderate-to-high volume."

What does the difference between 33 and 35 percent really mean? When you consider that the standard 12-needle TRUS prostate biopsy only samples 1 percent of prostate tissue, if more than 1/3 of your prostate biopsy is positive for cancer, there's probably a lot more cancer that the biopsy needles did not detect. In other words, there's a lot of cancer in your prostate.

Depending upon how much low-risk cancer is detected in the prostate biopsy, active surveillance may or may not be a smart treatment option. Patients with large amounts of low-risk prostate cancer are looking at emerging treatments (See **Figure 5.4** and **Chapter 6**) such as focal cryotherapy (freezing), focal brachytherapy (radioactive seed implantation), as well as various types of traditional treatments such as external beam radiation and surgery (See **Chapter 7**).

## SUCCESSFUL TREATMENT OPTIONS FOR LOW-RISK, MODERATE-TO-HIGH VOLUME PROSTATE CANCER

- Active Surveillance
- Freezing: Focal cryotherapy
- Radiation (External): Proton therapy, External Beam Radiation Therapy (EBRT), CyberKnife, and Intensity Modulated Radiation Therapy (IMRT)
- Radiation (Internal): Brachytherapy
- Surgery: Robotic, laparoscopic, or open radical prostatectomy

**MODERATE-RISK PROSTATE CANCER**

A cornered bobcat probably won't kill in its attempt to escape; however, it is likely to do some damage. The same is true of the prostate cancer Dr. Ripoll nick-named "Bobcat."

"Bobcat" describes a moderately aggressive, moderate-risk form of prostate cancer that is usually beyond the reach of active surveillance. Men with moderate-risk prostate cancer should seek definitive local treatment — usually surgery or some form of radiation.

**THERE ARE TWO TYPES OF MODERATE-RISK PROSTATE CANCER:**
1. Moderate Risk, Low-Volume
2. Moderate-Risk, Moderate-to-High Volume

**MODERATE-RISK LOW-VOLUME PROSTATE CANCER**

| MODERATE-RISK, LOW-VOLUME | |
|---|---|
| Cancer Stage | T2B |
| Gleason Score | 3+4 |
| PSA | 10-15 |
| % Cancer in Each Core | Less than 34% |

Figure 5.6 displays the basic clinical description for moderate-risk, low-volume prostate cancer.

The moderate-risk, low-volume sub-group is characterized by minimal amounts of cancer in 1-2 biopsy cores on one side of the prostate that have a Gleason Score of 3+4=7.

As **Figure 5.1** on **Page 114** suggests, patients in this sub-group can be treated as if they were low-risk, moderate-to-high volume patients, and all the same rules of treatment apply. It is very important that there is no Perineural Invasion (PNI), because PNI is a strong indicator that the cancer has spread (or is about to spread) outside the prostate.

Moderate-risk, low-volume prostate cancer is usually treated with a single type of therapy (surgery, radiation, or cryotherapy — See **Figure 5.7**).

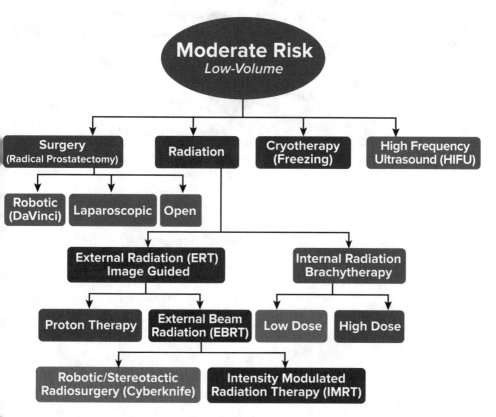

**Figure 5.7** displays the full spectrum of treatment options available for men with moderate-risk, low-volume prostate cancer. Note: In this figure and throughout this book, we use the words "surgery" and "radical prostatectomy" interchangeably.

## SUCCESSFUL (SINGLE) TREATMENT OPTIONS FOR MODERATE-RISK, LOW-VOLUME PROSTATE CANCER

- Freezing: Cryotherapy
- Radiation (External): EBRT, CyberKnife, Proton Beam, and IMRT
- Radiation (Internal): Brachytherapy
- Surgery: Robotic, Laparoscopic, or Open Radical Prostatectomy

As the cancer volume and other factors rise (See **Chapter 4** for all 12 factors), the disease becomes moderate-risk, moderate-to-high volume cancer. As this transformation occurs, doctors are more likely to combine treatments (dual-therapy approach) to ensure that all the cancer has been removed/destroyed (See **Figure 5.9**).

**MODERATE-RISK, MODERATE-TO-HIGH VOLUME PROSTATE CANCER**

| MODERATE-RISK, MODERATE-TO-HIGH VOLUME | |
|---|---|
| Cancer Stage | T2B |
| Gleason Score | 3+4 or 4+3 = 7 |
| PSA | 10-20 |
| % Cancer in Each Core | More than 34% |

Figure **5.8** provides a visual representation of the traditional prostate cancer information for Moderate-risk, Moderate-to-High volume prostate cancer. Please notice the difference between this graphic and **Figure 5.6.**

The dual treatment approach for moderate-risk, moderate-to-high volume prostate cancer is similar to the treatment of high-risk (Mountain Lion) cancer. The good news about moderate-risk, moderate-to-high volume prostate cancer is that it is treatable in the vast majority of cases. See **Chapter 8** for all the moderate-risk prostate cancer treatment success rates.

It is important to act quickly when treating both kinds of moderate-risk prostate cancer. The timing of treatment,

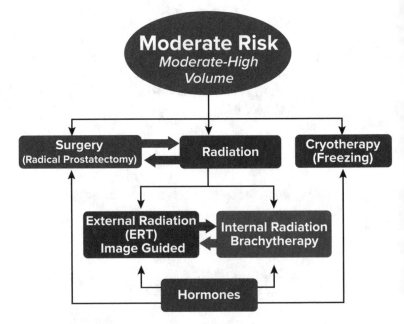

Figure **5.9** visually represents how combining different prostate cancer treatments (dual therapies) can be used to treat moderate-risk, moderate-to-high volume prostate cancer.

however, is not nearly as critical as it is with high-risk cancer, which should be treated right away.

## SUCCESSFUL (COMBINATION) THERAPIES FOR MODERATE-RISK MODERATE-TO-HIGH VOLUME PROSTATE CANCER

- Surgery + external radiation
- Surgery + hormone therapy
- External radiation + internal radiation
- External radiation + hormone therapy
- Internal radiation + hormone therapy
- Cryotherapy + hormone therapy

**HIGH-RISK PROSTATE CANCER**

| HIGH-RISK | |
|---|---|
| Cancer Stage | Greater than T2B |
| Gleason Score | 8-10 |
| PSA | Greater than 20 |

**Figure 5.10** lists the traditional prostate cancer information for high-risk prostate cancer. If any of these three scores (Cancer State, Gleason Score, or PSA) is elevated, you are automatically bumped into the high-risk category — regardless of the results from other prostate cancer tests/scans. That's just how it is.

Think of high-risk prostate cancer as metastatic disease in the making.

Dr. Ripoll's nick-name "Mountain Lion" speaks volumes about the dangers of high-risk local prostate cancer. Mature mountain lions look at people as food; the same is true of high-risk (Mountain Lion) prostate cancer.

If you try to keep a big cat cancer like that cooped up in a tiny space like your prostate, it is going to break out — and probably take you with it.

High-risk prostate cancer can be treated, but its deadly nature demands both respect and decisive action. The sooner you detect and remove/destroy this type of cancer, the better.

Because high-risk prostate cancer is so lethal, you have very little time to ponder treatment options once it is detected. Successful treatment of this kind of cancer requires swift action by a highly skilled medical team, a compliant patient (you), and an amazing support team.

High-risk prostate cancer also requires the use of multiple treatment modalities: some combination of radiation, hormone therapy, and other treatments.

This kind of cancer can be cured, although the 10-year survival rates are much lower than they are for low-risk and moderate-risk cancers (See **Chapter 8**).

### SUCCESSFUL (COMBINATION) TREATMENT OPTIONS FOR HIGH-RISK PROSTATE CANCER*

As with moderate-risk, moderate-to-high-volume cancer, the following treatment combinations for Mountain Lion cancer include

- External radiation + internal radiation
- External radiation + hormone therapy
- Internal radiation + hormone therapy
- Cryotherapy + hormone therapy
- Surgery + external radiation*
- Surgery + hormone therapy*

**NOTE**

*\* Today, surgery (radical prostatectomy) is not a preferred method of treatment for high-risk prostate cancer. It is NOT the first choice for combination therapy — even by the world's most renowned prostate cancer surgeons at the Johns Hopkins Hospital.*

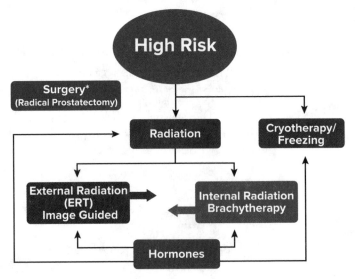

Figure 5.11 gives a visual representation of how traditional treatments can be combined to treat high-risk prostate cancer. Please note that hormone therapy can be used in conjunction with other treatments to create a local + systemic treatment approach. *Note that radical prostatectomy is not a recommended treatment.

## SYSTEMIC CONTROL

The type of treatments we have been talking about so far in this chapter are called "Local Control" (the treatment of local disease), which is best suited for treating prostate cancer that is still confined to the prostate.

Hormone therapy (also called "systemic therapy" or "systemic control") is the primary form of prostate cancer treatment for metastatic disease (cancer that has escaped prostate and spread to other areas).

Once cancer leaves the prostate, it is considered "systemic" or "metastatic" disease. Currently, hormone therapy is the best treatment for this type of cancer.

As previously discussed, hormone therapy can also be combined with other forms of treatment to create a full-spectrum (local plus systemic) approach to eradicating cancer that is still confined to the prostate. (See **Figures 5.9 and 5.11.**)

Doctors use hormone therapy to kill "floater" cancer cells that have escaped the prostate, preferably before these cells form a tumor in another part of your body. You can think of these floater cells like termites: They are much easier to exterminate *before* they colonize your home.

## METASTATIC DISEASE

The treatment of metastatic prostate cancer is a rapidly evolving field with new medications and innovative therapies going to clinical trial all the time.

We could literally write a separate book about all the changes that are occurring in the field of metastatic prostate cancer treatment; unfortunately, by the time the book was researched and written (1-2 years), much of the information in it would be out of date. That's how fast this field is changing.

If you have been diagnosed with metastatic prostate cancer (systemic disease), here is the basic information you need to know:

1. Metastatic disease begins when cancer escapes the membrane of the prostate and starts spreading to adjacent tissues.

2. The two most common metastatic pathways are perineural invasion and extracapsular extension. (See **Chapter 4** for more information.)

HORMONES

## METASTATIC DISEASE

| | Definition | Treatment |
|---|---|---|
| **Local** | • Early extension into the surrounding tissues such as prostate capsule and seminal vesicles<br>• Later into bladder wall and rectum | • Radiation and cloud effects can be used as either primary or additional treatment<br>• Additional hormone therapy |
| **Distant** | • Early extension into the lymph nodes and bones (spine, pelvis, and ribs)<br>• Later into liver and lungs | • Watchful waiting<br>• Constant hormone therapy<br>• Sequential hormone therapy<br>• Intermittent hormone therapy<br>• Second-line hormone therapy<br>• Radiation/quality of life care<br>• Chemotherapy<br>• Clinical trails |

Figure 5.12 provides a basic overview of the difference between local and distant metastatic disease and how they are treated. See **Chapter 7** for more information on metastatic disease and how hormone treatments are used to minimize its effects.

3. Although there are several ways to categorize metastatic prostate cancer, **Figure 5.12** looks at the treatment of metastatic cancer, based on whether the disease is "Local" (has only spread to the nearby lymph nodes and tissues) or "Distant" (spread beyond seminal vesicles and local lymph nodes).

If you compare **Figure 5.11** and **Figure 5.12**, you will notice that the treatment for "local" metastatic disease is similar to the way doctors often treat a more advanced case of high-risk cancer that is still confined inside the prostate.

Treatment for "distant" metastatic disease, however, is usually designed to limit cancer growth while maintaining quality of life. In addition to the treatments and therapies used to treat local metastatic disease, doctors also use additional medications and chemotherapy to control distant metastatic disease.

HORMONES

## THERE'S STRENGTH IN NUMBERS

*We recommend you bring someone (your spouse/partner, a family member, or a trusted friend) with you to your medical appointments to take notes, ask any questions that may have slipped your mind, and generally help you keep track of all the information and appointments.*

*If the idea of bringing someone to the doctor's office with you sounds childish, unnecessary, or weak — it's not.*

*The minute a doctor starts talking about cutting your abdomen open or blasting you with radiation, there's a good chance that your mind will go on vacation and you won't remember the details. Who would?*

*If you're like most men, confronting your own mortality is NOT a comfortable feeling. Having an ally in the room with you makes the whole experience a lot more bearable.*

*This recommendation is more of a request if you were diagnosed with High-Risk (Mountain Lion) prostate cancer. You are going to have to wade through a ton of medical information about treatments and complications, cope with a lot of heavy-duty emotions, decide on a treatment, and basically reshuffle your entire life — all within a couple of weeks.*

*Another good reason to bring a wife, friend, or family member with you to your medical appointments is that they are not "the patient"; therefore, they have a better chance of being more objective than you.*

*Having someone in the room who can help you "see" your interactions with your doctor from a different perspective (and advocate for you when necessary) is invaluable.*

*Maybe your current doctor is the ideal physician to help you heal from prostate cancer, and maybe he/she is not. When it come time to choose a doctor to perform a particular type of treatment, an objective voice in the conversation is a priceless asset.*

*We also recommend that you take a look at the "Doctor Selection Tips" in the* **Chapter 5** Digging Deeper *section.*

*Be smart and bring someone you trust with you to your appointments. You'll be glad you did.*

# Doctor Story
## DR. GEO ESPINOSA, ND, LAc

**Urology,
NYU Langone
Medical Center**

*Richard came to see me about a year and a half ago. He was freaking out because he was only 52 years old, he had a PSA of 5.2 — and his dad was undergoing treatment for advanced prostate cancer.*

*I recommended we measure the size of his prostate to check his PSA Density. It was pretty big (70 cc).*

*Because of Richard's elevated PSA and his family history of prostate cancer, I recommended we do a targeted MRI fusion biopsy. Out of 14 samples, two contained a small amount of Gleason 6 (low grade) cancer.*

*Because he had a large prostate and a small amount of low-risk disease, I told Richard that he was a good candidate for active surveillance. I explained to him that this would be an active process. He would go on my CaPLESS Method program (a comprehensive lifestyle overhaul that focuses on stress management, fitness, eating, and smart supplementation) and we would monitor his PSA every three months.*

*Richard knew his dad was dying, so he understood what could happen if his cancer "went crazy," but he decided to try the CaPLESS program.*

*Within a year, Richard's PSA had dropped to 3.2, and his dad passed away from prostate cancer. I asked Richard if he wanted to do another biopsy now, or wait six months. He wanted to wait because of how sad he was about losing his dad, and he just wasn't ready to look his own mortality in the face yet.*

*During those six months, his PSA fell again to 2.9.*

*His next targeted biopsy was negative — no detectable cancer! I might have been skeptical if we had done a randomized biopsy, but we were targeting the exact same area.*

*Richard was elated — hugging me and high-fiving me. "For the last year and a half, I felt like there was a dark cloud over my head, preventing me from living to the fullest," he told me. "Now I can live again."*

*He also had mixed feelings: he just took his life back from the disease that claimed his dad's.*

*I shared one of my favorite prayers with him: "Let me not die while I'm still alive."*

## LOOKING AHEAD

**CHAPTER 1:** You or your doctor is concerned about your prostate — We provide you with **Prostate 101**: where it lives, what it does, plus relevant statistics.

**CHAPTER 2:** Your doctor told you to **schedule a prostate biopsy** — We give you a **Prostate Biopsy Assessment Tool** to see if you actually need one, and what to expect if you do.

**CHAPTER 3:** You have a prostate biopsy — We explain the steps you need to take, whether you have a **negative biopsy or a positive biopsy**.

**CHAPTER 4:** You have a **positive prostate biopsy** — We provide you with a **Prostate Cancer Assessment Tool** to help you understand which kind of cancer you have.

**CHAPTER 5:** You need to select a prostate cancer treatment — We provide you with a summary of the most common types of treatment based on your **cancer risk type** (low-risk, moderate-risk, and high-risk).

**CHAPTER 6:** You have **low-risk, low-volume prostate cancer** and need to learn more about emerging treatments — We provide you with a summary of these treatments to help you understand the differences between focal, minimally invasive, alternative, whole gland, and traditional treatments.

**CHAPTER 7:** You have prostate cancer that is more advanced than low-risk, low-volume and need to know more about **whole-gland treatments** (both stand-alone traditional and combination treatments) — We provide you with a summary of these treatments.

**CHAPTER 8:** You want to know the **success and complication rates** for each type of treatment and for each cancer risk type (low-risk, moderate-risk, and high-risk) — We provide you with unbiased information to support your decision-making process.

**CHAPTER 9:** You feel **overwhelmed** by the news of a positive prostate biopsy — We give you the tools to surf this tidal wave of emotion and overcome the feeling of panic that almost always accompanies a positive biopsy report.

**CHAPTER 10:** You want to **use your cancer diagnosis as a springboard to better health** — We help you address your wellness goals with a proven plan that covers inflammation, diet, inactivity, stress, immune system, hormone optimization, structure, and removing toxic substances.

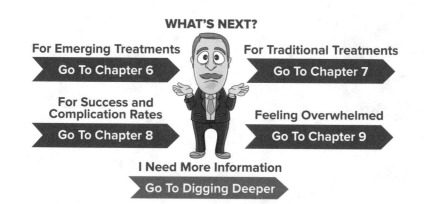

**WHAT'S NEXT?**

For Emerging Treatments
Go To Chapter 6

For Traditional Treatments
Go To Chapter 7

For Success and Complication Rates
Go To Chapter 8

Feeling Overwhelmed
Go To Chapter 9

I Need More Information
Go To Digging Deeper

# WELCOME TO THE TOOLBOX
# CHAPTER 5 **TOOLBOX**

**THIS TOOLBOX SECTION INCLUDES THE FOLLOWING TOOLS AND QUESTIONNAIRES TO HELP YOU UNDERSTAND WHICH TYPES OF TREATMENT BEST FIT THE KIND OF CANCER YOU HAVE :**

- Brief Explanation of Cancer Doctor Types
- General Questionnaire
- Urologist/Urologic Oncologist Questionnaire
- Radiation Oncologist Questionnaire
- Medical Oncologist Questionnaire
- Partin Tables

## *Doctor Types*

| | |
|---|---|
| **UROLOGIST** | A generalist who takes care of patients with urological diseases of the genitourinary system (the reproductive and the urinary systems). The primary physician to diagnose, treat, and follow-up with patients who have prostate cancer. Most urologists are capable of treating prostate cancer. Urologists are more likely to recommend surgery (radical prostatectomy). |
| **UROLOGICAL ONCOLOGIST** | Same training as a urologist, plus a fellowship in urological oncology. Treats all urological cancers: prostate, bladder, testicular, and kidney. |
| **RADIATION ONCOLOGIST** | Specializes in all types of radiation therapy. Many perform both internal and external types of radiation. A radiation oncologist is likely to recommend radiation therapy. |
| **MEDICAL ONCOLOGIST** | Medical oncologists treat cancer with chemotherapy. Unlikely to be involved with localized prostate cancer. Usually involved in the later stages and metastatic disease. |

TOOLBOX

## *General Questions for Doctors*

| QUESTIONS | ANSWERS |
|---|---|
| How much of your practice is dedicated to prostate cancer treatment? | |
| How current is your knowledge in the diagnosis and treatments of prostate cancer? | |
| Have you had special training in prostate cancer diagnosis and/or treatment? | |
| What type of prostate cancer do I have? | |
| What is my prostate cancer stage? | |
| What is my highest Gleason score? | |
| What is my highest PSA total? | |
| How many needles were used in my biopsy? | |
| How many biopsies needles were positive? | |
| What percent of the needles had cancer? | |
| Do I have perineural invasion (PNI)? | |
| Do I have seminal vesicle involvement? | |
| Do I have extra capsular extension? | |
| Do I have positive lymph nodes? | |
| Do I have prostate cancer in my bones? | |
| Will I need more tests? If so, which ones? | |
| How serious is my cancer? | |
| What are my chances of survival? | |
| Who would you recommend for a second opinion and why? (Write out the doctor's name and phone number.) | |
| Third opinion (write type of doctor and phone number) | |

TOOLBOX

## *Questions for Urologist or Urological Oncologist*

| QUESTIONS | ANSWERS |
| --- | --- |
| What treatments are most appropriate for my PSA, cancer stage, and Gleason score? | |
| What are the benefits and risks of each of these treatments? | |
| What treatment do you recommend? Would you recommend this for a family member? | |
| If you recommend a radical prostatectomy, which type would you recommend and why? Open (retropubic or perineal)? Laparoscopic? Robotic? | |
| What percent of your patients are continent after surgery (no diaper pads)? | |
| What percent of your patients are able to get and maintain full erections after surgery? | |
| Will I need to stay in the hospital for treatment? If so, for how long? | |
| How much pain will I have after surgery and how will you manage my pain? | |
| When can I return to work? | |
| When can I return to exercise? | |
| How long will it take before we know that the treatment worked? | |
| When do we schedule surgery? | |
| Will I also need hormone therapy? | |
| What are the complications from the hormone therapy that you recommend? | |
| What are the chances I will end up unable to urinate and require another procedure? | |

TOOLBOX

# Questions for Radiation Oncologist

| QUESTIONS | ANSWERS |
|---|---|
| What treatments are most appropriate for my PSA, cancer stage, and Gleason score? | |
| What are the benefits and risks of each of these treatments? | |
| Which treatment would be best for me? Would you recommend this treatment for a family member? | |
| Are these treatments experimental or established? | |
| What is the success rate of this protocol? | |
| Will it prolong my life? | |
| Will treatment affect my ability to have and maintain an erection? | |
| How will treatment affect my quality of life? | |
| Will I need to be in the hospital for treatment? If so, for how long? | |
| Will I have pain, and if so, how will you manage it? | |
| Will I experience symptoms such as nausea, vomiting, weight loss, hair loss, fatigue, and weakness? | |
| When can I return to exercise? | |
| When can I return to work? | |
| How is the treatment given? | |
| How long will each treatment session take? | |
| How many treatment sessions will I have? | |
| Any other complications I need to know about? | |
| Should a family member or friend come with me to my treatment sessions? | |
| How soon will I know if the treatments are working? | |
| How often will I have to do follow-ups? | |

TOOLBOX

## *Questions for Medical Oncologist*

| QUESTIONS | ANSWERS |
| --- | --- |
| Which treatments are most appropriate for the kind of cancer I have? | |
| What are the benefits and risks of each of these treatments? | |
| Which treatment(s) would you recommend to a family member ? | |
| Are these protocols experimental or established? | |
| What is the success rate of this treatment? | |
| Will it prolong my life? | |
| Will it affect my ability to have or maintain an erection? | |
| How will it affect my quality of life? | |
| Will I need to be in the hospital for treatment? If so, for how long? | |
| Will I have pain, and if so, how will you manage it? | |
| Will I experience symptoms such as nausea, vomiting, weight loss, hair loss, fatigue, and weakness? | |
| When can I return to exercise? | |
| When can I return to work? | |
| How is the treatment given? | |
| How long will each treatment session take? | |
| How many treatment sessions will I have? | |
| Any other complications I need to know about? | |
| Should a family member or friend come with me to my treatment sessions? | |
| How soon will I know if the treatment is working? | |
| How often will I have to follow up? | |

TOOLBOX

# PARTIN TABLE CALCULATOR

**http://urology.jhu.edu/prostate/partintables.php**

At the Web URL above, enter your own Gleason score, PSA, and clinical stage to predict the chances that your prostate cancer will:

1. *Remain inside the prostate (organ-confined)*
2. *Penetrate the capsule of the prostate (extracapsular extension)*
3. *Spread to the seminal vesicles (seminal vesicle involvement)*
4. *Spread to local lymph node (lymph node involvement)*

The information in quotations below comes directly from the James Buchanan Brady Urological Institute at the Johns Hopkins Medical Institute. For more information, please use this link (http://urology.jhu.edu/prostate/partintables.php) or visit their website (www.jhu.edu).

" *The Partin Tables use clinical features of prostate cancer – Gleason score, serum PSA, and clinical stage – to predict whether the tumor will be confined to the prostate. The tables are based on the accumulated experience of urologists performing radical prostatectomy at the James Buchanan Brady Urological Institute. For decades, urologists around the world have relied on the tables for counseling patients preoperatively and for surgical planning.*

*"Since PSA screening was introduced in the early 1990's, the extent of disease for men with prostate cancer has slowly changed over time. Also, subtle changes to the Gleason scoring system have made the system more accurate but were not considered in previous editions of the Partin tables. Earlier this year, the tables were updated using the experience of surgeons at the Brady performing radical prostatectomy from 2006-2011."*

TOOLBOX

**NOTES:**

TOOLBOX

# Emerging Treatments

" Just get your regular check-ups and PSAs and, if you're diagnosed, do everything you can to eradicate the disease. I think we are fortunate to have the best doctors in the world in this country. If you're not satisfied with the diagnosis and prognosis, then get another couple of opinions. But, in the final analysis, you need to do what it takes to get rid of the cancer and get on with your life.

*— Arnold Palmer*

# Patient Story

## GENE

*After reviewing my journey with prostate cancer, I have a few things to say:*

**The Good** *: I had "cancer light."*

*At age 58, my prostate cancer was barely detectable during a digital rectal exam and my PSA was normal.*

*Eventually, I chose to undergo CyberKnife treatment, which was nearly painless and without any complications. A little daily Cialis helps with continence and ED. I still long for my glory days, but I have found that making today full of glory is where I need to focus my attention.*

**The Bad:** *Professional jealously & insurance companies.*

*I was about to receive my first external beam radiation treatment (before I opted for CyberKnife), when my first urologist told me, "You know, this will give you cancer." I wanted to plant a right hook squarely on his jaw.*

*I had done the research. I knew about the possible complications, so why was he reiterating the long-term effects of radiation? At my age and with low-risk cancer, I wanted to skip the prostatectomy and keep my body more or less intact. I still feel like I won that battle.*

*The other train wreck was my insurance company. I would like to know the name of the genius who, after giving the OK for a CyberKnife procedure, decided to claim the procedure was "experimental" — a full 3 months after the treatments were over. The appeal process was demeaning and sucked the life out of me.*

*If I had anything to do over, I would make sure I had a legally binding written document from my insurance company. My trust in the health insurance industry will forever remain zero. My disease & treatment were less toxic than dealing with my insurance company.*

# chapter
## SIX
# summary

In **Chapter 6**, we introduce you the world of "emerging" prostate cancer treatments. (We will do the same for traditional prostate cancer treatments in **Chapter 7**.)

This chapter intended to be a point of departure for your journey to find the best prostate cancer treatment for you. It is NOT the final word on emerging treatments.

In order to give you a good idea of what types of emerging treatments are available, we will start with the simplest treatments and move on to the more complicated ones.

*If you know that you're only interested in traditional prostate cancer treatments, please skip ahead to* **Chapter 7**.

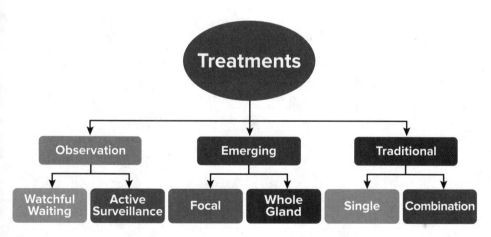

**Figure 6.0** gives you a general overview of the types of prostate cancer treatments. We will cover observation and emerging treatments in this chapter. We will cover traditional treatments in **Chapter 7**.

## VOCABULARY

See Glossary for Definitions

4KScore

Active Surveillance

Alternative Treatment

Apoptosis

Combination Treatment

Cryotherapy (Cryoablation)

CyberKnife

Da Vinci (Robotic Surgery System)

Digital Rectal Exam (DRE)

External Beam Radiation Therapy (EBRT)

Focal Treatment

High Dose Radiation

High Intensity Focused Ultrasound (HIFU)

Hyperthermia

Intensity-Modulated Radiation Therapy (IMRT)

Interstitial Ablation

Irreversible Electroporation

Laparoscopic Prostatectomy

Laser Ablation

Low Dose Radiation

Lumpectomy

Lymph Nodes

Microwave Ablation

Minimally Invasive Treatment

Minimal Disease

MRI

Multi-focal

Mutation

NanoKnife

Non-Invasive Treatment

Observation

Organ-Confined Cancer

Outpatient

Perineal

Photodynamic Therapy

Prostate Biopsy

Prostatic Urethra

PSA

Radiation Therapy

Radical Mastectomy

Radical Prostatectomy

Radiofrequency Ablation

Retropubic

Traditional Treatment

Transrectal Ultrasound

Urologist

Watchful Waiting

Whole Gland Treatment

DEBUNKING MYTHS

## "DON'T GO THERE!"

*That's what Mark's first urologist told him about emerging prostate cancer treatments. The doctor's message was simple: Why risk your life on some new type of treatment that isn't supported by 20 years worth of data about survival rates?*

*When Mark asked the doctor about complications from robotic radical prostatectomy (the type of surgery this doctor recommended), the doctor replied that he was 90 percent sure that Mark would NOT need to wear diapers or pads for the rest of his life, and he was 65-70 percent sure that Mark would still be able to have an erection with Viagra.*

*You can understand why, at age 46 with low-risk, low-volume cancer, these were not compelling arguments for surgery (robotic or otherwise).*

*That conversation occurred in 2006. Since then, the world of prostate cancer research has mushroomed. So has the development of emerging prostate cancer treatments — which are the topic of* **Chapter 6.**

*After consulting with five doctors, Mark opted for a comprehensive active surveillance program that included a monthly consultation with his doctor. In three months, his cancer was undetectable by biopsy or MRI and his other cancer markers improved (PIN disappeared, and PSA was cut in half). More importantly, 10 years later, the cancer remains undetectable.*

## WHAT DOES "EMERGING TREATMENT" MEAN?

What are the differences between **emerging, focal, minimally invasive**, and **alternative** treatments?

For the purposes of this book, we will use the term **"emerging"** to cover a wide range of prostate cancer treatments that are quickly gaining acceptance as legitimate alternatives to surgery and external beam radiation. Emerging treatments include techniques adopted from other types of cancer treatment (focal cryotherapy, for example) and innovative treatments that have great short-term success rates — but lack the long-term data (irreversible electroporation, for example).

**Focal** prostate cancer treatments center on small areas of the prostate — as opposed to the "whole gland."

These treatments are to the prostate what the lumpectomy is to the breast (removing a small tumor but leaving the rest of the prostate — or breast — intact).

What can be confusing about "**focal** treatment" is that in some cases (cryotherapy and brachytherapy, for example), the same type of treatment can be used for either a focal or "whole gland" procedure. It all depends on which kind and how much cancer the patient has.

"**Minimally invasive**" is a difficult term to define. For the purpose of this book, we will use these guidelines to define minimally invasive prostate cancer treatment:

- Does NOT cause long-term damage to the body
- Complications are rare or non-existent
- Side-effects seldom occur
- Treatment is done as an outpatient procedure
- A day or two of recovery is all that is required

## RECENT TRENDS IN PROSTATE CANCER TREATMENT

Originally, **"alternative"** meant a form of prostate cancer treatment other than surgery. Today, "alternative" can be used to describe many non-traditional prostate cancer treatments. We prefer the term "**emerging,**" however, because one doctor's "alternative" is another's "bread and butter." Over time, the term "alternative" has lost some of its meaning. For example, treatments that are generally accepted as "traditional" today (cryotherapy and brachytherapy) were once considered "alternative" as little as 15 years ago.

Also, thanks to tests like PSA screening, 4KscoreTest, PCA3, SelectMDx, and ConfirmMDx (and the increase in early prostate cancer detection these tests provide), there has been a movement towards focal/minimally invasive/emerging treatments for men who have low-risk, low-volume prostate cancer.

For these prostate cancer patients, focal/minimally invasive/emerging treatments have success rates similar to traditional surgery and external radiation. More importantly, they have lower complication rates, which help preserve a man's quality of life (see **Chapter 8**).

Both active surveillance and focal treatments are considered "minimally invasive," with active surveillance being the de-facto definition of a "non-invasive" treatment.

Focal and minimally invasive treatments are the leading edge of prostate cancer research; however, they lack the 20-year follow-up studies and scientific analyses to make definitive claims about their long-term effectiveness (see **Chapter 8**). They should only be used with low-risk, low-volume disease as part of a program that includes regular follow-ups and testing.

On the other hand, traditional treatments (see **Chapter 7**) have well-established 20+ year success rates, which makes them a good match for patients in the following categories who need definitive treatment:

- Low-risk, moderate-to-high-volume cancer
- Moderate-risk prostate cancer
- High-risk cancer

## EMERGING TREATMENTS

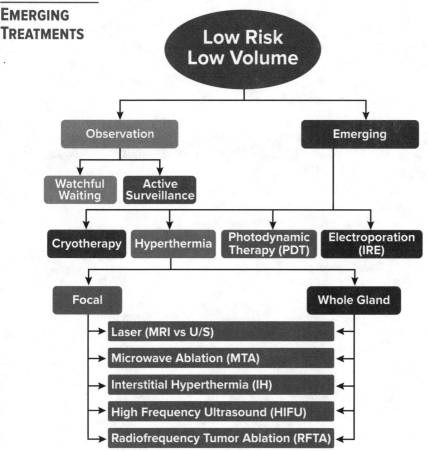

Figure 6.1 displays the emerging treatments discussed in **Chapter 6**.

## WHOLE GLAND VERSUS FOCAL TREATMENTS

*Prostate cancer treatment is evolving in the same direction as breast cancer treatment.*

*Thirty years ago, the gold standard of breast cancer treatment was the radical mastectomy (complete removal of the breast and underarm lymph nodes).*

*A 2014 study in the Journal of American Medicine showed that 2/3 of women with early stage breast cancer in one breast opted NOT to have a total mastectomy. Instead, they had a lumpectomy (removing the tumor, while leaving the breast mostly intact) plus radiation to kill any residual cancer.*

*Thankfully, new "focal" treatments for low-risk, low-volume prostate cancer do NOT require removing or destroying the entire prostate gland — the male equivalent of a female lumpectomy.*

*Selecting the right patients, and then pairing them the right focal treatment, is crucial to treatment success.*

*As with active surveillance patients, focal therapy patients should have regular follow-ups to make sure there are no signs that the cancer has returned. If the cancer does come back, these patients should be treated with a definitive whole-gland treatment (where the entire prostate is removed, frozen, or destroyed by radiation).*

*Please see **Chapter 7** to learn more about these types of treatments.*

| Focal | Whole Gland |
|---|---|
| • Works best for low-risk, low-volume patients with minimal disease in only one half of the prostate. | • Is a definitive treatment of the entire gland, and it will treat all cancers within it, including cancers that have more than one tumor (multi-focal). |
| • In 50-76% of cases, prostate cancer has multiple tumors. Focal treatment may miss these undetected tumors. | • Has the potential for more (and more severe) complications depending on the modality chosen. |
| • Complications are minimal, if at all, which makes focal treatment very attractive. | • In general, follow-up doctor visits require fewer tests, unless PSA starts going up. |
| • Focal treatment is an ideal bridge between active surveillance and definitive treatment; it provides a proactive feeling of "doing something." | • Emotionally easier to put prostate cancer behind you and move on with less anxiety about a potential recurrence of cancer. |
| • Like active surveillance, focal treatment leaves the door open for whole-gland treatment if cancer is detected after additional tests or scans. | |

Figure 6.2 displays the differences between focal and whole-gland prostate cancer treatments.

As we mentioned on **Page 142**, many emerging treatments can be used to treat a portion of the prostate (focal therapy) or the entire prostate (whole gland). These focal and whole-gland treatments are essentially the same treatment; they are used differently depending upon how much and what type of cancer a patient has.

For example, cryotherapy can be used to freeze the entire prostate, which destroys all the cells in the prostate (and usually creates permanent erectile dysfunction — ED), or it can also be used to freeze tumors the size of a pea (without ED). In both cases, the treatment process is similar, however, the application is different.

The two most popular types of emerging prostate cancer treatment are cryotherapy and brachytherapy. Since these types of treatment are also used extensively as traditional treatments, we felt it would be less confusing to discuss them in detail in **Chapter 7** (instead of giving you a little bit here and a little bit there). For more information about brachytherapy, turn to **Page 171**; for more information about cryotherapy turn to **Page 177**.

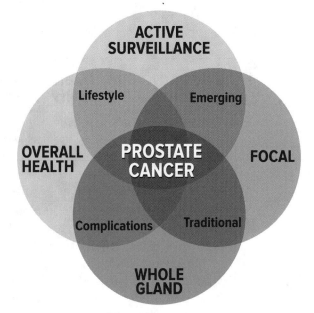

**Figure 6.3** illustrates the interconnectedness between prostate cancer treatments, possible complications, and your overall health.

As with focal cryotherapy and brachytherapy, both robotic and laparoscopic prostate cancer surgeries are much less invasive than traditional "open" radical prostatectomies; however, robotic and laparoscopic surgeries fail to meet the guidelines for emerging treatments we gave on **Page 142**. For more information about these surgery options, see **Chapter 7**.

The decision about whether to select a focal (emerging) treatment over of a whole gland (traditional) treatment is driven by your cancer numbers (See **Chapter 4**) and what those numbers say about the kind of cancer you have. (See the **Prostate Cancer Assessment Tool** in the **Chapter 4 Toolbox** as well as **Chapter 8** about possible treatment complications.)

## WATCHFUL WAITING

Watchful waiting is best suited for patients who are too frail to undergo treatment, too old (and, therefore, likely to pass away long before prostate cancer becomes a significant health issue), or who have other health problems that are more likely to limit their life expectancy.

Some people refer to watchful waiting as a "hands-off" or "non-treatment" approach, because if you opt for a watchful waiting strategy, your doctor will not actively treat you for prostate cancer.

---

### EMERGING TREATMENTS: WHO SHOULD CONSIDER THEM AND WHY?

*The good news about focal/minimally invasive prostate cancer treatments is they are less likely to cause unwanted complications. The bad news about these treatments is they are relatively new, so there are fewer studies about their long-term success and complication rates.*

*Because we don't have this information, emerging treatments should be reserved for patients with minimal disease (low-risk, low-volume) who are willing to have regular follow-ups and adhere to a strict active surveillance program. As we mentioned earlier, definitive (traditional) treatment can be performed at the first hint that the cancer has progressed.*

*For more information about targeted therapies, see the* **Chapter 6** Digging Deeper *Section.*

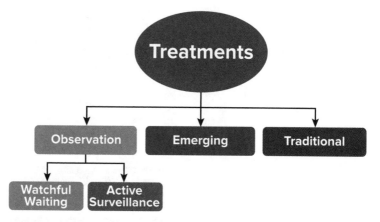

**Figure 6.4** highlights the two types of observation treatment: watchful waiting and active surveillance. If it sounds strange that there are two types of observation, these two treatments are actually quite different.

**ACTIVE SURVEILLANCE**

Active surveillance is NOT the same thing as watchful waiting.

As the name implies, active surveillance is an active form of treatment that involves regular follow-up visits with your doctor coupled with dramatic lifestyle reforms designed to reverse the unhealthy environment that allowed prostate cancer to develop in the first place. (See **Chapter 10** and Chapter 10 **Toolbox** for more information on active surveillance lifestyle changes.)

Originally practiced in Europe, active surveillance is only recommended for low-risk, low-volume prostate cancer patients. Patients are frequently monitored with tests such as DRE, PSA velocity, 4Kscore, PCA3, SelectMDx, MRI, prostate biopsy, ConfirmMDx, and others.

As with most prostate cancer treatments, active surveillance protocols vary depending on the needs of the individual patient. Likewise, active surveillance protocols vary from clinic to clinic and doctor to doctor.

Recent medical studies by well-respected researchers in the United States and elsewhere have shown that selecting the right patients is the key to a successful active surveillance program. Also, prompt treatment for patients whose cancer shows signs of progress is vital to patient longevity. For more information about active surveillance, go to the **Chapter 5 Digging Deeper** section.

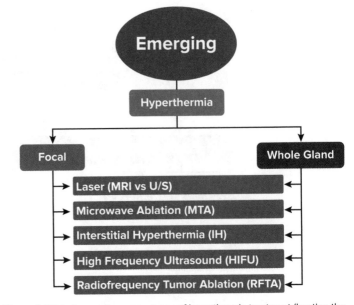

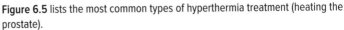

Figure 6.5 lists the most common types of hyperthermia treatment (heating the prostate).

## HYPERTHERMIA (HEAT THERAPY)

Hyperthermia is a way to turn up the heat on prostate cancer, improve the success of radiation and chemotherapy treatments, as well as reduce the complications of radiation treatments. It is a relatively non-invasive method of increasing tumor temperature to stimulate blood flow and increase oxygenation — which sounds like just the opposite of what you want to do to get rid of prostate cancer.

Hyperthermia, however, makes tumor cells more sensitive to radiation, therefore easier to treat. Also, the increased blood flow is believed to improve the immune system's ability to penetrate tumors and destroy the cancer.

In Europe, hyperthermia is used as a stand-alone treatment or in combination with radiation. By adding hyperthermia to radiation treatments, radiation oncologists can maximize the destruction of cancer tumor cells, while minimizing damage to healthy tissue surrounding the prostate.

Focal hyperthermia for prostate cancer involves inserting a probe in one of three places:

1. In the tissues next to the prostate
2. In the urethra
3. In the rectum

The closer the probe is to the tumor(s) inside the prostate, the more successful the hyperthermia treatment is. This is why putting the probe in the interstitial space right next to the prostate is the preferred placement.

There are many types of hyperthermia used to treat prostate cancer; the following five are the most common methods used in United States:

1. **High-Intensity Focused Ultrasound (HIFU)** uses the energy of sound waves to superheat and destroy small tumors. HIFU uses MRI scans and sometimes transrectal ultrasound to pinpoint the tumor location. HIFU is an attractive treatment because it is relatively noninvasive. In 2015, the Food and Drug Administration (FDA) approved HIFU for use in the United States. HIFU does have complications like urinary incontinence and urethral scaring; however, these complications are more common with whole-gland HIFU treatments than when HIFU is used as a focal therapy.

2. **MRI-Guided Focal Laser Ablation** of prostate cancer has the advantage that it can be performed under local anesthesia (the same kind that is used during a prostate biopsy). As the name indicates, the procedure is done with the help of MRI guidance. Laser ablation uses a needle to place an optical fiber laser directly into the area that contains the cancer. After the laser heats the treatment area, killing the cancer, a contrast dye is injected to make sure the treatment is complete.

3. **Interstitial Ablation** is similar to brachytherapy in that the patient is under general anesthesia (or an epidural), and the standard brachytherapy needle template is used to place the electrodes that heat the prostate, and kill the cancer. This procedure is done with the help of a transrectal ultrasound to guide the electrodes.

4. **Microwave Ablation** is performed by inserting a needle into the prostate (and/or the nearby tissue) or by inserting a very thin antenna into the prostatic urethra. This type of treatment essentially cooks small sections of the prostate (focal treatment) or larger sections (whole-gland treatment).

5. **Radio Frequency Tumor Ablation** destroys tumors inside the prostate by heating them to over 180° F (80° C) with high-frequency radio waves. Radio frequency tumor ablation of prostate cancer is

- Minimally invasive (no incision)
- Effective for small tumors
- Minimal risks and complications
- Procedure can be repeated if cancer returns

## PHOTODYNAMIC THERAPY

Photodynamic therapy uses a light-sensitive drug (porfimer sodium or Photofrin), which is activated by a low-power laser to cause a cascade of cell death inside the prostate (including the cancer cells).

Once activated by the laser, the light-sensitive drug triggers the formation of a highly reactive form of oxygen (called "singlet oxygen"), which destroys all the cells that come in contact with it.

## IRREVERSIBLE ELECTRO-PORATION

Irreversible electroporation (also known as NanoKnife) is a unique type of cancer treatment that does NOT use heat or radiation to destroy cancer cells. Instead, irreversible electroporation uses very thin needles as electrodes to create tiny, but extremely powerful, electrical fields that open permanent holes in the cell membranes of healthy and cancerous cells. These holes quickly lead to cell death (apoptosis).

Irreversible electroporation can also be used without causing permanent damage to surrounding tissues such as the urethra, bladder, rectum, and the neurovascular bundle of the prostate (which is critical to maintaining healthy sexual function).

Compared to the other ablation treatments, the lack of heat or radiation, combined with no damage to surrounding tissues, makes irreversible electroporation an excellent choice for a focal/minimally invasive treatment.

**NOTE**

*The perfect cancer treatment doesn't exist (not yet, anyway), or you wouldn't be reading this book. Instead, your doctor would have written you a prescription to fill at your local pharmacy, injected you with a virus that seeks out and destroys prostate cancer cells, or given you an immunotherapy drug that kills all the cells in your body with a particular mutation (and leaves the rest of the cells alone). Sometime in the not-too-distant future, this is how we'll treat prostate cancer.*

*For now, however, rest in the knowledge that prostate cancer treatments are improving rapidly, creating better success rates with fewer complications.*

**FISHING FOR SALMON IN ARIZONA?**

As a general rule, it is better to think globally but shop locally for a doctor to help you with prostate cancer. The same is true for your treatment options. There are three main reasons why this statement is true:

**1. Health Insurance**

Many health insurance plans will not pay for procedures done outside your service area, which is often the borders of your state.

**2. Out-of-Pocket Expenses**

If you choose to have treatment outside your service area, expect to pay BIG out-of-pocket expenses. In addition to the cost of treatment, there will be charges for assisting doctors and nurses, other medical staff, transportation, lodging, and meals. You could easily spend $30,000 – $50,000.

**3. Success Rates**

The success rates for all the major definitive treatments are similar (the success rates for emerging treatments vary), so often the decision comes down to which doctor in your coverage area has the best success rate and the lowest complication rate.

That said, there are legitimate reasons for looking outside your health insurance coverage area.

For example, if you want to follow an active surveillance protocol (which is relatively inexpensive), and you cannot find a doctor in your network, then it's time to start looking for one in the nearest major metropolitan area.

Your search for the best possible care may lead you to large metropolitan medical centers in cities like New York, Los Angeles, or Houston.

The same holds true for cryotherapy, brachytherapy, or robotic surgery — although these treatments cost much more than active surveillance, so your out-of-pocket expenses would be significant.

# Doctor Story
## DR. JAMES WOLACH, MD

Urology
Banner Health
Greeley, Colorado

*Practicing urology for 20 years in the same rural town helps you to see your patients as unique individuals — instead of people with a diagnosis.*

*I met my patient, John, about five years ago when his primary care physician referred him to me to evaluate an elevated PSA. I didn't think much about why he had missed several appointments, until I finally met him.*

*He was a lot more nervous and agitated than other patients, and he wasn't able to sit still during the appointment. He paced the room, walked out of the room several times, so I had to keep the door open during our consultation.*

*John waited until the end of our appointment before he told me about the near-death experience that made him claustrophobic.*

*Twenty years earlier, he worked for a pipe company. He was down in a hole on a construction site when the walls collapsed, burying him alive.*

*Since that accident, he couldn't stand being in a doctor's office or a hospital. For a long time, it was hard for him just to leave his house.*

*John's elevated PSA led to a prostate cancer diagnosis. First, however, I had to understand his claustrophobia before I could schedule his surgery and hospital stay. It was the first time he had been in a hospital since his accident.*

*Five years later, John remains prostate cancer free, and he can sit in my exam room with the door closed. In return, he taught me that my patients are people who come to me with their own individual struggles and needs.*

## LOOKING AHEAD

**CHAPTER 1:** You or your doctor is concerned about your prostate — We provide you with **Prostate 101**: where it lives, what it does, plus relevant statistics.

**CHAPTER 2:** Your doctor told you to **schedule a prostate biopsy** — We give you a **Prostate Biopsy Assessment Tool** to see if you actually need one, and what to expect if you do.

**CHAPTER 3:** You have a prostate biopsy — We explain the steps you need to take, whether you have a **negative biopsy or a positive biopsy**.

**CHAPTER 4:** You have a **positive prostate biopsy** — We provide you with a **Prostate Cancer Assessment Tool** to help you understand which kind of cancer you have.

**CHAPTER 5:** You need to select a prostate cancer treatment — We provide you with a summary of the most common types of treatment based on your **cancer risk type** (low-risk, moderate-risk, and high-risk).

**CHAPTER 6:** You have **low-risk, low-volume prostate cancer** and need to learn more about emerging treatments — We provide you with a summary of these treatments to help you understand the differences between focal, minimally invasive, alternative, whole gland, and traditional treatments.

**CHAPTER 7:** You have prostate cancer that is more advanced than low-risk, low-volume and need to know more about **whole-gland treatments** (both stand-alone traditional and combination treatments) — We provide you with a summary of these treatments.

**CHAPTER 8:** You want to know the **success and complication rates** for each type of treatment and for each cancer risk type (low-risk, moderate-risk, and high-risk) — We provide you with unbiased information to support your decision-making process.

**CHAPTER 9:** You feel **overwhelmed** by the news of a positive prostate biopsy — We give you the tools to surf this tidal wave of emotion and overcome the feeling of panic that almost always accompanies a positive biopsy report.

**CHAPTER 10:** You want to **use your cancer diagnosis as a springboard to better health** — We help you address your wellness goals with a proven plan that covers inflammation, diet, inactivity, stress, immune system, hormone optimization, structure, and removing toxic substances.

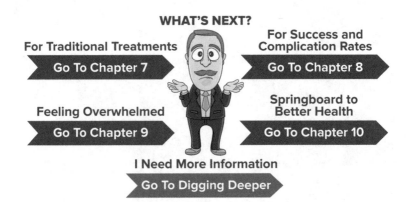

**WHAT'S NEXT?**

For Traditional Treatments
**Go To Chapter 7**

For Success and Complication Rates
**Go To Chapter 8**

Feeling Overwhelmed
**Go To Chapter 9**

Springboard to Better Health
**Go To Chapter 10**

I Need More Information
**Go To Digging Deeper**

# WELCOME TO THE TOOLBOX
# CHAPTER 6 **TOOLBOX**

---

**THIS TOOLBOX SECTION INCLUDES THE FOLLOWING TOOLS AND RESOURCES TO HELP YOU UNDERSTAND WHAT "EMERGING TREATMENTS" ARE AND IF YOU WOULD BE A GOOD CANDIDATE FOR ONE:**

- Low-Risk, Low-Volume Treatment Candidates List
- Emerging Treatments Candidates List

---

Men who have low-risk, low-volume prostate cancer are fortunate because they can be treated successfully with a variety of treatments (See **Chapter 8**). From active surveillance to focal hyperthermia to focal versions of cryotherapy and brachytherapy to traditional treatments, men with low-risk, low-volume cancer have the luxury of choice.

We include the **Low-Risk, Low-Volume Treatment Candidates List** in the **Chapter 6 Toolbox** to help men with this type of cancer start the treatment selection process.

The **Emerging Treatments Candidates List** refines the treatment selection process for men with low-risk, low-volume prostate cancer by providing a side-by-side look at the seven emerging treatments discussed in **Chapter 6**.

We include these two lists because, as we mentioned in **Chapter 5**: For some men, the biggest challenge with a low-risk, low-volume cancer diagnosis is making up their mind about a treatment plan.

TOOLBOX

# Low-Risk, Low-Volume Cancer Treatments

TOOLBOX

|  | DESCRIPTION | WOULD YOU BE A GOOD CANDIDATE? |
|---|---|---|
| WATCHFUL WAITING | • WW is generally suitable for men with other significant health issues.<br>• Commonly used when life expectancy is less than 5 years.<br>• Usually does NOT involve prostate cancer follow-up appointments or curative treatment.<br>• Treatment is palliative (relieving pain and alleviating symptoms). | |
| ACTIVE SURVEILLANCE | • Works best for low-risk, low-volume patients.<br>• It involves close monitoring and regular testing with the following (whichever is available to you and your physician): PSA free and total, PSA density, PSA velocity, PCA3, 4Kscore Test, SelectMDx, MRI scans, prostate biopsies, and ConfirmMDx.<br>• Active surveillance may lead to definitive treatment if cancer progress is indicated by any of the above tests. | |
| FOCAL TREATMENT | • Works best for low-risk, low-volume patients with minimal disease in only one half of the prostate<br>• It has the potential of local recurrence in another area of the prostate due to the fact that prostate cancer is multi-focal in 50-76% of cases.<br>• It has minimal if any complications, which makes it attractive to many people.<br>• It helps people feel they have done something to treat their cancer, and it is a perfect type of treatment between active surveillance and definitive (traditional) treatment.<br>• Follows the guidelines for active surveillance and may lead to definitive (traditional) treatment. | |
| WHOLE GLAND TREATMENT | • It is definitive treatment of the entire gland and will treat all cancers within it, including all the multi-focal ones.<br>• Depending on the modality chosen, it generally has more complications.<br>• Follow-up is more relaxed and biopsies are not required.<br>• Emotionally it is easier to put prostate cancer behind you and move on with less anxiety. | |

## Emerging Treatments

| EMERGING TREATMENTS | DESCRIPTION | WOULD YOU BE A GOOD CANDIDATE? |
|---|---|---|
| HIGH FREQUENCY ULTRA SOUND (HIFU) | • This procedure was approved for use in the United States by the FDA in 2015.<br>• It does have relatively high complication rates for urinary incontinence and urethral scaring.<br>• These complications are more common with whole-gland HIFU treatments and less common when HIFU is used as a focal therapy. | |
| LASER ABLATION | • Laser can be performed under local anesthesia (the same one that is used during a prostate biopsy).<br>• Done with either an ultrasound or with MRI guidance.<br>• Uses a needle to place an optical fiber laser directly into the area that contains the cancer.<br>• At the end of the procedure, a contrast dye is injected into the treatment area to make sure the treatment is complete. | |
| INTERSTITIAL HYPERTHERMIA (IH) | • (IH) is similar to brachytherapy in that the patient is under general anesthesia (or an epidural), and the standard brachytherapy needle template is used to place the electrodes that heat the prostate.<br>• This procedure is done with the help of a transrectal ultrasound to guide the electrodes. | |
| MICROWAVE ABLATION | • Microwave is performed by inserting a needle into the prostate (and/or the nearby tissue) or by inserting a very thin antenna into the prostatic urethra.<br>• This type of treatment essentially cooks small sections of the prostate (focal treatment) or larger sections (whole-gland treatment). | |
| RADIO FREQUENCY (RFTA) | • RFTA destroys tumors inside the prostate by heating them to over 180° F (80° C) with high-frequency radio waves.<br>• Minimally invasive (no incision)<br>• Effective for small tumors<br>• Minimal risks and complications<br>• Procedure can be repeated if cancer returns. | |

TOOLBOX

## Emerging Treatments - Continued

| EMERGING TREATMENTS | DESCRIPTION | WOULD YOU BE A GOOD CANDIDATE? |
|---|---|---|
| **PHOTODYNAMIC THERAPY (PDT)** | PDT uses a light-sensitive drug (porfimer sodium), which is activated by a low-power laser to cause a cascade of cell death inside the prostate (including prostate cancer cells). Activated by the laser, the light-sensitive drug triggers the formation of a highly reactive form of oxygen (called "singlet oxygen"), which destroys all the cells that come in contact with it. | |
| **IRREVERSIBLE ELECTROPORATION (IRE)** | IRE, also known as NanoKnife, is a unique type of cancer treatment that does NOT use heat or radiation to destroy cancer cells. Instead, it uses very thin needles as electrodes to create tiny, but extremely powerful, electrical fields that open permanent holes in the cell membranes of healthy and cancerous cells. These holes quickly lead to cell death (apoptosis). It has minimal, if any, effect on surrounding tissues such as the urethra, bladder, rectum, and the neurovascular bundle of the prostate (which is critical to maintaining healthy sexual function). | |

TOOLBOX

☐ HISTORY OR FAMILY HISTORY OF HEART DISEASE?

☐ DIABETES?

☐ HIGH BLOOD PRESSURE?

☐ HIGH CHOLESTEROL?

☐ CIGARETTE SMOKING?

**Answering YES to any one of these can affect which ADT you should be on. Talk to your doctor about these serious risk factors before starting therapy.**

# WHEN STARTING ADT,
## SOME THINGS ARE WORTH TALKING ABOUT

 Some commonly prescribed androgen deprivation therapies (ADTs) include a warning about an increased risk of heart attack, sudden cardiac death, and stroke (cardiovascular diseases), as well as diabetes.[1]

 Tell your doctor if you have a family history of heart disease, have had a previous heart attack or stroke, have diabetes, or have other cardiovascular risk factors, such as high blood pressure, high cholesterol, or cigarette smoking.

 If you have any concerns about which ADT you have been prescribed, please discuss your treatment options with your doctor.

 **TALK TO YOUR DOCTOR TODAY ABOUT YOUR RISK FACTORS AND WHICH ADT IS RIGHT FOR YOU. VISIT ADTCHOICES.COM TO LEARN MORE.**

Reference: 1. Food and Drug Administration. FDA drug safety communication: update to ongoing safety review of GnRH agonists and possible increased risk of diabetes and certain cardiovascular diseases. http://www.fda.gov/Drugs/DrugSafety/ucm229986.htm. Accessed November 16, 2016.

# chapter SEVEN
# Traditional Treatments

" When cure is possible, is it necessary?
When cure is necessary, is it possible?

*— Dr. Willet Whitmore (1917-1995)*
*"The Dean of Urologic Oncology"*

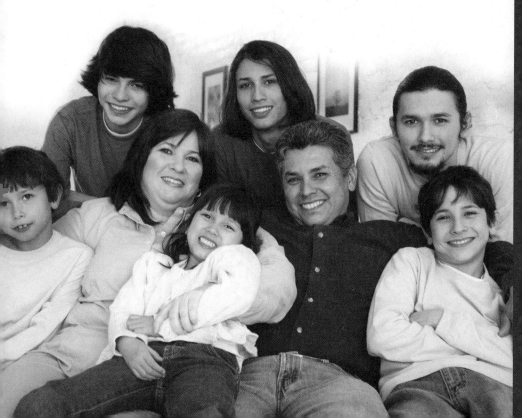

# Patient Story

## MIKE

*My first piece of advice to anyone dealing with prostate cancer is to educate yourself. A number of books exist on the subject, but one that I found most helpful in negotiating my way through treatment options is "Dr. Patrick Walsh's Guide to Surviving Prostate Cancer."*

*I would then recommend that you meet with several medical practitioners about treatment options. As the patient, you need to find a comfort zone for yourself and the option you determine will work best.*

*Depending on how advanced your cancer is, understand that not every treatment option is open to you. The major decision facing any prostate cancer patient is probably whether surgery is or is not desired. Your medical advisor(s) can tell you if the treatment you want to undergo is appropriate for your condition.*

*Also, know that some medical practitioners only advocate surgery, and that may NOT be your best option. Find a medical provider in whom you have confidence and who is in agreement with the treatment option you desire. Remember that this is a cancer that in the majority of cases can be overcome — or at least held in abeyance for years to give you more of the life and lifestyle you want to live.*

# chapter
## SEVEN
# summary

Chapter 7 introduces you to traditional prostate cancer treatments — from single treatments to combinations of single treatments plus hormone therapy.

By no means is this chapter the final word on traditional treatments. It is intended as a starting point for educated discussions with your doctors and loved ones.

To keep this chapter informative yet easy to follow, we will start with the simplest types of traditional treatment and progress to more complicated treatment combinations.

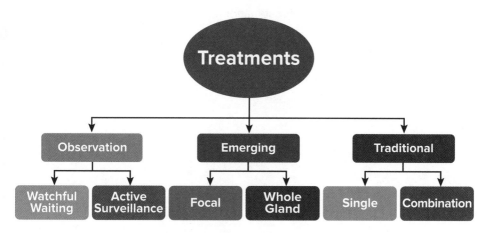

**Figure 7.0** gives you a simple overview of the types of prostate cancer treatment. **Chapter 7** focuses on traditional treatments — both single treatments and treatment combinations.

## VOCABULARY

See Glossary for Definitions

4Kscore Test

Active Surveillance

Alternative Treatment

Cryotherapy (Cryoablation)

CyberKnife (stereotactic radio-surgery)

Da Vinci (Robotic Surgery System)

Digital Rectal Exam (DRE)

Distant Metastatic Disease

Dual Therapy

External Beam Radiation Therapy (EBRT)

External Radiation Therapy (ERT)

Focal Treatment

High Dose Radiation

Image-Guided Radiation Therapy (IGRT)

Intensity-Modulated Radiation Therapy (IMRT)

Laparoscopic Prostatectomy

Local Metastatic Disease

Low Dose Radiation

Lymph Nodes

Metastatic Disease

Minimal Disease

Minimally Invasive Treatment

MRI

Mutation

NanoKnife

Non-Invasive Treatment

Organ-Confined Cancer

Perineal

Photodynamic Therapy

Photon

Prostate Biopsy

Proton

PSA

Radiation Therapy

Radical Prostatectomy

Rectal Fistula

Retropubic

Robotic-assisted Laparoscopic Radical Prostatectomy (RALRP)

Traditional Treatment

Urologist

Watchful Waiting

Whole Prostate Treatment

**DEBUNKING MYTHS**

# TESTOSTERONE AND PCA

*Despite what you may have heard or read, recent medical research reveals that the male hormone testosterone does NOT cause prostate cancer!*

*If it did, the following three conditions would occur:*

1. *"Twenty something" men, who have the highest testosterone levels, would also have the highest rates of prostate cancer — **but they have the lowest**.*

2. *Dozens of peer-reviewed medical studies would have found a strong connection between testosterone levels and prostate cancer — **but none have been found**.*

3. *The most aggressive forms of prostate cancer would occur in men with the highest testosterone levels— **but the opposite is true; the most aggressive forms of prostate cancer occur in men with the lowest levels of testosterone**.*

## What Does This Information Tell Us?

*That medical dogma from the last 60 years about high testosterone levels causing prostate cancer is incorrect.*

*Dr. Abraham Morgentaler and his colleagues at Harvard Medical School have demonstrated that when testosterone levels are low, both healthy and cancerous prostate cells absorb testosterone like a sponge. However, healthy and cancerous prostate cells reach a saturation point for testosterone at the low end of normal range for adult men. Once the prostate cells reach this saturation point, they quit absorbing testosterone.*

## Wait! What?

*If this information runs counter to everything you thought you knew about prostate cancer, we empathize with your confusion.*

*To make matters even more confusing, "Hormone Therapy" (which deprives prostate cancer patients of testosterone) is part of the preferred treatment for advanced prostate cancer — everything from moderate-risk, moderate-volume cancer to metastatic disease.*

*To learn more about how testosterone affects prostate cancer, see the **Chapter 7 Digging Deeper** section.*

## TRADITIONAL TREATMENTS/ LOCAL DISEASE

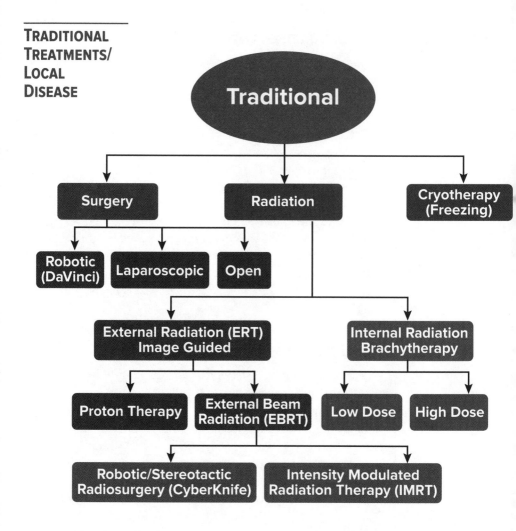

Figure 7.1 illustrates how traditional prostate cancer treatments are divided into three main categories: 1. Surgery (radical prostatectomy), 2. Radiation (internal and external), and 3. Cryotherapy (freezing). There are three types of surgery and eight different kinds of radiation therapy. Whole-gland cryotherapy freezes the entire prostate. This type of treatment is generally reserved for older men who are either impotent already or cannot undergo other types of treatment.

## WHEN TRADITIONAL TREATMENTS MAKE THE MOST SENSE

Single traditional treatments (also called "conventional," "curative," or "definitive," treatments) are used to either remove the prostate gland or destroy all the tissue inside of it. The goal of traditional treatments is to eliminate any "organ-confined" cancer (cancer that is still within the prostate). Obviously, if the cancer has spread outside the prostate, removing or destroying the gland will not prevent cancer from spreading to other parts of the body. That horse has already left the barn, so to speak.

Traditional treatments can be used for any kind of prostate cancer; however, emerging treatments (**Chapter 6**) are usually performed when patients have low-risk, low-volume cancer because the complication rates are much lower (**Chapter 8**).

As we mentioned in **Chapter 6**, prostate cancer treatment is moving in the same direction as breast cancer treatment — towards "minimally invasive" procedures.

That's not to say that you couldn't have a radical prostatectomy for low-risk, low-volume cancer — you could.

In fact, many men do because they want that diseased gland out of their body for good! (And who can blame them.) However, the lower rates of incontinence and impotence with emerging treatments make them a more attractive treatment option for many low-risk, low-volume patients.

Single traditional treatments are well suited for low-risk, moderate-to-high volume and moderate-risk patients. Combinations of traditional treatments are the best course of action for moderate-risk, moderate-to-high volume patients and high-risk patients, regardless of the cancer volume.

## RADICAL PROSTATECTOMY

Today, doctors and their prostate cancer patients are opting for minimally invasive procedures such as active surveillance and focal treatments. Even the open radical prostatectomy (ORP), once considered the gold standard of prostate cancer treatment, has given way to less-invasive prostatectomies such as laparoscopic radical prostatectomy (LRP) and robotic-assisted laparoscopic radical prostatectomy (RALRP). (See **Figure 7.2** for more information.)

## WHAT'S SO "RADICAL" ABOUT A RADICAL PROSTATECTOMY?

*In this context, the word "radical" means the complete removal of the prostate.*

*A "simple prostatectomy," on the other hand, is a procedure that helps men with an enlarged prostate (BPH) to urinate normally. This procedure removes the inside of the prostate, which allows for better flow of urine. A simple prostatectomy is NOT a treatment for prostate cancer.*

Both of these techniques offer doctors more precision, which decreases the risk of unwanted complications like incontinence and impotence and provides patients with a faster recovery and shorter hospital stay.

Both LRP and RALRP are technically demanding surgeries that require a significant learning curve for the surgeon, so the transition to these less-invasive surgeries takes longer for doctors who treat fewer patients.

For example, studies have shown that surgeons who are new to LRP may require 80 to 100 cases in order to attain proficiency of this technique (let alone mastery). For urologists who do NOT have a high volume of laparoscopic patients, it may take a decade to complete this learning curve — which is bad news for their first 80-100 patients!

Looking ahead, it may take a generation (or two) of technically trained urologists coming into the field to shift the balance away from open radical prostatectomies (which is still considered the gold standard of prostate cancer care at many non-academic hospitals) to laparoscopic and robotic surgical treatment.

Also, open perineal prostatectomies are performed less frequently (5 percent) than open retropubic prostatectomies (95 percent) because impotence and incontinence are more common complications of perineal surgeries, and it is difficult to remove the nearby lymph nodes (should that be necessary). However, a perineal prostatectomy is a shorter surgery and an option for men who are unable to get or maintain an erection or have been told not to have abdominal surgery by their doctor. (See **Figure 7.3** on **Page 170**.)

# Pros & Cons of 3 Types of Prostatectomies

| RRP | Advantages | Disadvantages |
|---|---|---|
| **Open (ORP)** | • In experienced hands, open radical prostatectomy (ORP) remains the gold standard | • 71% remain potent (age dependent)<br>• 94% maintain continence (defined as 1 pad/per day or less)<br>• Longer recovery time<br>• Longer hospitalization<br>• More pain medication |
| **Laparoscopic (LRP)** | • Improved ability to see small structures<br>• Decreased blood loss<br>• Minimally invasive incisions<br>• Less post-operative pain<br>• Less pain medication required | • Potency 76% (age dependent)<br>• Continence 69% (defined as 1 pad/per day or less)<br>• 2-8% end up as an open prostatectomy (ORP)<br>• Longer operative times: 4-5 hours<br>• Technically difficult<br>• Average blood loss 400 cc<br>• Not a good fit for patients with:<br>  – Previous pelvic surgery<br>  – Previous TURP (BPH surgery)<br>  – Large prostate glands<br>  – Metastatic disease |
| **Robotic (RALRP)** | In hands of experienced robotic urologists:<br>• 2-3 hour surgery<br>• Relatively small amount of blood loss (100 cc)<br>• Short hospital stay (24 hour)<br>• 0-1% end up as an open prostatectomy (ORP)<br>• 60% of all radical prostatectomies performed in the United States in 2007 were done using robotic assistance. This number is growing every year. | • Potency 76.5% (age dependent)<br>• Continence 97% (defined as 1 pad/per day or less)<br>• Not a good fit for patients with:<br>  – Previous pelvic surgery<br>  – Previous TURP (BPH surgery)<br>  – Large prostate glands<br>  – Metastatic disease |

**Figure 7.2** displays the data about the pros and cons of the three most common types of radical prostatectomy. This data comes from the world's best surgical centers. So it may **NOT** accurately reflect the outcomes of the doctors and hospitals in your area. If you are considering having a radical prostatectomy, we encourage you to talk with your doctor(s) about their success and complications rates. Also, ask them to tell you how many laparoscopic and robotic prostatectomies they have performed. This information is vital to your final treatment decision. In addition, we recommend you write down any questions about radical prostatectomies in the Notes section at the end of this chapter, so you won't forget to ask them during your next appointment.

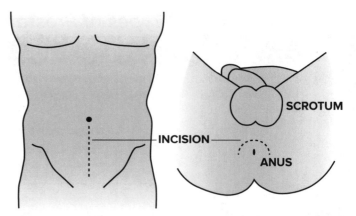

**Figure 7.3** displays the two ways to do an open radical prostatectomy: retropubic on the left (95% of all open radical prostatectomies) and perineal on the right (5% of all open radical prostatectomies). The outcomes of these two types of prostatectomies are similar; however, perineal prostatectomies have a higher incidence of erectile dysfunction.

## IT'S ALL ABOUT THE SURGEON

The truth is that when studies compare the long-term success and complication rates of open radical prostatectomies with laproscopic radical prostatectomies or robot-assisted laparoscopic radical prostatectomies, it's all about the surgeon.

In the hands of an experienced open radical prostatectomy surgeon, the long-term outcomes are equivalent with laproscopic and robotic surgeries.

Regardless of which type of prostate cancer treatment you choose, always pick the best/most experienced doctor possible. This recommendation is especially true for radical prostatectomy.

If you decide to have a radical prostatectomy, we strongly suggest you select the best/most-experienced surgeon (urologist) in your area. And don't allow yourself to be swayed by new technology — unless, of course, it

---

### NERVE-SPARING PROSTATECTOMIES

*The vast majority of radical prostatectomies performed today are the nerve-sparing variety, which preserves the nerves responsible for normal sexual function. The standard of practice in all urological training institutions in the United States is to teach nerve-sparing prostatectomies. If you decide to have a radical prostatectomy, please make sure it is a nerve-sparing one.*

is being used by the best/most experienced surgeon in your area. And even then, be sure to ask for this doctor's personal success and complication rates — NOT the results for an entire hospital or medical center.

## INTERNAL RADIATION (BRACHY-THERAPY)

Brachytherapy has evolved from an alternative treatment that raised lots of eyebrows to one of the premier prostate cancer treatments.

**THERE ARE TWO FORMS OF INTERNAL RADIATION THERAPY (BRACHYTHERAPY):**
1. **Permanent Low Dose Radiation (LDR, seed implants)**
2. **Temporary High Dose Radiation (HDR)**

**Permanent Low Dose Radiation (LDR)** or "seed implantation" places 80 to 120 very small radioactive seeds inside your prostate gland — the number of seeds depends on the size of the prostate. A computer program guides the needles that contain the radioactive seeds, so each seed is deposited in precisely the right spot. The seeds remain behind when the needle is removed.

The accuracy of seed implantation has been improved significantly in the last decade with real-time implants and computer-imaging programs. These innovations have improved outcomes and reduced complication rates. (See **Chapter 8** for more information about success and complication rates.)

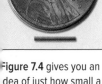

Figure 7.4 gives you an idea of just how small a brachytherapy seed is.

Permanent seed implantation is used as a single prostate cancer treatment for patients with low-risk cancer and in combination with either hormone therapy or external beam radiation for moderate-to-high-risk patients who have cancer that is confined to their prostate.

The survival rate for permanent seed implantation brachytherapy is similar to those for External Beam Radiation Therapy (EBRT) or surgery (radical prostatectomy). Permanent seed implantation is a less invasive treatment option than radical prostatectomy — with fewer complications. The treatment is usually done as an outpatient procedure with patients returning to their normal routines in a couple of days.

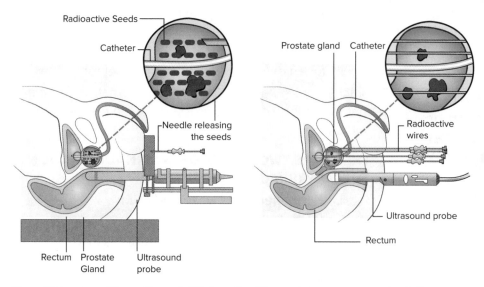

**Figure 7.5** (courtesy of Cancer Research UK) shows the difference between permanent brachytherapy (seed implantation, on the left) and temporary brachytherapy (on the right).

**Temporary High Dose Radiation (HDR)** therapy involves inserting thin tubes directly into the prostate. These tubes contain a radioactive material that delivers a short blast of high-dose radiation to the prostate gland.

When the prostate receives the right therapeutic dose of radiation, the tubes are removed. Unlike seed implantation, this type of brachytherapy does NOT leave any radioactive seeds inside your body. Different protocols use different exposure times and number of treatments. The exposure times can vary between 15 and 30 minutes and the number of treatments between 2 and 6, depending on the patient, the doctor, and the institution.

For patients with low-risk, low-volume prostate cancer, the outcomes for Temporary High Dose Radiation (HDR) brachytherapy are similar to the outcomes for seed implantation (LDR); however, for reasons that are not entirely clear, it is used less often than permanent seed implantation. As with low-dose seed implantation, high-dose radiation is also used to "boost" other single therapies: For example, to shorten a course of External Radiation Therapy (ERT).

For brachytherapy success, survival, and complication rates, turn to **Chapter 8.**

# Permanent versus Temporary Brachytherapy

| BRACHYTHERAPY | Advantages | Disadvantages |
|---|---|---|
| Permanent Low Dose (LDR) | • One-time outpatient procedure<br>• Minimal seed migration with the strands of seeds used today. | • Radiation protection precautions<br>• Seed migration with loose seeds (seldom used today) |
| Temporary High Dose (HDR) | • No hardware left in the body<br>• No seed migration | • Possible overnight hospitalization<br>• Usually 2-4 treatment of 15 minutes each. Total time for each treatment: 4-5 hours. |

**Figure 7.6** compares and contrasts the advantages and disadvantages of permanent (LDR) versus temporary (HDR) brachytherapy.

## THE CLOUD EFFECT

*An interesting benefit of permanent low-dose brachytherapy (seed implantation) is what doctors call "the Cloud Effect." The Cloud Effect refers to the ability of seed implantation to have a therapeutic benefit in patients whose cancers have probably spread outside the prostate — without damaging the surrounding tissue, particularly the rectum.*

*Unfortunately, the Cloud Effect does not occur after surgical procedures like a radical prostatectomy (open, laparoscopic, or robotic). That's why some patients may require some form of external beam radiation therapy (EBRT) after surgery to treat "positive margins" (when there isn't a big enough cushion of healthy tissue between the tumor and the edge of prostate).*

## EXTERNAL RADIATION THERAPY (ERT)

Unlike brachytherapy, where the source of radiation is implanted inside your body, the radiation in External Radiation Therapy (ERT) comes from a source outside your body.

Like brachytherapy, technological advancements are moving this field of radiation therapy rapidly towards smaller, more precise, imaging-guided, and robot-assisted treatments. The goal of these innovations is to increase the radiation delivered to areas where it is desired (cancer tumors) and reduce the radiation exposure everywhere else (the healthy tissue surrounding your prostate).

**There are two types of External Radiation Therapy:**
- Photon (x-rays, also called External Beam Radiation Therapy or EBRT)
- Protons (charged particles)

**Photon Therapy (EBRT) can be further divided into:**
- Intensity-Modulated Radiation Therapy (IMRT)
- Stereotactic Radiosurgery (CyberKnife)

Please see **Figures 7.1 & 7.7** for more information about the differences between these types of radiation therapy.

Most forms of ERT use photon beam radiation, including IMRT and CyberKnife. You can think of this kind of radiation like X-rays that travel in waves (called photons). The principal difference between these two types of EMRT is the number and intensity of treatments.

**Intensity Modulated Radiation Therapy (IMRT)** uses lower doses, but requires more treatments to eradicate the cancer — approximately 40-44 treatments.

**CyberKnife (Stereotactic Radiosurgery)** delivers higher doses of radiation, but requires fewer treatments — approximately 4-5 treatments.

**PHOTON VS. PROTON THERAPY**

Unlike photon therapy, proton therapy uses microscopic charged particles (called protons) that deliver microscopic packets of energy (radiation) at the end of their 3-D pathway, instead of all along their path (as with EBRT).

This delivery of radiation "all along the path" is the major disadvantage of EBRT, as the photons have to pass through the healthy tissue surrounding your prostate cancer (skin, bladder, rectum, urethra, the nerves that control erections, and healthy prostate tissue) before it reaches the cancer. For this reason, modern EBRT treatments use multiple beams of relatively low dose radiation that intersect at exactly the same spot to deliver a highly effective dose of radiation with minimal damage to the surrounding tissues.

Theoretically, proton therapy reduces the radiation exposure to healthy tissue, while allowing higher doses of radiation to reach the intended target. This idea is somewhat controversial, and results suggest that both particle (proton) and beam (photon) radiation treatments have very similar long-term success and complication rates.

## IMAGE-GUIDED RADIATION THERAPY

Unless you live in Timbuktu, most forms of external radiation therapy are guided by images of your prostate such as an MRI, CT, or PET scan, hence the name, Image-guided radiation therapy (IGRT). Multiple scans are repeated many times during each treatment. These images are processed by computers every few seconds to identify the precise location of the prostate and the tumor(s). These calculations allow for adjustments in the patient's position or the amount of radiation being delivered. Still, "motion management" issues remain a challenge.

**NOTE of CAUTION**

*It is rare these days to find a healthcare institution that does NOT use imagery to guide their external radiation treatments. If you are a patient of a doctor who does external radiation therapy WITHOUT guided imagery, we recommend you have a conversation with your doctor and find out why.*

# 3 TYPES OF EXTERNAL BEAM RADIATION (ERT)

| ERT | ADVANTAGES | DISADVANTAGES |
|---|---|---|
| Proton | • Very precise<br>• Proton technology (theoretically fewer complications)<br>• Higher radiation doses | • Expensive technology<br>• Few centers in the United States<br>• 5 days per week for 7 weeks<br>• Placement of fiducial markers |
| Intensity Modulated Radiation Therapy (IMRT) | • Very precise<br>• Beam technology | • 40-44 treatments<br>• Lower doses per treatment |
| Stereotactic Radiosurgery (CyberKnife) | • Very precise<br>• Beam technology<br>• 4-5 treatments | • Placement of fiducial markers<br>• Higher doses per treatment |

**Figure 7.7** contrasts the major differences between the three most common types of external beam radiation (ERT): Proton, IMRT (photon), and CyberKnife (photon). All three types of external beam radiation use some form of imagery to guide the radiation. So all three are considered Imagery-guided radiation therapy (IGRT).

# OVERVIEW OF 4 TYPES OF TREATMENTS

| | ADVANTAGES | DISADVANTAGES |
|---|---|---|
| **External Beam Radiation** | • Outpatient procedure<br>• No interruption of work/employment during treatment<br>• Very low risk of significant bleeding<br>• No anesthesia required<br>• No pain medication required<br>• No urinary catheter needed<br>• Can be used in patients who are taking blood thinners.<br>• Acceptable for religious practices that do not allow blood transfusions | • 40-44 treatments for IMRT, 35 treatments from proton therapy, and 5 treatments for CyberKnife<br>• Incomplete pathologic staging<br>• PSA follow up more difficult to interpret<br>• Temporary rectal irritation |
| **Brachytherapy** | • Outpatient procedure<br>• No need for extended use of urinary catheters<br>• Minimal post-operative pain (over-the-counter pain relievers)<br>• Can return to work after 2-3 days | • Patients who have an IPSS of less than 10 or are on hormone therapy have a slight chance (2%) of urinary retention. (See **Chapter 8 Toolbox.**)<br>• Patients who have an IPSS of greater than 20 should NOT consider brachytherapy due to a 20% increased risk of urinary retention.<br>• Prostates larger than 60 cc are too big for seed implantation.<br>• Minimal incontinence, impotence, and rectal injuries when done by experienced doctors.<br>• Incontinence is rare; however, it may occur in patients who have had a TURP. |
| **Cryotherapy** | • Outpatient procedure<br>• No risk of significant bleeding<br>• Can be used in patients who are taking blood thinners.<br>• Acceptable for religious practices that do not allow blood transfusions | • Catheter required<br>• High (75-95%) impotence rate with whole-gland treatments<br>• Prostates larger than 40 cc are too big for cryotherapy.<br>• Avoid patients with prior TURP<br>• Incontinence rate is approximately 5%. |
| **Radical Prostatectomy** | • Allows for post-operative staging<br>• PSA is a better predictor of recurrence<br>• Quicker recovery with laparoscopic and robotic procedures | • Hospitalization required<br>• Catheter required<br>• Blood transfusion may be required<br>• Rare complications such as blood clots in the legs and lymph pooling may occur. |

**Figure 7.8** displays a brief overview of the advantages and disadvantages of the four most common types of traditional prostate cancer treatment.

**CRYOTHERAPY**

Cryotherapy or "cryoablation" for prostate cancer is the controlled freezing of the prostate gland. The freezing destroys cancer cells but is not cancer specific, that is; it kills all cells and tissues it comes in contact with — not just cancer.

Cryotherapy is flexible and can be used in three ways:

1. Focal treatment (for low-risk, low-volume cancer)
2. Single therapy for localized prostate cancer
3. Salvage procedures for patients who have failed other types of treatment

In the past, cryotherapy was used primarily as a single treatment for the entire prostate; however, the incidence of impotence was so high that it was reserved for elderly patients or men who had lost their sexual function.

Today, cryotherapy is used as a focal treatment with minimal complications and is rarely associated with impotence. In fact, some patients report better sexual function after focal cryotherapy.

The freezing is done with the help of special needles called "cryoprobes" that are placed inside the prostate through the perineal area (See **Figure 7.9**). This procedure is done either under spinal or general anesthesia.

Argon gas inside the cryoprobes creates an "ice ball" that kills all the cells in the area. These ice balls vary in size depending on the size and shape of the tumor(s), as well as the anatomy of the prostate.

Constant monitoring via minute temperature probes inserted in and around the prostate ensure that the rectal wall, the nerve bundle that controls erections, and the urinary sphincter are unaffected. This monitoring helps prevent incontinence and the formation of a rectal fistula (a hole between the rectum and prostate). A urethral warming catheter also prevents the urethra from freezing, thus minimizing damage to normal tissues.

There are usually two freezing cycles. Between them, the prostate is allowed to thaw passively or actively, using helium or argon gas.

Freezing starts at the front of the prostate, then the middle, and finally the back. Constant monitoring by

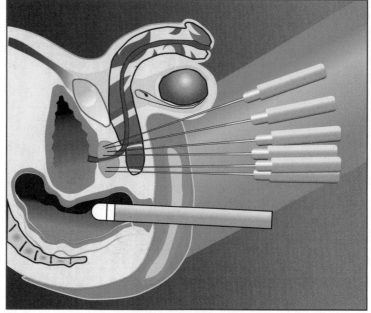

**Figure 7.9** displays a cutaway view of a cryotherapy procedure, including an ultrasound probe inside the rectum and the needles used to freeze a portion or the entire prostate, depending upon the risk level and volume of the cancer.

ultrasound allows doctors to sculpt the ice balls into the desired shape and size.

A suprapubic catheter (a drainage tube that runs from the bladder and out the lower belly) is inserted at the end of the procedure. This allows draining of the bladder until the patient can urinate normally (1-2 weeks). Once that happens, the catheter is removed.

With today's high-tech imaging technology, intra-operative computer programs, temperature probes, and urethral warming catheters, the freezing is well controlled and excellent results are obtained with minimal complications (if any).

The entire procedure usually takes less than two hours.

## HORMONE THERAPY & METASTATIC DISEASE

### SYSTEMIC CONTROL

Except for a brief mention of hormone therapy at the end of **Chapter 5**, this book has focused on the diagnosis and treatment of local prostate cancer (cancer that is still inside the prostate). This section, however, is a brief discussion of hormone therapy and metastatic disease.

## WHAT IS HORMONE THERAPY?

When most people hear the words, "hormone therapy," they think of athletes doping or guys taking hormones like testosterone to improve their sex lives. With prostate cancer, it's just the opposite.

Another name for the type of hormone therapy that prostate cancer patients undergo is "Androgen Deprivation Therapy." "Androgens" is the medical term for male sex hormones — testosterone, DHT (dihydrotestosterone), DHEA, and others. "Deprivation" is to deprive someone of something. So androgen deprivation therapy either stops the production of testosterone and other male hormones or blocks the body's ability to use androgens.

Thankfully, "local" prostate cancer (also called "organ-confined disease") accounts for 90 percent of all prostate cancer cases diagnosed in the United States today. That

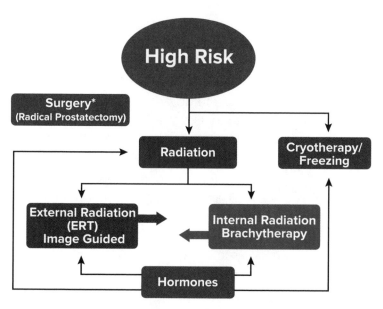

**Figure 7.10** (a repeat of **Figure 5.11**) provides a visual representation of how traditional treatments can be combined to treat moderate-to-high volume "local" prostate cancer. It's also important to notice that hormone therapy can be used in conjunction with other treatments to create a "local + systemic" approach to eliminating the cancer. *Please note that "Surgery" (radical prostatectomy) is not a preferred treatment type for high-risk prostate cancer, even by the world's most renowned prostate cancer surgeons at Johns Hopkins Hospital.

day. That number (90%) is a true blessing because local prostate cancer is much easier to treat successfully. (See "Success Rates" in **Chapter 8**.) Once cancer spreads outside the prostate, it is harder to eliminate and difficult to control.

"Local control" (what we have been discussing through-out this book) is ideal for low-to-moderate risk patients.

Once cancer crosses over an invisible threshold and becomes moderate-risk, moderate-to-high volume disease, doctors begin to combine traditional treatments (local controls) with hormone therapy (systemic control) to make sure they destroy all of the cancer.

As **Figure 7.10** illustrates, there are several ways to combine local and systemic controls. The final decision depends upon the patient, the kind of cancer he has, and the type of medicine that the lead doctor practices.

## HOW DOES HORMONE THERAPY WORK?

Male hormones contribute to the initiation, promotion, and progression of prostate cancer. Without testosterone and other male hormones, metastatic prostate cancer goes into remission, often for several years.

Hormone therapy is virtually a requirement when treating high-risk local disease. It is also the first line of defense for metastatic disease (cancer that has spread outside the prostate).

Unfortunately, hormone therapy is not a silver bullet. It is NOT a stand-alone treatment for prostate cancer, because some kinds of prostate cancer are resistant to hormone therapy. These types of cancer do not require male hormones to grow and thrive.

Also, starving a male body of male hormones can cause some kinds of prostate cancer to adapt to an "andro-gen-free" environment. Doctors call this kind of cancer, "Androgen Independent Cancer."

However, hormone therapy is the treatment of choice when it comes to killing nomadic "micro-metastatic" cancer cells (called "floaters") that have escaped the prostate.

Hormone therapy can be combined with all types of tradi-tional treatments to give men with advanced local prostate cancer the best shot at eliminating all of the disease.

The advantage of combining hormone therapy with traditional treatments (See **Figure 7.10)** is that traditional treatments go after the cancer inside the prostate, and hormone therapy creates a toxic environment for "floaters" outside the prostate.

Given enough time, these floaters will establish new cancer tumors (lesions) elsewhere in the body: lymph nodes, seminal vesicles, bones, organs, and eventually the entire body.

**Local Control**   +   **Hormone Therapy**   =   **Combination Therapy**

*Traditional Treatments*   +   *Systemic Control*   =   *Combined Treatments*

## LOCAL VS. DISTANT METASTATIC DISEASE

|  | Definition | Treatment |
|---|---|---|
| Local | • Early extension into the surrounding tissues such as prostate capsule, seminal vesicles<br>• Later into bladder wall and rectum | • Radiation and cloud effects are either primary or additional treatment<br>• Additional hormone therapy |
| Distant | • Early extension into the lymph nodes and bones (spine, pelvis and ribs)<br>• Later into liver and lungs | • Watchful waiting<br>• Constant hormone therapy<br>• Sequential hormone therapy<br>• Intermittent hormone therapy<br>• Second-line hormone therapy<br>• Radiation/quality-of-life care<br>• Chemotherapy<br>• Clinical trails |

**Figure 7.11** gives a basic overview of the differences between how doctors treat local and distant metastatic disease. What's important to understand is that local metastatic disease (also called "invasive cancer") and distant metastatic disease are different diseases with different treatments and objectives. Local metastatic disease is a treatable condition. Treatment for distant metastatic disease is designed to extend the patient's life and make him as comfortable as possible.

You can think of these nomadic cells circulating in the blood stream like termites. A colony of termites buzzing around the outside of your house is a clear threat to your home. However, once those termites burrow into the structure of your home, your condition goes from a "threat" to a complex and difficult problem to solve.

As with termites, floaters are a lot easier to exterminate before they start setting up colonies (tumors) inside your house. Hormone therapy is less effective over time, so if you have high-risk local prostate cancer, it is important to begin hormone therapy as soon as you can.

## CONTINUOUS HORMONE THERAPY VERSUS INTERMITTENT HORMONE THERAPY

The goal of continuous hormone therapy varies depending upon the kind of cancer and the type of treatment.

For example, men with moderate-risk, moderate-to-high volume prostate cancer may receive continuous hormone therapy for six months to one year as part of "dual therapy" approach to curing their cancer. (Dual therapy means that the hormone therapy is used in conjunction with some other form of treatment — usually a type of surgery or radiation.)

Men with metastatic disease are often given continuous hormone therapy to keep their cancer in check (as much as possible) and provide them with the best possible quality of life. Quality of life, however, is a big issue for most men on continuous hormone therapy because this type of therapy causes a kind of erectile dysfunction that includes a loss of libido, which drugs like Viagra cannot correct.

Recent studies indicate that intermittent hormone therapy (a type of hormone therapy that allows men to go off the therapy for periods of time), is equally effective as continuous hormone therapy — and allows men to periodically regain their normal sexual function.

For more information about intermittent hormone therapy, see **the Chapter 7 Digging Deeper** section on **Page 350**.

# Doctor Story

## DR. DAVID CRAWFORD, MD

Urology, Urologic Oncology
University of Colorado Hospital
Aurora, Colorado

*For almost 20 years, my team and I took care of a patient with castrate resistant prostate cancer. Our patient's longevity with this kind of cancer speaks volumes about our ability to understand and treat this disease.*

*He was first diagnosed in 1996 with Gleason 7 prostate cancer. He had surgery to remove his prostate (radical prostatectomy); after treatment, his cancer was upgraded to Gleason 9. Unfortunately, the cancer returned, and he had a surgical castration along with chemotherapy and radiation.*

*We were able to keep his metastatic cancer (cancer that has spread outside the prostate — which, in his case, he no longer had) under control until 2009. At that time, he started showing signs that the cancer was actively growing in his body.*

*He had received a variety of innovative treatments and therapies that produced brief periods of remission, but the cancer always came back. Nevertheless, these therapies allowed us to prolong his life 19 years after his initial diagnosis of Gleason 9 prostate cancer! He eventually passed away from pneumonia at the age of 94 — not prostate cancer.*

*Thanks to the autopsy that this patient's family requested, we were able to learn that he was harboring an area of Gleason 10 prostate cancer in the lymph nodes in his pelvis. We also gained a clearer understanding about the connection between the lab tests we utilized and this patient's particular cancer burden. It was a little like cracking part of an elaborate code between the disease and our ability to detect certain aspects of it.*

*Most importantly, despite this aggressive form of prostate cancer, our patient was able to live a long and happy life — which goes to show that even with one of the most aggressive forms of this disease, doctors are able to provide care that extends both the years of a man's life and the life within those years.*

## LOOKING AHEAD

**CHAPTER 1:** You or your doctor is concerned about your prostate — We provide you with **Prostate 101**: where it lives, what it does, plus relevant statistics.

**CHAPTER 2:** Your doctor told you to **schedule a prostate biopsy** — We give you a **Prostate Biopsy Assessment Tool** to see if you actually need one, and what to expect if you do.

**CHAPTER 3:** You have a prostate biopsy — We explain the steps you need to take, whether you have a **negative biopsy or a positive biopsy**.

**CHAPTER 4:** You have a **positive prostate biopsy** — We provide you with a **Prostate Cancer Assessment Tool** to help you understand which kind of cancer you have.

**CHAPTER 5:** You need to select a prostate cancer treatment — We provide you with a summary of the most common types of treatment based on your **cancer risk type** (low-risk, moderate-risk, and high-risk).

**CHAPTER 6:** You have **low-risk, low-volume prostate cancer** and need to learn more about emerging treatments — We provide you with a summary of these treatments to help you understand the differences between focal, minimally invasive, alternative, whole gland, and traditional treatments.

**CHAPTER 7:** You have prostate cancer that is more advanced than low-risk, low-volume and need to know more about **whole-gland treatments** (both stand-alone traditional and combination treatments) — We provide you with a summary of these treatments.

**CHAPTER 8:** You want to know the **success and complication rates** for each type of treatment and for each cancer risk type (low-risk, moderate-risk, and high-risk) — We provide you with unbiased information to support your decision-making process.

**CHAPTER 9:** You feel **overwhelmed** by the news of a positive prostate biopsy — We give you the tools to surf this tidal wave of emotion and overcome the feeling of panic that almost always accompanies a positive biopsy report.

**CHAPTER 10:** You want to **use your cancer diagnosis as a springboard to better health** — We help you address your wellness goals with a proven plan that covers inflammation, diet, inactivity, stress, immune system, hormone optimization, structure, and removing toxic substances.

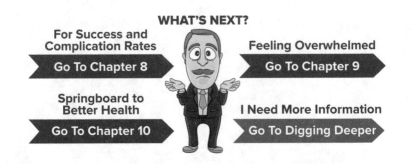

**WHAT'S NEXT?**

For Success and Complication Rates
Go To Chapter 8

Feeling Overwhelmed
Go To Chapter 9

Springboard to Better Health
Go To Chapter 10

I Need More Information
Go To Digging Deeper

# WELCOME TO THE TOOLBOX
# CHAPTER 7 **TOOLBOX**

**THIS TOOLBOX SECTION INCLUDES THE FOLLOWING TOOLS AND RESOURCES TO HELP YOU UNDERSTAND WHAT "TRADITIONAL TREATMENTS" ARE AND IF YOU WOULD BE A GOOD CANDIDATE (WHAT WORKS FOR YOU?):**

- Side-by-Side Analysis of Traditional Treatments

## *Analysis of Traditional Treatments*

| | DESCRIPTION | WHAT WORKS FOR YOU? |
|---|---|---|
| **Open Radical Prostatectomy** | • Potency 71% (age dependent)<br>• Continence 94% (defined as 1 pad per day or less)<br>• Longer recovery time<br>• Longer hospitalization<br>• More pain medication | |
| **Laparoscopic Radical Prostatectomy** | • Improved vision of minute details<br>• Decreased blood loss<br>• Minimally invasive incisions<br>• Less postoperative pain<br>• Less pain medication required<br>• Continence 69% (defined as 1 pad per day or less)<br>• Potency 76% (age dependent)<br>• 2-8% end up as an open prostatectomy (ORP)<br>• Longer operative times: 4-5 hours<br>• Technically difficult<br>• Average blood loss 400 cc<br>• Not a good fit for patients with:<br>  – Previous pelvic surgery<br>  – Previous TURP (BPH surgery)<br>  – A large prostate gland<br>  – Metastatic disease | |

TOOLBOX

## Analysis of Traditional Treatments – Continued

| | DESCRIPTION | WHAT WORKS FOR YOU? |
|---|---|---|
| Robotic Assisted Laparoscopic Radical Prostatectomy | • 2-3 hour surgery<br>• Relatively small amount of blood loss (100 cc)<br>• Short hospital stay (24 hours)<br>• 0-1% end up as an open prostatectomy (ORP)<br>• Potency 76.5% (age dependent)<br>• Continence 97% (defined as 1 pad per day or less)<br>• Not a good fit for patients with:<br>  – Previous pelvic surgery<br>  – Previous TURP<br>  – Large prostate glands<br>  – Metastatic disease | |
| Brachytherapy (Permanent) | • One-time outpatient procedure<br>• Minimal seed migration with strands<br>• Seed migration possible with loose seeds<br>• Radiation protection precautions needed for the first few weeks | |
| Brachytherapy (Temporary) | • No hardware left in the body<br>• No seed migration<br>• No radiation exposure to others<br>• Possible overnight hospitalization<br>• Usually 2-4 treatments (15 min each)<br>• Total time for each treatment: 4 -5 hours. | |
| External Beam Radiation | • Outpatient procedure<br>• No interruption of work/employment during treatment<br>• Very low risk of significant bleeding<br>• No anesthesia required<br>• No pain medication required<br>• No urinary catheter needed<br>• Can be used in patients who are taking blood thinners.<br>• Acceptable for religious practices that do not allow blood transfusions | |

TOOLBOX

## *Analysis of Traditional Treatments – Continued*

| | DESCRIPTION | WHAT WORKS FOR YOU? |
|---|---|---|
| Proton Radiation | • Very precise<br>• Theoretically fewer complications<br>• High radiation doses<br>• Expensive technology<br>• Few centers in the United States<br>• 5 days per week for 7-9 weeks<br>• Requires fiducial markers | |
| Intensity-Modulated Radiation Therapy (IMRT) | • Beam technology (photon)<br>• Very precise<br>• Requires fiducial markers<br>• Lower doses per treatment<br>• 40-44 treatments | |
| Stereotactic Radiosurgery (CyberKnife) | • Beam technology (photon)<br>• Very precise<br>• Requires fiducial markers<br>• Higher doses per treatment<br>• Only 4-5 treatments | |
| Cryotherapy | • Freezes prostate tissue, causing cancer cells (and healthy cells) to die.<br>• It can be used in three ways:<br>  1. Focal treatment<br>  2. Single therapy for localized prostate cancer<br>  3. Salvage procedure for patients who have failed other types of treatment<br>• As a whole-prostate treatment, it has a high incidence of impotence, so it is mostly used with elderly patients or men who have very low sexual function.<br>• As a focal treatment, it has minimal complications and is rarely associated with impotence. | |

TOOLBOX

**NOTES:**

TOOLBOX

chapter EIGHT

# Success Rates and Side Effect/ Complication Rates

> It ain't what you don't know
> that gets you in trouble,
> it's what you know that
> just ain't so.
>
> — *Mark Twain*

# Patient Story

## WILLIAM

*What I learned from this whole ordeal is that you have to be proactive. In the age of the Internet, you really have no excuse.*

*The thing that really bugs me about my prostate cancer experience is that once I decided on a treatment path, the cancer center that I went to originally kept sending me threatening letters saying, if I didn't come down there and get treated by them, then I was going to die. It was pretty crazy. Each letter became more insistent. It was beyond a high-pressure sales pitch.*

*What's even crazier, once I decided to have HIFU treatment, my personal physician refused to do my pre-op physical, because I wasn't being treated at the prostate cancer center that she sent me to. She told me to go back and see them because they were nice guys. Can you believe that?*

*My PSA was as high as 4.7, and three other tests (PSA free, MRI, and PCA3) indicated that I needed treatment.*

*I had the HIFU procedure in Cancun, Mexico where it was performed by North American doctors. The procedure went very well. My wife and I joke that our 20-minute walk on the beach cost $30,000 — because my insurance wouldn't cover anything.*

*About 30 days after the HIFU, my urethra tissue clogged up and sealed shut. So I had a catheter for a couple of weeks, then I had a TURP, which opened everything up.*

*From that point on (4 years ago as of this writing), my PSA has been undetectable, and I am fully functional with no incontinence.*

# chapter
## EIGHT
# summary

**Chapter 8** is about including success rates and complication rates into your treatment decision.

All treatments, hospitals/medical centers, and doctors have success and complication rates. You should know what these numbers are before you make your final decision.

The goal of **Chapter 8** is to help you know which questions to ask so you can make accurate side-by-side comparisons of treatments, treatment facilities, and doctors (See the **Chapter 8 Toolbox**).

For example, if you think you'd never sleep knowing there is some kind cancer in your prostate, then surgery may be a good treatment option for you. On the other hand, if the thought of wearing diaper pads every day for the rest of your life sounds unbearable, then some form of radiation therapy would be a better match.

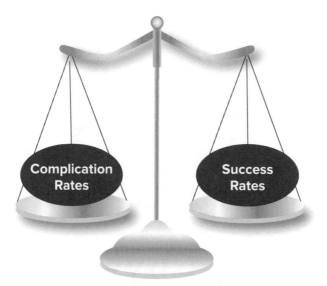

**Figure 8.0** illustrates the balancing act between treatment success and treatment complication rates. In general, the more invasive the treatment, the more complications it creates. If you know what kind of cancer you have (**Chapter 4**) and the types of treatment that are best suited for this kind of cancer (**Chapters 5, 6, & 7**), then evaluating success and complication rates is the next step in your treatment decision process.

**DEBUNKING MYTHS**

# PICKING THE RIGHT DOCTOR

*All doctors are NOT created equal. Picking the right doctor is the most important decision you will make in this healing journey from a prostate cancer diagnosis to living a long and healthy life.*

*From architects to attorneys, electricians to educators — some people are just better at what they do than others.*

*It should come as NO surprise that the same is true of doctors. However, there is something about healing the sick and saving lives that protects doctors from the same level of public scrutiny that other professions receive.*

*After interviewing several doctors and recording their treatment recommendations, your challenge now becomes one of sorting through these potential health partners and selecting the one who is right for you. This is NO small task. Finding the right mix of skill, knowledge, experience, personality, and bedside manner can be tricky business.*

*Unfortunately, www.doctormatch.com has yet to be invented. Despite all the consumer review websites available online, the Internet is little help when selecting a doctor. The problem with online doctor reviews is that they tend to fall into two camps:*

*1. I love my doctor*
*2. I'll never go back there again*

*People who feel satisfied with their medical care but not "over the moon" usually don't bother writing online medical reviews.*

*So how do you pick the right doctor?*

*We suggest you go to the **Doctor Selector Questionnaire** in the **Chapter 8 Toolbox.** This worksheet guides you through the process of finding the doctor who is right for you. We also suggest the **Doctor Selection Tips** in the **Chapter 5 Digging Deeper** section.*

**NOTE**

*One of the challenges with the type of information presented in Figures 8.1-8.4 is how wide the ranges are. For example, in Figure 8.1, there is a 32 percent difference in the success rate of cryotherapy with low-risk prostate cancer patients — that's crazy! There is an ocean of difference between a 60 percent success rate and a 92 percent one.*

*This difference is due to data coming from multiple doctors working at different hospitals and medical centers. In addition to some doctors being more proficient than others, as the Debunking Myth on the opposite page suggests, some treatment facilities produce better results than others. Exploring these differences is what this chapter is all about.*

**WHAT CAN TREATMENT SUCCESS AND COMPLICATION RATES TELL YOU?**

A lot!

Once you know the kind of prostate cancer you have **(Chapter 4)** and which options would best fit the kind of cancer you have **(Chapters 5, 6, & 7)**, the next step is to look at treatment success and complication rates. (By complication rates, we mean unwanted side effects that occur as part of the procedure. The three major complications are impotence, incontinence, and rectal bleeding, but others are important too.)

Making a side-by-side comparison of treatment success

and complication rates is the best way to make sure that you know how effective a particular type of treatment is and how likely you are to have a diminished quality of life after this type of treatment.

## BEFORE WE DIVE INTO THE DATA

The success rate percentages you see in **Figure 8.1 - 8.4** are based on data from Dr. John C. Rewcastle and his collaborators as well as several other studies. These numbers come from medical studies that looked at 10-year prostate cancer success rates.

The researchers selected the best studies in each treatment category that represented the most scientifically sound information from the available medical literature. This level of scrutiny allowed the researchers to make side-by-side comparisons of the success rates for each type of treatment.

Likewise, the complication-rate information presented in **Figures 8.9 - 8.12** compares the complications from four types of prostate cancer treatment: robotic radical prostatectomy (RRP, a from of surgery), external beam radiation (Beam RT), brachytherapy (seed implantation), and cryotherapy (freezing of the prostate). As you look at the complication rates, keep in mind that these figures indicate how many men HAD the complication in question — NOT how many did not.

**SUCCESS RATES**

The success rates in **Figures 8.1 - 8.4** describe men who had definitive prostate cancer treatment and remained alive and disease free for at least 10 years.

These figures look at the data by treatment type (robotic surgery, cryotherapy, brachytherapy, Beam RT, IMRT, and combination therapy) and by cancer risk group (low-risk, moderate-risk, and high-risk). It's also important to notice that **Figures 8.1 - 8.3** are divided by risk type, and Figure 8.4 is a summary of **Figures 8.1 - 8.3**.

In **Chapter 5**, we mention that low-risk prostate cancer patients usually receive a single type of treatment, moderate-risk patients often receive two types of treatment (combination therapy), and high-risk patients frequently receive two or more types of treatment (also combination therapy).

As we discussed in **Chapter 6**, combining therapies (surgery plus radiation, internal radiation plus external radiation, cryotherapy plus radiation) is very effective at eliminating prostate cancer; however, it also increases the risk of complications.

**TRENDS**

While the numbers in **Figures 8.1 - 8.4** are interesting all by themselves, there are some trends we would like you to pay attention to when comparing the success rates of different treatments for different kinds of prostate cancer.

### 1. OVERALL, LOW-RISK CANCER HAS THE BEST TREATMENT SUCCESS RATES

If you look at **Figure 8.4**, you'll see that the success rates are better for low-risk patients than patients in the other two risk categories. The success rates for low-risk patients are also roughly equal from treatment to treatment (especially at the top end of the treatment success range).

What does this tell us?

Basically, treatment outcomes are going to be successful in the vast majority of cases. What low-risk cancer patients need to consider are the long-term complications associated with each type of treatment and how those complications will impact them for the rest of their lives (See **Figures 8.9 - 8.12**).

### 2. THE MODERATE-RISK CATEGORY CONTAINS THE WIDEST RANGE OF CANCER OF THESE THREE CATEGORIES

Some of the cancers in the moderate-risk category behave like low-risk cancer and others behave like high-risk cancer. In general, they tend to behave more like low-risk cancers; however, some patients (especially high-volume patients) may require combination therapy to achieve success rates that come close to those of low-risk cancer patients.

### 3. COMBINATION THERAPY HAS THE HIGHEST SUCCESS RATE FOR PATIENTS WITH MODERATE-RISK AND HIGH-RISK PROSTATE CANCER

**Figure 8.4** illustrates this the key point from the medical literature — the treatment of moderate-risk and high-risk cancer is most effective when treatments are combined.

**Figures 8.1 - 8.4** shed some light on prostate cancer treatment success rates. The data used in these figures comes from many sources. Please note the following trends:

1. Combination therapy is the most effective type of treatment for all risk categories. This trend is more pronounced for the moderate-risk and high-risk patient groups.
2. When treatments are combined, they effectively ratchet the cancer risk down a category (high-risk to moderate-risk, moderate-risk to low-risk).
3. The wide range of success rates within some treatment types points to data coming from different treatment facilities (hospitals and medical centers).

| SUCCESS RATE FOR LOW-RISK PROSTATE CANCER | | | | | | |
|---|---|---|---|---|---|---|
| RISK | RRP | CRYOTHERAPY | BRACHYTHERAPY | BEAM RT | IMRT | COMBO |
| LOW | 76-90% | 60-92% | 78-89% | 76-87% | 81-86% | 95% |

Figure 8.1 demonstrates that low-risk prostate cancer success rates are the best of any risk category. Low-risk prostate cancer is easier to treat successfully. Also, the type of treatment is not as critical as it is with moderate-risk or high-risk cancer.

| SUCCESS RATE FOR MODERATE-RISK PROSTATE CANCER | | | | | | |
|---|---|---|---|---|---|---|
| RISK | RRP | CRYOTHERAPY | BRACHYTHERAPY | BEAM RT | IMRT | COMBO |
| MODERATE | 37-77% | 61-89% | 66-82% | 51-85% | 26-60% | 90-95% |

Figure 8.2 shows that the type of treatment is more important when treating moderate-risk cancer than it is with low-risk disease. Combination therapy still has a very high treatment success rate, but all the individual therapies are all less effective than they are with low-risk prostate cancer.

| SUCCESS RATE FOR HIGH-RISK PROSTATE CANCER | | | | | | |
|---|---|---|---|---|---|---|
| RISK | RRP | CRYOTHERAPY | BRACHYTHERAPY | BEAM RT | IMRT | COMBO |
| HIGH | 11-61% | 36-89% | 45-65% | 21-43% | 19-25% | 80-85% |

Figure 8.3 demonstrates why combination therapy (also called "multi-modal therapy") is essential to the successful treatment of high-risk prostate cancer.

| SUMMARY OF SUCCESS FOR ALL PROSTATE CANCER RISK CATEGORIES | | | | | | |
|---|---|---|---|---|---|---|
| RISK | RRP | CRYOTHERAPY | BRACHYTHERAPY | BEAM RT | IMRT | COMBO |
| LOW | 76-90% | 60-92% | 78-89% | 76-87% | 81-86% | 95% |
| MODERATE | 37-77% | 61-89% | 66-82% | 51-85% | 26-60% | 90-95% |
| HIGH | 11-61% | 36-89% | 45-65% | 21-43% | 19-25% | 80-85% |

Figure 8.4 provides a summary of success rates for all six treatments across the three cancer risk groups.

For example, when moderate-risk prostate cancer patients received combination therapy, their treatment success rates were similar to those of low-risk patients.

The same is true for high-risk cancer patients when two or more treatments are combined: their treatment success rate approach that of the moderate-risk cancer group. High-risk patients, however, don't achieve the same level of treatment success as moderate-risk patients, which speaks to the challenge of treating high-risk disease.

You may be saying to yourself, *if that's true, then why doesn't everyone have "combo" therapy?*

The truth is not everyone needs to combine treatments, especially low-risk patients. As you'll see in the second half of this chapter, no treatment (not even active surveillance) is free from complications. As a general rule, increasing the number of treatments also increases the potential for complications (unwanted side effects).

## 4. HIGH-RISK PATIENTS HAVE THE LOWEST SUCCESS RATE

Overall, patients who have high-risk prostate cancer have much lower success rates than patients in the other two categories. For high-risk patients, combining two or more types of therapy is essential for treatment success. If you have high-risk prostate cancer, using a single form of therapy may actually be putting your life at risk.

**A CLOSER LOOK AT LOW-RISK PROSTATE CANCER SUCCESS RATES**

Low-risk prostate cancer is by far the largest category of prostate cancer diagnosed in the United States (85-90 percent). This category of cancer responds well to single treatment modalities from active surveillance to more invasive procedures (See **Chapter 6**).

Because such a high percentage of the prostate cancer diagnosed in the United States is low-risk cancer, it makes sense to take a closer look at treatment success and complication rates for this cancer risk group.

Figures **8.5 - 8.7** display some interesting information about the 10-year success rates of watchful waiting and active surveillance, which can be successful in treating low-risk prostate cancer. The point of including non-invasive treatments like watchful waiting and active surveillance is to use their effectiveness as a baseline, because they have the lowest complication rates of all prostate cancer treatments.

**Figures 8.6 & 8.7** compare the 10-year success rates for watchful waiting and active surveillance with two well-studied traditional treatments, radical prostatectomy and external beam radiation. (Unfortunately, **Figure 8.7** lumps watchful waiting/active surveillance together into the one type of treatment, even though they are not.)

**CLARIFYING TERMS**

In **Chapter 6**, we made a clear distinction between "Watchful Waiting" and "Active Surveillance."

Watchful waiting is essentially a non-treatment recommended by doctors for men who are too frail, old, or sick to undergo prostate cancer treatment.

Active surveillance, on the other hand, is an effective form of treatment for men who have low-risk, low-volume prostate cancer. It requires a lifestyle overhaul in the following seven areas: diet, inactivity, stress, immune system, hormones, structure, and toxic substances.

Although we have made a clear distinction between watchful waiting and active surveillance, two of the studies we mention in this chapter did not.

For the purposes of our discussion of the information in **Figures 8.5 - 8.7**, it is important to be clear about how these three studies use the terms: "Watchful Waiting" and "Active Surveillance."

**Figure 8.5 & 8.7**: Watchful waiting and active surveillance are considered the same treatment. So the terms are used interchangeably.

**Figure 8.6**: Active surveillance is considered its own form of treatment — separate from watchful waiting.

**Figure 8.5** uses information from a SEER Study (Surveillance, Epidemiology, and End Results) to compare the 10-year mortality rates of Medicare prostate cancer patients that chose active surveillance/watchful waiting with Medicare patients that received a different type of treatment. This study also divided patients by their cancer risk factor: low-risk, moderate-risk, and high-risk.

| ACTIVE SURVEILLANCE/WATCHFUL WAITING | | |
| --- | --- | --- |
| 14,516 PATIENTS | 10-YEAR RISK OF DYING OF OTHER CAUSES | 10-YEAR PROSTATE CANCER SPECIFIC MORTALITY |
| LOW-RISK | 60% | 8.3% |
| MODERATE-RISK | 57% | 9.1% |
| HIGH-RISK | 57% | 25.6% |

Figure 8.5 uses data from the SEER study of more than 14,500 prostate cancer patients to illustrate three key points: 1. Active surveillance/watchful waiting works best with low-risk prostate cancer patients. 2. High-risk patients should only use active surveillance/watchful waiting as a last resort. 3. Low-risk, moderate-risk, and high-risk prostate cancer patients all have a similar risk of dying from other causes.

As you can see in the second column of **Figure 8.5**, the 10-year mortality rates for causes of death other than prostate cancer are approximately the same for the three cancer-risk categories: 60, 57, 57 percent, respectively. The difference between these categories is statistically insignificant (meaning that with a group of 14,500 men, the 3 percent difference between these categories could be attributed to random chance).

The third column is where the information starts to get interesting. The 10-year death rate from prostate cancer is similar for the low-risk and moderate-risk cancer patients (8.3 and 9.1 percent, respectively). The 0.8 percent difference between these groups is statistically insignificant.

The 10-year death rate from high-risk prostate cancer, however, is three times higher than the low-risk group (25.6 vs. 8.3 percent). That is significant!

This dramatic difference speaks volumes about why it is so important to aggressively treat high-risk prostate cancer with a combination of treatments.

The difference also takes us back to a concept we discussed in **Chapter 5**: You don't want to use a flyswatter to treat high-risk prostate cancer when you need a sledgehammer; likewise, you also don't want to treat low-risk prostate cancer a sledgehammer when a flyswatter will get the job done.

**Figure 8.6** highlights information from a Swedish study of nearly 7,000 men with low- and moderate-risk prostate cancer. The important take away from this study is how small the difference is in 10-year mortality (death rates) for low- and moderate-risk prostate cancer patients who received three different kinds of treatment: active surveillance, radical prostatectomy, and external radiation.

The biggest difference (between active surveillance and radical prostatectomy) is less than 1.5 percent — an insignificant difference given the size of the study.

Active surveillance is also the treatment of choice for many European men who already have other significant health problems. So this group of men *may* contain individuals who were already ill before being diagnosed, so their death rates would naturally be higher.

In addition, when you factor in complications like impotence, incontinence, and rectal problems, the 3.6 percent mortality rate for active surveillance looks more attractive when compared to the other two treatments, which have much higher complication rates (See **Page 202 - 207**).

**Figure 8.7** is a summary of the PIVOT-1 study (also called the VC-CSP-407 study). This study is one of the few "randomized" studies done in the PSA era that compares treatment success side-by-side between watchful waiting/active surveillance and radical prostatectomy.

| ACTIVE SURVEILLANCE VS. OTHER TYPES OF TREATMENT | | |
|---|---|---|
| 6,849 PATIENTS (LOW-RISK AND MODERATE-RISK ) | NUMBER OF PATIENTS | 10-YEAR PROSTATE CANCER MORTALITY |
| ACTIVE SURVEILLANCE | 2,2021 | 3.6% |
| RADICAL PROSTATECTOMY | 3,399 | 2.4% |
| RADIATION THERAPY | 1,429 | 3.3% |

Figure 8.6 compares the prostate cancer death rates for low- and moderate-risk patients who received three types of treatment. In this study of approx. 7,000 men, the 10-year mortality rates from prostate cancer are roughly the same: there is NO significant difference in the death rates of men who received these treatments.

"Randomized" means that the men who volunteered for this study were randomly assigned either watchful waiting or radical prostatectomy, so there was no bias by the researchers about which men received watchful waiting or prostatectomy.

This study of about 730 men under the age of 75 examined the 10-year death rate from "all causes" (second column) and death from "prostate cancer" (third column).

The most interesting detail to emerge from this study occurs when the data is divided into two groups by PSA total: Group 1 — PSA total is less than 10; Group 2 — PSA total is more than 10.

| WATCHFUL WAITING VS. RADICAL PROSTATECTOMY | | |
|---|---|---|
| 731 PATIENTS | ALL-CAUSE MORTALITY | PROSTATE CANCER MORTALITY |
| WATCHFUL WAITING | 50% | 8.4%[1] |
| RADICAL PROSTATECTOMY | 47% | 5.8%[1] |

**Figure 8.7** is a random study (PIVOT 1) that compares the death rates between watchful waiting and radical prostatectomy in men younger than 75 years old.

A PSA of less than 10 is generally considered low-risk-prostate cancer, and a PSA of more than 10 is considered moderate-to-high-risk disease.

**NOTE**

*When the men in the PIVOT-1 study were separated into two groups by PSA, those with a PSA of less than 10 (low-risk patients) had the same prostate cancer mortality rate with watchful waiting and radical prostatectomy.*

In Group 1 (men who had a PSA of less than 10), the difference in prostate cancer mortality between the watchful waiting patients and the radical prostatectomy patients **is statistically insignificant.** In other words, there was NO significant difference in the rate of death from prostate cancer between the patients who followed a watchful waiting protocol and the patients who had a radical prostatectomy.

In Group 2 (men who had a PSA of more than 10), the 10-year prostate cancer death rate is significantly higher for men who followed a watchful waiting protocol than for men who had a radical prostatectomy.

The takeaway from this study is that for men with low-risk prostate cancer, the 10-year survival rates for watchful waiting/active surveillance and radical prostatectomy are essentially the same.

**COMPLICATIONS** The survival rates discussed in **Figures 8.5 - 8.7** do NOT take complications from treatment into account, which are much higher for all forms of surgery and radiation than watchful waiting or active surveillance.

The biggest "complication" for men who choose active surveillance is that 20-25 percent of these patients have higher-grade tumors than those seen in their prostate biopsy. Genomic testing of a positive prostate biopsy sample (see **Chapter 3**) can prevent this type of under-staging, so men who have more aggressive cancer can be identified and treated appropriately.

There are two types of complications from definitive prostate cancer treatment: short-term and long-term.

Immediate post-treatment complications are very common and considered short-term. They can last up to two months and usually resolve on their own.

Long-term complications could continue indefinitely and require additional forms of treatment, medications, or management to bring men back to their pre-treatment baseline.

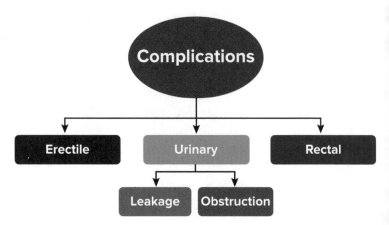

Figure 8.8 illustrates the three major kinds of complications: erectile, urinary, and rectal. No one wants any of these complications; however, being able to rank these complications (knowing which of these you could/could NOT live with) may be part of making your final treatment decision (see the **Chapter 8 Toolbox**).

The most common complications are:

1. Erections (impotence and erectile dysfunction)
2. Urinary (incontinence and urinary retention)
3 Rectal damage (bleeding, diarrhea, and fistula)

## IMPOTENCE AND ERECTILE DYSFUNCTION (ED)

Impotence is the inability to achieve and/or maintain an erection. It can be both a short-term and long-term complication. A patient's age and ability to have an erection before treatment have the biggest impact on impotence rates for prostate cancer patients. Age is often a better predictor of long-term ED than the type of treatment.

Also, if a patient has ED before treatment, in most cases, this condition becomes worse after treatment — not better.

Because older men tend to have more major health issues, doctors often advise older patients to have some form of radiation therapy instead of surgery, because radiation therapy is less likely to cause major complications.

As these older patients follow their doctors' recommendations and choose radiation therapy, their choice raises the impotence (and incontinence) rates for radiation therapy — skewing the complication-rate data somewhat.

On the other hand, younger (healthier) patients are often encouraged to undergo a radical prostatectomy because surgery is considered to be a more permanent solution.

| IMPOTENCE (cannot have or maintain an erection) | | | | |
|---|---|---|---|---|
| | RRP | BEAM RT | BRACHYTHERAPY | CRYOTHERAPY |
| AVERAGE | 14-96% | 6-84% | 0-40% | 53-93% |
| MEDICARE STUDY (101,604 PATIENTS) | 60% no erections 90% no erections sufficient for intercourse | 20-50% | 15-30% | Not Discussed in This Study |

**Figure 8.9** compares impotence rates for prostate cancer patients who had one of the four treatments. The more than 100,000 men in this Medicare study could fill a major college football stadium. This information comes from several different institutions across the country; therefore, it represents a large cross-section of hospitals, medical centers, providers, and men who have been treated for prostate cancer. Throughout this book, we define "impotence" as when a man cannot have or maintain an erection. However, some of the studies in this meta study used different definitions for impotence, which complicates a simple side-by-side comparison. That said, the information in this figure is still compelling.

COMPLICATIONS

For example, 95 percent of men in their 40s who undergo a traditional (open) nerve-sparing radical prostatectomy will regain sexual function adequate for intercourse; whereas, only half the men in their 70s will regain the same function.

## URINARY COMPLICATIONS

The two major types of urinary complications are the inability to hold your urine (incontinence) and being unable to urinate (urinary retention). Urinary incontinence can be both a short- and long-term complication. Long-term incontinence can be a depressing and life-altering problem. Urinary retention is usually a short-term problem.

The two biggest causes of urinary incontinence are a weak urinary sphincter and an excessively muscular bladder (also called "bladder hypertonicity"). Both of these conditions may go unnoticed before treatment. If they are present, they will increase the risk of post-treatment incontinence regardless of the treatment.

Also, incontinence after prostate cancer treatment often depends upon the type of treatment. For example, patients who undergo a radical prostatectomy are the most likely to have incontinence issues.

## INCONTINENCE (LEAKING URINE)

In general, older men have higher rates of incontinence than younger men. The same is true of prostate cancer

| INCONTINENCE (leaking urine) | | | | |
|---|---|---|---|---|
| | RRP | BEAM RT | BRACHYTHERAPY | CRYOTHERAPY |
| AVERAGE | 15-52% | 0-15% | 0-18% | 1.3-7.5% |
| MEDICARE STUDY (101,604 PATIENTS) | 30% required pads or clamps 63% complained of wetness | 7% | Not Reported | Not Reported |
| SINGLE HOSPITAL (1,000 PATIENTS) | 20% | 3.5% | Not Reported | Not Reported |

Figure 8.10 compares incontinence rates by treatment type. The large numbers in this Medicare study come from multiple hospitals and medical centers. Also, one of the challenges in discussing incontinence rates after prostate cancer treatment is that different studies define incontinence differently: "no wetness," "1 pad per day," and "up to 2 pads per day"... We have seen all of these different definitions for "incontinence" in the literature.

COMPLICATIONS

survivors, regardless of which type of treatment they choose. It is important to note that the incontinence percentages in **Figure 8.10** do not take the age of the patient into account. Also, these percentages do not consider the level of "continence" prior to receiving treatment. In addition, men who have had a TURP procedure for an enlarged prostate prior to prostate cancer treatment are more likely to leak urine.

However, the difference in the incontinence rates in **Figure 8.10** between the RRP (robotic surgery) group and the Beam RT (external radiation) group is significant.

**NOTE**

*The lack of a standard definition for incontinence makes discussing complication rates difficult. In some medical studies, "incontinence" is defined as any sort of leakage. Other studies define "incontinence" by the number of diaper pads a man uses per day: no pads, 1 pad, 2 pads .... Leaking any amount of urine should be considered incontinence. It doesn't matter how many pads or what causes the leakage to occur.*

## URINARY RETENTION (CANNOT URINATE)

This painful condition is usually caused by some sort of obstruction: an enlarged prostate, urinary stricture (scar tissue in the urethra), bladder stones, or a swelling of any part of the urinary tract after prostate cancer treatment.

Sudden (acute) urinary retention is a serious medical problem that requires prompt attention. If patients do not receive help with urinary retention, urine backs up from the bladder into the kidneys where it can wreak all sorts of havoc.

Fortunately, urinary retention after prostate cancer treatment is usually a short-term complication that can be resolved by medications and the temporary use of a Foley catheter until normal urinary function returns (a couple of days to a couple of weeks depending upon what is causing the problem).

Hospitalization is usually not required for urinary retention; as it can be treated in a doctor's office or at home.

COMPLICATIONS

| URINARY RETENTION (cannot urinate) | | | | |
|---|---|---|---|---|
| | RRP | BEAM RT | BRACHYTHERAPY | CRYOTHERAPY |
| URINARY STRICTURES | 17% | 7% | 2-10% | 1-4% |
| RETENTION | 9% | > 1% | 4-6% | 13-22% |

**Figure 8.11** compares Urinary Stricture and Urinary Retention rates for patients who have undergone four types of prostate cancer treatment.

There is an increased risk of urinary retention in the following patients:

- Older men — age is the #1 risk factor for acute urinary retention after prostate cancer treatment
- Patients who have urinary retention issues prior to treatment
- Type 2 diabetics
- Smokers — past and present
- Men with coronary artery disease

## RECTAL COMPLICATIONS

Rectal complications (also called "rectal morbidity") can occur after prostate cancer treatment. Fortunately, these complications are usually short-term.

There are four major kinds of rectal complications from prostate cancer treatment:

**Fistula:** An abnormal connection that forms between the rectum and the bladder. This "channel" allows urine to leak into the rectum and feces to travel into the bladder.

**Urgency:** The need to go to the bathroom (#2) right now that does not usually involve diarrhea.

**Diarrhea:** Soft, watery stools often accompanied by intestinal cramping.

**Bleeding:** Usually occurs from an inflammation of the intestinal lining (proctitis) or an injury that leads to bleeding. Both proctitis and rectal injury occur from treatment that is too close to the rectum, which can happen when prostate cancer is close to the margin of the prostate.

As you can see in **Figure 8.12**, the rectal complication rates for external beam radiation are higher than the other types of treatment listed. These complications occur

| RECTAL MORBIDITY (problems pooping) | | | | |
|---|---|---|---|---|
| | RRP | BEAM RT | BRACHYTHERAPY | CRYOTHERAPY |
| FISTULA | 1-3% | 0-1% | 0-3% | 0-0.5% |
| URGENCY | 6-16% | 19-43% | 4-9% | Not Reported |
| BLEEDING | 1-3% | 13-17% | 4-11% | 2% |
| DIARRHEA | 6-19% | 12-42% | 4-9% | Not Reported |

Figure 8.12 compares/contrasts the most common rectal complications after prostate cancer treatment.

more frequently with external radiation because it also impacts the healthy tissue surrounding the prostate.

**Figure 8.13** (on the following page) compares the major treatment complications for radical prostatectomy and external beam radiation. The huge amount of data in this study (more than 100,000 Medicare patients) is a good baseline for results and complication rates for patients treated in the United States.

## HORMONE THERAPY COMPLICATIONS

Hormone therapy uses chemicals to shut down male hormone production or block the absorption of male hormones. Hormone therapy is different than surgical castration, which is rarely done in modern medicine.

Although hormone therapy is not used as a single therapy to treat localized prostate cancer (cancer that is confined inside the prostate), it is the primary treatment for cancer that has spread outside the prostate (metastatic disease).

Hormone therapy is used in combination with other treatments for moderate- to high-risk prostate cancer.

How long an individual patient receives hormone therapy, whether it is used continuously or intermittently, or is used in conjunction with other therapies like chemotherapy is a hot topic of debate among the world's top urologists.

Truthfully, how hormone therapy is used to treat advanced metastatic prostate cancer depends (in large part) on your doctor, where he/she practices, how much of the cancer has spread outside the prostate, how far it has spread (local vs. distant disease), and how aggressive the cancer is.

COMPLICATIONS

## TREATMENT COMPLICATIONS FROM SURGERY AND EXTERNAL RADIATION FOR MEDICARE PATIENTS

| MEDICARE STUDY (101,604 PATIENTS) | RRP (Radical Prostatectomy, AKA: Surgery) | EXTERNAL RADIATION THERAPY (Generally older patients who have more health problems overall) |
|---|---|---|
| TREATMENT MORTALITY | 0.5% | None |
| RE-HOSPITALIZATION RATE | 4.5% | Hospitalization not required |
| MAJOR COMPLICATION RATE | 12-28% | None Reported |
| INGUINAL HERNIA | 7-21% | None Reported |
| FECAL INCONTINENCE | 4% | None Reported |
| BOWEL FUNCTION/ FREQUENT BOWEL MOVEMENTS | 3% | 10% |
| NEED FOR SECONDARY TREATMENT WITHIN 4 YEARS | 28% | 24% |
| PENILE SHORTENING | 3.7% (avg. 1-2 cm) | None Reported |
| IMPOTENCE | 90% could NOT have an erection firm enough for intercourse 60% could NOT have or maintain an erection | 67% |
| URINARY INCONTINENCE | 30% of men required pads or clamps 63% of men complained of wetness | 7% |

COMPLICATIONS

The first word you should pay attention to in **Figure 8.13** is "Medicare." More than 85 percent of this population are men 65 and older, and older men tend to have more complications from prostate cancer treatment than younger men. If you are younger than 65, this data still provides an accurate comparison of surgery and radiation complication rates. Perhaps the most interesting finding of this study is that 90% of men who underwent radical prostatectomy were unable to have an erection firm enough for intercourse.

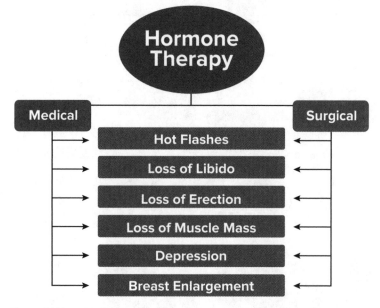

Figure 8.14 lists the most common complications of both medical and surgical castration. (Medical castration is another name for hormone therapy; surgical castration is rarely performed anymore.)

If a patient is given hormone therapy for less than one year, most of the complications listed in **Figure 8.14** are reversible, unless the patient is elderly or had very low testosterone levels before receiving hormone therapy.

Also, the longer men stay on hormone therapy past their first year, the more permanent these complications become.

In the **Chapter 8 Digging Deeper** section, we have created a blank "Action Plan" that allows you input all your prostate cancer information — including success and complication rates.

COMPLICATIONS

# Doctor Story
## DR. CURTIS CRYLEN, MD

Urology
Banner Health
Greely, Colorado

*"D.A." was 59 years old when he was diagnosed. He had his first PSA and it came back significantly elevated: 50 ng/mL (normal for his age is less than 4.0 ng/mL). His biopsy returned Gleason 4+5=9 prostate cancer in all cores.*

*He had a CT scan of his abdomen and pelvis and a nuclear medicine bone scan to look for any spread of the disease, and these did not show any obvious evidence of spread or metastases.*

*After a long discussion about the various treatment options for a man with "locally advanced" prostate cancer, he elected to proceed with a plan for aggressive, multi-modal therapy (a combination of different treatments). D.A. planned to have surgery (a radical prostatectomy) with pelvic lymph node sampling to see if any of the cancer had spread there.*

*We discussed several possible treatment scenarios if any cancer found in the lymph nodes.*

*Traditionally, this would mean stopping the operation and NOT removing the prostate, proceeding with hormonal therapy, and possibly radiation therapy.*

*Recent data, however, has demonstrated the effectiveness of using radical prostatectomy followed by radiation therapy and hormone therapy. This type of treatment can produce long-term cancer control for patients with "micro-metastatic" disease in lymph nodes.*

*During D.A.'s prostatectomy, a single lymph node was detected that contained a very small amount of prostate cancer. We proceeded with the surgical removal of his prostate. After D.A. recovered from surgery, he had external beam radiation therapy as well as long-term hormonal therapy.*

*D.A.'s PSA remains undetectable six years since his surgery, and he feels well. He continues to golf several times every week and enjoys spending time with several new grandchildren.*

## LOOKING AHEAD

**CHAPTER 1:** You or your doctor is concerned about your prostate — We provide you with **Prostate 101**: where it lives, what it does, plus relevant statistics.

**CHAPTER 2:** Your doctor told you to **schedule a prostate biopsy** — We give you a **Prostate Biopsy Assessment Tool** to see if you actually need one, and what to expect if you do.

**CHAPTER 3:** You have a prostate biopsy — We explain the steps you need to take, whether you have a **negative biopsy or a positive biopsy**.

**CHAPTER 4:** You have a **positive prostate biopsy** — We provide you with a **Prostate Cancer Assessment Tool** to help you understand which kind of cancer you have.

**CHAPTER 5:** You need to select a prostate cancer treatment — We provide you with a summary of the most common types of treatment based on your **cancer risk type** (low-risk, moderate-risk, and high-risk).

**CHAPTER 6:** You have **low-risk, low-volume prostate cancer** and need to learn more about emerging treatments — We provide you with a summary of these treatments to help you understand the differences between focal, minimally invasive, alternative, whole gland, and traditional treatments.

**CHAPTER 7:** You have prostate cancer that is more advanced than low-risk, low-volume and need to know more about **whole-gland treatments** (both stand-alone traditional and combination treatments) — We provide you with a summary of these treatments.

**CHAPTER 8:** You want to know the **success and complication rates** for each type of treatment and for each cancer risk type (low-risk, moderate-risk, and high-risk) — We provide you with unbiased information to support your decision-making process.

**CHAPTER 9:** You feel **overwhelmed** by the news of a positive prostate biopsy — We give you the tools to surf this tidal wave of emotion and overcome the feeling of panic that almost always accompanies a positive biopsy report.

**CHAPTER 10:** You want to **use your cancer diagnosis as a springboard to better health** — We help you address your wellness goals with a proven plan that covers inflammation, diet, inactivity, stress, immune system, hormone optimization, structure, and removing toxic substances.

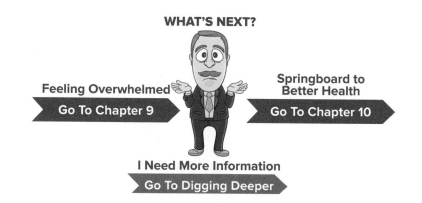

**WHAT'S NEXT?**

Feeling Overwhelmed
**Go To Chapter 9**

Springboard to Better Health
**Go To Chapter 10**

**I Need More Information**
Go To Digging Deeper

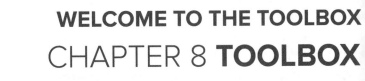

# WELCOME TO THE TOOLBOX
# CHAPTER 8 **TOOLBOX**

**THIS TOOLBOX SECTION IS DESIGNED TO HELP YOU SELECT THE BEST DOCTOR AND TYPE OF TREATMENT FOR YOU AND THE KIND OF CANCER YOU HAVE:**

- Possible Treatment Complications List
- Concerns about Complications
- Doctor Selector Questionnaire
- Tips for Finding the Right Doctor

## *Possible Treatment Complications*

| Can I live with... | YES | NO |
|---|---|---|
| Decreased Vitality | | |
| Pain | | |
| Impotence | | |
| Incontinence | | |
| Retrograde Ejaculation | | |
| Fertility | | |
| Catheter | | |
| Blood Transfusion | | |
| Male Menopause | | |
| Loss of Control | | |
| Loss of Masculinity | | |
| Loss of Family | | |
| Loss of Job/Income | | |
| Loss of Privacy | | |
| Loss of Social Status | | |

TOOLBOX

# Concerns About Complications

| | RANK 0-10<br>0 = No Concern<br>10 = Huge Concern | RANK CONCERNS FROM<br>HIGHEST TO LOWEST |
|---|---|---|
| Death | | |
| Pain | | |
| Impotence | | |
| Incontinence | | |
| Retrograde Ejaculation | | |
| Fertility | | |
| Radiation | | |
| Surgery | | |
| Anesthesia | | |
| Catheter | | |
| Blood Transfusion | | |
| Hormones | | |
| Loss of Control | | |
| Loss of Masculinity | | |
| Loss of Family | | |
| Loss of Job/Income | | |
| Loss of Privacy | | |
| Loss of Social Status | | |

T O O L B O X

# *DOCTOR SELECTOR QUESTIONNAIRE*

*Use the answers to the following 10 questions to
help guide your decision process:*

1. What is your doctor's treatment specialty
   (surgery, external radiation, brachytherapy, and so on)?

2. What are his/her 5- 10- 15- 20-year prostate cancer success rates?

3. What are his/her complication rates?

4. What are the national success and complication rates for the
   type of treatment your doctor uses?

5. What are the success and complication rates for the treatment
   center(s) that your doctor uses?

6  What do local prostate cancer support groups have to say about
   your doctor?

7. What do local prostate cancer support groups have to say about
   the treatment center(s) he or she uses?

8. Ask your doctor for the names of other prostate cancer doctors
   who he/she would recommend you consult with that specialize in
   different types of treatment.

9. Do you feel like your doctor is trying to pitch you on a particular
   type of treatment?

10. Is your doctor annoyed by your questions?

TOOLBOX

# THREE TIPS FOR FINDING THE RIGHT PROSTATE CANCER DOCTOR

1. **Narrow the field of treatments based on the kind of cancer you have:**  Use treatment success and treatment complication rates of several "good fit" treatments. Seek out physicians who perform those treatments.

2. **Listen to what different doctors have to say:** Consult with doctors who specialize in different types of treatment for prostate cancer. Compare their information with what you've heard from doctors who specialize in other treatments.

3. **Use the Doctor Selector Questionnaire (previous page):** Keep track of the doctors you've consulted with, what they told you, and your reactions.

For additional information, see the "Doctor Selection Tips" in the **Chapter 5 Digging Deeper** Section.

TOOLBOX

**NOTES:**

TOOLBOX

# chapter NINE
# Coping with a Prostate Cancer Diagnosis

> “Fear is the mind-killer
>
> — *Frank Herbert, Dune*

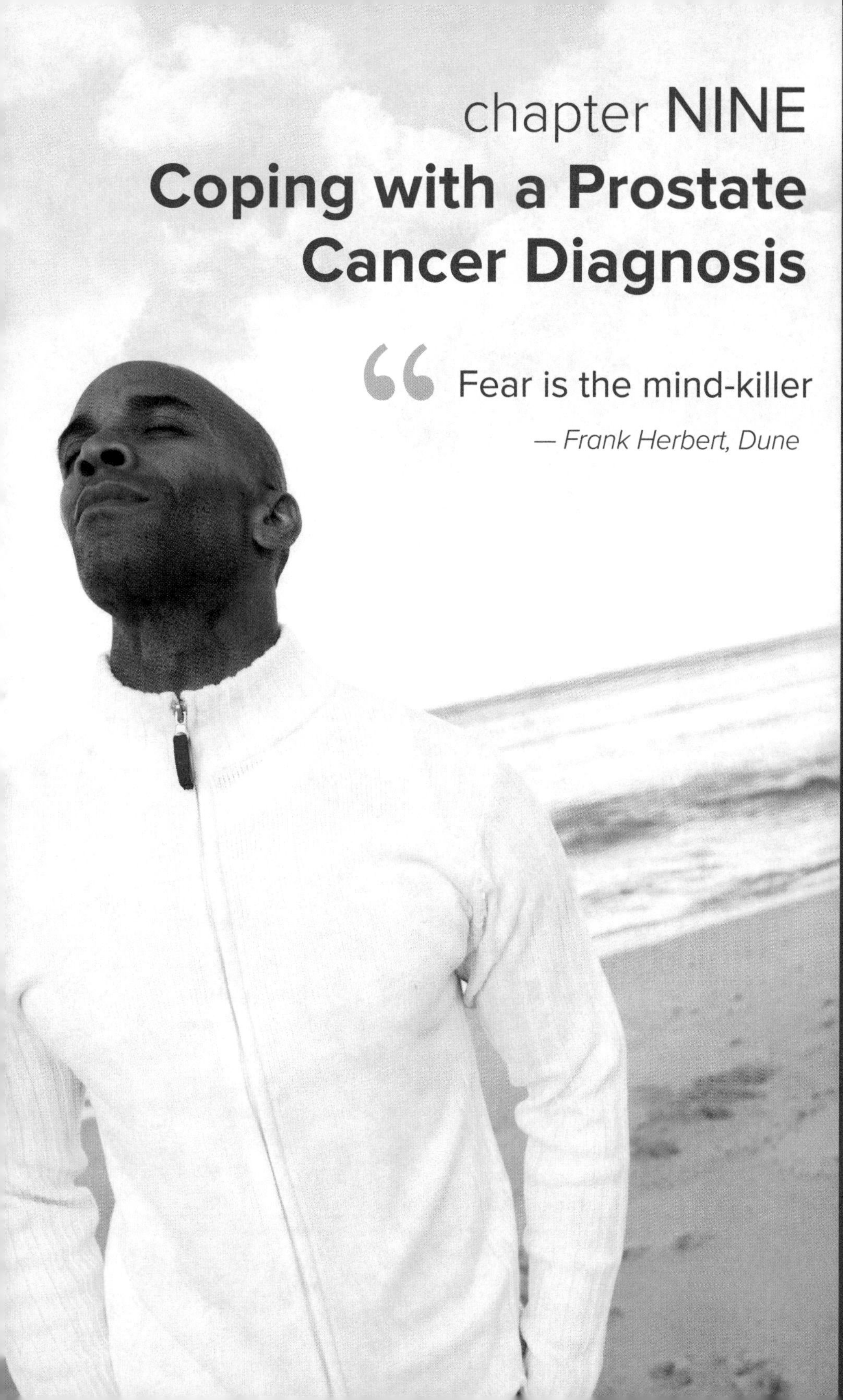

# Patient Story

## JOHN

*For those with this diagnosis, know that fear is the problem. Fear and the accompanying stress push our internal organs and systems to extremes. Abandon fear, find love both inside yourself and share it with your loved ones and friends. It does no harm to others and gives the body strong messages.*

*The love I feel is a sustaining force in my recovery from prostate cancer. The love I share with others, especially my wife, has been the ultimate reason to survive cancer.*

*Also, educate yourself about prostate cancer. Both Western medicine and alternative methods have helped me understand what cancer is. Each discipline has engendered hope, while helping my body respond favorably to treatment.*

*Cancer is a natural occurrence that becomes a threat when our bodies are out of balance; use this knowledge as a tool in your recovery. I binged on sugar, fried foods, chips, and junk food for years. That was normal for me. My diet also lacked essential vitamins and nutrients, which are vital now to my health.*

*The power of constant devoted prayer (religious or non-religious meditation) were a key factor during my operation, my other treatments, and as a lifestyle. Pray for others and find the inner peace of giving the energy that we all share. My body listened and believed it was healed — and then it was.*

*I have also faced the final issue all mortals must face. The death we all know is coming. This is sobering. Death is a personal event for all of us — and even though we may survive our cancer treatment, none of us lives forever, and no one gets out of this world alive.*

# chapter
## NINE
# summary

**Chapter 9** is about helping you (and your support team) surf the tidal wave of panic and fear that often accompanies a prostate cancer diagnosis.

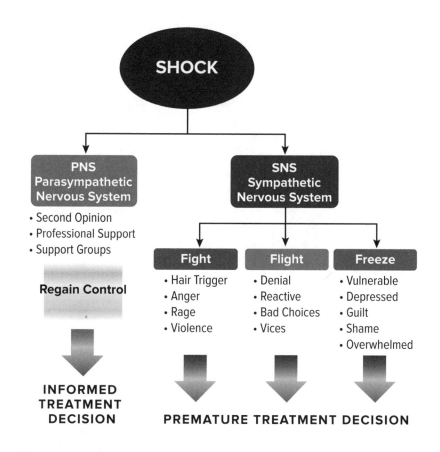

Figure 9.0 gives you a general overview of how panic and fear lead to premature treatment decisions (the right-hand side of the figure), and how feeling calm and grounded in the face of a cancer diagnosis (the left-hand side) leads to more informed decisions. Common sense dictates that more-informed decisions lead to better treatment outcomes.

**DEBUNKING MYTHS**

## DEVELOPING PROSTATE CANCER IS YOUR FAULT (THE CANCER BLAME GAME)

*There is a stigma of failure around receiving a prostate cancer diagnosis. It's a feeling of:*

*I must have done something wrong.*

*I should have....*

*If only ...*

*Bottom line: Beating yourself up over something you did or didn't do in your past is counterproductive and leads nowhere; besides, there's nothing you can do about the past — except learn from it.*

*Making yourself wrong about having cancer only drags you further down the rabbit hole of depression and despair.*

*So let's agree to skip "The Cancer Blame Game," shall we?*

*If you find yourself recycling this kind of mental anguish, simply say to yourself, "That was then; this is now. Now is the only time I really have. Today, I choose health."*

*If all of us could keep this mantra in mind as we go through life, our days would be a lot more forgiving.*

*Infants and little children develop cancer all the time. What did they do to cause or deserve their diseases? The answer is obvious:* nothing.

*Since there are no do-overs in life, the best thing (the only thing) you can do to improve your health is to learn from your mistakes, start making healthier choices, and stick with them. (More on this concept in* **Chapter 10.***)*

---

**VOCABULARY**

See Glossary for Definitions

| | |
|---|---|
| Adrenaline (epinephrine) | System |
| Cortisol (hydrocortisone) | Shock |
| Panic | Stress Hormones |
| Panic Attack | Sympathetic Nervous System |
| Parasympathetic Nervous | |

Every man who has heard the words: "You have prostate cancer," goes into some form of shock. That's normal. You've just been told that you have a potentially fatal disease. A strong emotional reaction, which includes panic and fear, happens to almost everyone. We would be far more concerned if you **didn't** feel like the rug had just been pulled out from under you.

As Dr. Ripoll puts it, "No matter how optimistic I am when I tell a man that he has prostate cancer, I see the same thing happen: His eyes glaze over, and I know my patient has checked out mentally. When I see that look, I know he can't absorb any more information."

Here's how a few of Dr. Ripoll's patients describe being told that they had prostate cancer:

- It felt like the ground was coming out from under me

- Everything just went numb

- I thought I was going to puke

- After Dr. Ripoll said, "You have cancer," I was gone. I don't remember a word she said after that.

The vacant stare that Dr. Ripoll sees in the eyes of her patients is a telltale sign of shock. Once you go into shock, you stop listening, the higher functioning areas of your brain shut down, and panic takes over.

When you panic, your animal instincts (the fight, flight, or freeze responses) kick in, and logic goes out the

---

### A SHORT LIST OF PANIC SYMPTOMS:

- *Heart racing*
- *Sweating*
- *Feeling dizzy, woozy, faint, weak, or like you're about to vomit*
- *Shortness of breath*
- *Tingling/numbness in your fingers and hands*
- *Feeling terrified and out of control*

*These are all normal reactions to being told you have cancer. People who are in this state of shock often feel overwhelmed by panic and the desire to run away from everyone and everything in their lives.*

window. You can't see the forest for the trees. You feel isolated, vulnerable, and alone — and your mind is consumed with finding the quickest way out of this rat maze. Feeling "panicked" can turn into a full-blown panic attack when you realize that have no idea which way to run.

Clearly, this is NOT the time to make a complex medical decision with potential lifelong consequences — like deciding which type of treatment is best for you!

It doesn't matter if you thought a prostate cancer diagnosis was coming down the pike, receiving that news is still a major emotional shock. For the next couple of weeks (or months), you may not be the same person — even if you manage to make it into work the next day. Your logical mind and your emotions are at cross-purposes.

## LOGIC AND PANIC DON'T SPEAK THE SAME LANGUAGE

They're not speaking the same language because the part of your brain that looks at things objectively and makes rational decisions is being trampled by your survival instincts.

Simply by receiving a prostate cancer diagnosis, your body starts pumping out stress hormones like adrenaline and cortisol to jump start your brain and prepare for the fight of your life.

The problem lies within: You are preparing to do battle with an opponent that lives inside your body.

**NOTE**

*Regardless of the type of prostate cancer a man is diagnosed with, anyone who has ever heard the words, "You have prostate cancer," will tell you it feels like the floor is being ripped out beneath you and the walls are closing in. The experience is both frightening and surreal.*

For more information on how to regain your normal life, please see the **Chapter 9 Toolbox**.

The first order of business is to get your nervous system to calm down. You cannot make a good decision about your treatment options until the emotional roller coaster about having prostate cancer comes to a stop.

And that takes "a tincture of time."

# How to Get Over the Shock and Panic of a Prostate Cancer Diagnosis

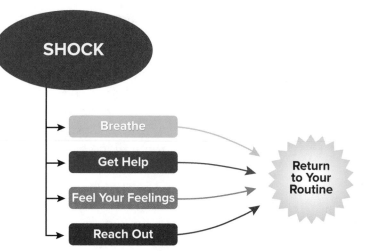

**Figure 9.1** points out that getting over the shock and panic of a prostate cancer diagnosis is more complicated than getting up and going to work the next day. You've just received shocking news, and it takes time to emotionally integrate that information. You can't force it, but you can ease yourself back into your normal routine, which has an amazingly calming effect on your nervous system. Having a predictable schedule and doing things you enjoy will help you adjust to this "new normal."

How much time? It varies from man to man. It takes time for the stress hormones to wear off and for your brain to start hitting on all cylinders again. Most of Dr. Ripoll's patients report that it takes between two weeks and two months before they are back to thinking clearly again.

We also recognize that these first couple of weeks may be the scariest time in your life, and all you can think about is, "Get this cancer out of my body — NOW!"

We totally get it; however, before you jump into kicking-prostate-cancer's-butt mode, you need to take care of the man who has the cancer first.

*That's why we strongly recommend you put off making a decision about your treatment options until you have read* **Chapters 4 through 8** *of this book.*

Right now, your #1 job is to move out of fight, flight, or freeze thinking (where you are reacting on pure animal instinct), and shift into a more rational state of mind where the higher functioning parts of your brain are working in harmony with your survival skills.

**NOTE**

*If you have been diagnosed with advanced localized cancer (high-risk cancer that is still confined to your prostate), you do NOT have the luxury of waiting until your emotional storm has passed before you decide on a treatment option. You need to begin treatment as soon as possible. If you have advanced local prostate cancer, we recommend that you assemble your support team to help you get through the eye of the hurricane.*

### How to Get Through the First Few Weeks after a Prostate Cancer Diagnosis

The following five suggestions (and the "Happy, Healthy, and Strong" list in the **Chapter 9 Digging Deeper** section) are designed to calm your mind, enliven your body, and assemble the right kind of support so you can shift into decision-making mode and select the best treatment plan for you.

### 1. BREATHE

When you find yourself slipping into panic, terror, fear, worry, anxiety, anger, rage, tears, even thoughts of suicide — simply close your eyes and take 10 deep breaths. This practice may feel ridiculous at first, but it will quickly help you step off the emotional roller coaster you've been riding and stand still with your feet firmly planted in the here and now. *Even if the sense of calm only lasts for a moment.*

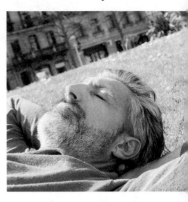

We recommend you take 10 of these breaths in a row, but if you only have time for 5, that will still help calm your nervous system.

This breathing practice is more than some yoga trick. Deep breathing shifts your nervous system away from the fight, flight, or freeze of the sympathetic nervous system into the safety and security of the parasympathetic nervous system.

This simple shift allows you to micro-manage your nervous system so you can, as the Brits say, "Keep Calm and Carry On."

All you have to do is close your eyes and take a nice, easy, full breath — followed by a gentle exhale when your body tells you it's ready. If closing your eyes makes you feel uncomfortable (or if you're driving a car, at a business meeting, and so on), just leave them open.

Do this practice as often as you need to. Air is free, and as far as we know, there's no limit to the number of deep relaxed breaths you can take.

*The magic happens on the exhale. Your mind slows down, your body softens — even if just for a moment.*

## 2. GET PROFESSIONAL HELP FOR SUICIDAL FEELINGS

If you're feeling suicidal, you need to get professional help — NOW!

Killing yourself because you have prostate cancer would be like joining cancer's team. We recommend that you embrace life instead.

---

**National Suicide Prevention Hotline**

**1 (800) 273-8255**

**1 (800) 273-TALK**

*Counselors are available in English and Spanish (24/7/365)*

---

If you don't know a mental health professional (therapist or counselor) in your area, ask your doctor to recommend some. If you need help right away, call **The National Suicide Prevention Lifeline** (See above).

If calling a suicide prevention hot line feels uncomfortable, call a friend, family member, or religious advisor and tell them what's going on. Share what you're going through. You'll be surprised how fast the feeling of hopelessness goes away.

The rate of suicide increases dramatically for men who recently received a prostate cancer diagnosis. This risk persists for about three months. For more information about suicide rates after a prostate cancer diagnosis (as if the diagnosis itself wasn't bad enough), please turn to the **Chapter 9 Digging Deeper** section.

*Don't reserve getting professional help just for when you're feeling suicidal. A prostate cancer diagnosis brings up all sorts of feelings that you probably didn't anticipate dealing with this week: sadness, depression, despair, hopelessness, isolation, anger, feeling victimized, rage, shame ... you name it.*

### 3. FEEL YOUR FEELINGS

This suggestion may sound like the opposite of Suggestion #2, but it's not.

Giving yourself permission to feel your feelings is one of the best ways to allow old emotional baggage to work its way through your nervous system. Otherwise, this invisible luggage tends to get "stuck" somewhere in your body (See **Chapter 10**).

Trying to move forward when you're emotionally stuck is like rowing a boat upstream: it's slow going. Instead, it's time to open up, feel the feelings, and start rowing with the river.

Sometimes it doesn't feel safe to let yourself experience the full weight of your emotions. Again, this is where family, friends, religious leaders, and professional counselors come into play. Make some calls and get help from as many different sources as feels right to you. If you're having a crisis, OWN IT! There's no shame in that.

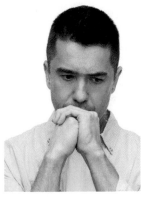

*A prostate cancer diagnosis can definitely be a catalyst for lots of old emotional junk coming to the surface where it can be healed. And that's a good thing. The challenge is this old "stuff" lands right on top of an ongoing health crisis — and that's not such a good thing. As Winston Churchill once said, "If you're going through Hell, keep going."*

## 4. REACH OUT — STRENGTH IN NUMBERS

Opening up to your community of family, friends, loved ones, teammates, people you do activities with, people you worship with, and mental health professionals is a natural extension of allowing your emotions to simply "be." The benefits of talking with the people closest to you during your time of need are enormous. These people are your greatest sources of support.

During this challenging time, you'll quickly figure out who can be there for you in a non-judgmental way — and keep your health information confidential. These people are worth their weight in gold. Cherish them.

**NOTE of CAUTION**

*Keep in mind that cancer scares the life out of some people. It brings up all their issues about death and dying, and even though they really want to be there for you, they just can't.*

*Also bear in mind that certain people in your inner circle have preconceived ideas about what you should/ shouldn't do to treat your prostate cancer. Their opinions are often based on what other men they know have done and information they saw on the 6 o'clock news. Some of this information may be useful; much of it is not. Accept the well-intended opinions of others as information: nothing more, nothing less.*

*It's probably best to avoid talking about your diagnosis at work, at least initially. The gossip and rumors generated by people at work far outweigh any benefits that come from confiding in your work friends.*

### HUMOR AND HEALTH OUTSIDE THE BOX

*While laughter may not be "the best medicine," it certainly helps. Norman Cousins, the author of "Anatomy of an Illness," is a great example. Cousins literally laughed himself back to health from heart disease and arthritis with a steady diet of Three Stooges short films and Marx Brothers movies. Cousins' experience says a lot about maintaining a sense of humor in the middle of a healing crisis. Even though you just received some bad news about your health, it's still OK to laugh — in fact, it's healthy.*

## 5. RETURN TO YOUR ROUTINE AND DO THINGS THAT MAKE YOU FEEL GOOD

We are all creatures of habit, and there is comfort in our familiar routines.

The simple act of feeling comfortable in your surroundings releases hormones and neurotransmitters that support happiness and chase the blues away. As a general rule, the more you stimulate the release of these chemicals in your body, the better you feel.

Your pelvic floor also relaxes, which helps eliminate congestion in your prostate.

After a man receives a prostate cancer diagnosis, there's a tendency to stop laughing, hunker down, and solve the problem. Problem solving — that's what men do best, right?

In this search for a solution, however, men often put off enjoying life until they've cracked the cancer code and figured out what to do. This type of "delayed gratification" is a critical mistake. Now is the time to reach out and connect with the people who love and care about you. We invite you to risk laughter, enjoy life, and have fun!

You don't have to figure it all out. That's what your doctors (and this book) are for. **Chapters 5-8** will help you explore which treatment options are right for you based on the kind of cancer you have. As you learn all you can about your condition and consult with your medical team, see if you can integrate one (or more) of these suggestions:

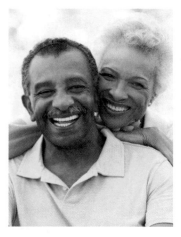

- Play with your kids, grandkids, or your friend's kids

- Take your dog (or your neighbor's dog) for long walks

- Call up old friends and tell them what you're going through

- Invite people over for dinner, to play cards, watch sports on TV, work on projects, or just hang out.

## ONCE THE TIDAL WAVE OF EMOTIONS HAS PASSED

Your diagnosis just gave you a legitimate excuse to connect with the people, animals, and activities that bring you the most joy. We highly recommend that you continue to do the activities that give your life purpose and pleasure.

We also encourage you to explore new ones. Give yourself permission to do something you've always wanted to try. Allow yourself to have fun. It's OK. In fact, it's healthy!

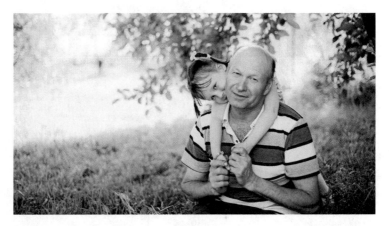

When you postpone pleasure for the sake of solving the prostate cancer puzzle, you deprive yourself of enjoying life, which restricts your supply of the healthy hormones and neurotransmitters and isolates you from the very people who have the most to offer in your time of trouble.

You'll recognize when you start feeling like your old self again. The people closest to you will, too. You'll smile more often, engage with other people, feel a little lighter, and look up at the sky more.

When you're ready, it's time to revisit **Chapters 4-8** and figure out the kind of prostate cancer you have and which treatment plan is right for you. Now that you have a sense of calm about you, we know you're going to make a better decision.

# Doctor Story

## DR. KELLY SIMPSON, MD

Radiation Oncology
Colorado CyberKnife
Lafayette, Colorado

*Oliver was a very active man in his mid-60s when he was diagnosed with prostate cancer. He had a PSA of 11.5 and a Gleason score of 7 (3+4).*

*When I met with Oliver and his wife for a second opinion, we discussed his treatment options: brachytherapy, intensity modulated radiation therapy (IMRT), surgery, and CyberKnife. I explained that the latter is a shorter, noninvasive treatment with a higher daily dose of radiation than IMRT.*

*We also discussed possible side effects: increased urinary frequency, feeling like he could not empty his bladder completely — plus a minor risk of erectile dysfunction and an even smaller one for short-term rectal irritation.*

*Oliver liked the fact that CyberKnife treatment had slightly better results than surgery but did not involve cutting, and it could all be done in a week. Oliver lived in an adjacent state and traveled a lot for work.*

*After taking a few days to weigh his options, Oliver decided to go with CyberKnife.*

*His treatment was straightforward. He did develop a slow urine stream and increased urinary frequency, which were treated successfully with an oral medication (Flomax).*

*I checked in with Oliver by phone regularly. His side effects resolved after a few months, and we monitor his PSA every three months. Two years after treatment, it was down to 0.26. He's recently started a new job in a different state and continues to be extremely active.*

*Oliver's wife was so happy with his results that when she ran into a friend at the grocery store whose husband had recently been diagnosed with prostate cancer, she recommended CyberKnife to her. We have subsequently seen this patient and treated him, too.*

## LOOKING AHEAD

**CHAPTER 1:** You or your doctor is concerned about your prostate — We provide you with **Prostate 101**: where it lives, what it does, plus relevant statistics.

**CHAPTER 2:** Your doctor told you to **schedule a prostate biopsy** — We give you a **Prostate Biopsy Assessment Tool** to see if you actually need one, and what to expect if you do.

**CHAPTER 3:** You have a prostate biopsy — We explain the steps you need to take, whether you have a **negative biopsy or a positive biopsy**.

**CHAPTER 4:** You have a **positive prostate biopsy** — We provide you with a **Prostate Cancer Assessment Tool** to help you understand which kind of cancer you have.

**CHAPTER 5:** You need to select a prostate cancer treatment — We provide you with a summary of the most common types of treatment based on your **cancer risk type** (low-risk, moderate-risk, and high-risk).

**CHAPTER 6:** You have **low-risk, low-volume prostate cancer** and need to learn more about emerging treatments — We provide you with a summary of these treatments to help you understand the differences between focal, minimally invasive, alternative, whole gland, and traditional treatments.

**CHAPTER 7:** You have prostate cancer that is more advanced than low-risk, low-volume and need to know more about **whole-gland treatments** (both stand-alone traditional and combination treatments) — We provide you with a summary of these treatments.

**CHAPTER 8:** You want to know the **success and complication rates** for each type of treatment and for each cancer risk type (low-risk, moderate-risk, and high-risk) — We provide you with unbiased information to support your decision-making process.

**CHAPTER 9:** You feel **overwhelmed** by the news of a positive prostate biopsy — We give you the tools to surf this tidal wave of emotion and overcome the feeling of panic that almost always accompanies a positive biopsy report.

**CHAPTER 10:** You want to **use your cancer diagnosis as a springboard to better health** — We help you address your wellness goals with a proven plan that covers inflammation, diet, inactivity, stress, immune system, hormone optimization, structure, and removing toxic substances.

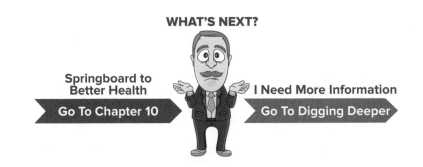

**WHAT'S NEXT?**

**Springboard to Better Health**

**Go To Chapter 10**

**I Need More Information**

**Go To Digging Deeper**

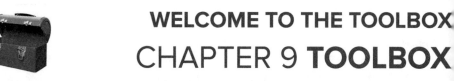

# WELCOME TO THE TOOLBOX
# CHAPTER 9 **TOOLBOX**

**THIS TOOLBOX SECTION INCLUDES THE FOLLOWING TOOLS AND RESOURCES TO HELP YOU COPE WITH THE EMOTIONAL ASPECTS OF A PROSTATE CANCER DIAGNOSIS:**

- Coping Strategies List
- Dominant Emotions List
- Dominant Fears List
- Regaining Control Strategies
- Doctor's Office Visit Suggestion List

## *Coping Strategies*

| SUGGESTIONS | RATE 0-10 (10 means you are most likely to do it) | RANK ACTIVITIES FROM HIGHEST TO LOWEST RATING |
|---|---|---|
| Get Out of the House, Walking, Jogging | | |
| Outdoor Sports | | |
| Gym or Rec. Center | | |
| Qigong, Yoga, or Pilates | | |
| Movies, Television, or Sports | | |
| Games, Videos, or Cards | | |
| Read and/or Write | | |
| Music: Listen, Play, Dance | | |
| Art, Photography, Drawing, Painting | | |
| Bath, Shower | | |
| Massage | | |
| Gardening | | |
| Private Time | | |

TOOLBOX

# Negative Emotions

| EMOTIONS | RATE 0-10 *(10 means your most dominant emotion **today**)* | RANK EMOTIONS FROM HIGHEST TO LOWEST |
|---|---|---|
| Shock | | |
| Fear | | |
| Confusion | | |
| Anger | | |
| Numbness | | |
| Depression | | |
| Disbelief | | |
| Guilt | | |
| Sadness | | |
| Grief | | |
| Hopelessness | | |
| Uncertainty | | |
| Frustration | | |
| Worry | | |
| Rage | | |

TOOLBOX

## Dominant Fears

| FEARS | RATE 0-10 (10 means that it is at the top of your list) | RANK FEARS FROM HIGHEST TO LOWEST |
|---|---|---|
| Death | | |
| Pain | | |
| Impotence | | |
| Incontinence | | |
| Retrograde Ejaculation | | |
| Fertility | | |
| Radiation | | |
| Surgery | | |
| Anesthesia | | |
| Catheter | | |
| Blood Transfusion | | |
| Hormones | | |
| Loss of Control | | |
| Loss of Masculinity | | |
| Loss of Family | | |
| Loss of Job or Income | | |
| Loss of Privacy | | |
| Loss of Social Status | | |

TOOLBOX

# Regaining Control

*The Regaining Control worksheet gives you a space to use the information from the Coping Strategies, Negative Emotions, and Dominant Fears worksheets. Select the two highest scores from each of the previous worksheets and list them here.*
*Are you willing to work on any of these items?*

| Worksheets | Your 2 Highest Scores |
|---|---|
| Coping Strategies | |
| Negative Emotions | |
| Dominant Fears | |

## Doctor's Office Visit Suggestion List

| Problem | Strategies |
|---|---|
| Trouble Staying Present | Bring a family member or friend to your appointments to help you stay focused. |
| Trouble Remembering | Record doctor conversation (phone apps or digital recorder), take notes. |
| Trouble Understanding | • Bring a list of questions.<br>• Ask your doctor to slow down and use non-medical language when appropriate.<br>• Ask your doctor for medical information that you can read/review on your own.<br>• If all else fails, make another appointment to ask additional questions. |

TOOLBOX

**NOTES:**

TOOLBOX

**NOTES:**

TOOLBOX

chapter **10**

# Using Your Diagnosis as a Springboard to Better Health

" *To find health should be the object of the doctor. Anyone can find disease.*

*Dr. Andrew Taylor Still, MD*
*Father of Osteopathic Medicine*

# Patient Story

## JEFF

*I am one of the fortunate people who have overcome prostate cancer and now live a cancer-free life. While cancer is not a journey that I would wish on anyone, I do feel that it has taught me 10 profound lessons.*

### 1. The diagnosis can be overwhelming

*It doesn't matter what type, what stage, or at what age, getting cancer is no fun. One day you're feeling fine, life is normal, and the next day your doctor tells you that you have cancer — and that's just the beginning: Doctor visits, expensive tests, treatment options, big decisions, and a wicked learning curve in "doctor speak" — and that's just the physical side. Cancer is also mentally, emotionally, and spiritually draining.*

### 2. Some things are beyond our control

*Cancer affects people from all walks of life. You can minimize the risk of cancer, but you can't control what life throws your way. You can, however, control how you deal with those curve balls.*

### 3. It's a wake-up call

*If being told you have a disease that could kill you doesn't make you take stock of your life, then I don't know what will. Cancer made me realize that life is precious and not to be taken for granted. It made me think about my purpose on this planet, the life I want to live, the people I want to touch, and the legacy I want to leave.*

### 4. Cancer doesn't define me

*Yes, I am a cancer survivor, but that label doesn't define me. I am more than a disease. I was a vibrant person before being diagnosed, and am even more so now.*

### 5. Cancer is a gift

*It might sound cliché, but I see my cancer as a gift. It has brought me closer to my kids and deepened my relationship with my wife. I have received love and compassion from unexpected people and in unexpected ways. It has opened me up to feeling more empathy for others.*

### 6. Cancer knows no boundaries

Cancer can affect anyone at any time; I know athletes in peak physical shape, children, grandparents, and people from all walks of life who have been diagnosed.

When I was diagnosed, I was in great shape, ate a healthy diet, exercised regularly, and did not have a single symptom. My dad had prostate cancer, so I knew that I had a higher chance of getting it.

### 7. Appreciate the little things in life

Not long after my diagnosis, I remember pulling off to the side of the road to watch a flock of birds overhead. I remember stopping in the middle of a bike ride to pet and feed a horse. It wasn't until after I had cancer that I really started to take notice of the finer things in life, things that I was either too busy to notice or took for granted.

### 8. Life is short

Cancer woke me up to how short a run we have on this planet. Prior to cancer, I hadn't thought about my mortality. Cancer changed that. I realize that I had an end date, and no matter which life I wanted to create, the time to act was now.

### 9. It raised my level of empathy

Surviving cancer made me a more empathetic person. I am a lot less judgmental after I realized that I have no idea what path other people are on, or what they have to endure every day.

### 10. I am not alone

According to the American Cancer Society, the lifetime risk of developing cancer for men in the United States is slightly less than 1 in 2, for women a little more than 1 in 3. These numbers tell us how close to home cancer actually is, and they have prompted an unprecedented level of research, care, treatment, and understanding of this disease.

Unknowingly, my cancer journey has been a path of personal growth. It has had a huge impact on my quality of life and my ability to appreciate how blessed my life truly is.

## VOCABULARY

See Glossary for Definitions

Bladder

Bio-individuality

BPH (Benign Prostatic Hyperplasia)

Brainspotting

Chi Gong

Cortisol

Craniosacral Therapy

Digital Rectum Exam (DRE)

DHEA (Dehydroepiandrosterone)

DHT (Dihydro-testosterone)

DNA (Deoxyribonucleic acid)

EMDR (Eye Movement Desensitization and Reprocessing)

Emotional Freedom Technique

Estrogen

Heart Math

Hormones

Functional Medicine Doctor

Gene

Gleason Score

GMO: Genetically Modified Organisms

Gyrotonics

Insulin

Metastatic cancer

Muscle Activation Technique

Mutation

Neurokinetic Therapy

Neuromodulation Technique

Non-GMO

Pelvic Floor

Pilates

PIN (Prostatic Intraepithelial Neoplasia)

Prostate Biopsy

Prostate Cancer

Prostate Zones

PSA (Prostate Specific Antigen)

PSA Testing

Rectum

Rolfing

Sacroiliac

Standard American Diet

Structural Integration

Testosterone

The Smile

Trans Fat

Touch for Health

Urethra

Urinary Retention

Urinary Sphincter

Western Diet

# chapter
## TEN
# summary

We included **Chapter 10** because we know how important it is to have everyday tools that improve your prostate health, by improving the health of the body your prostate lives in.

Regardless of the kind of prostate cancer you have, the seven sections of **Chapter 10** act like springboards to better health — better prostate health and better overall health.

We highly recommend that you use the information in this chapter to jump-start your journey back to wellness.

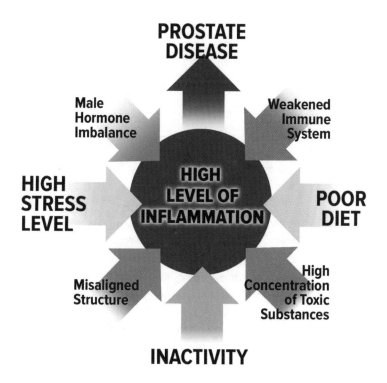

Figure 10.0 is an easy way to visualize how interconnected the seven health factors mentioned in this chapter are. They can either work together to promote prostate cancer (as in this diagram) or to promote prostate health (as in **Figure 10.2**).

# 7 FACTORS THAT DECREASE INFLAMMATION AND REDUCE THE RISK OF PROSTATE CANCER

**1. Diet**    **2. Inactivity**    **3. Stress**    **4. Structure**
**5. Immune System**    **6. Hormones**    **7. Toxic Substances**

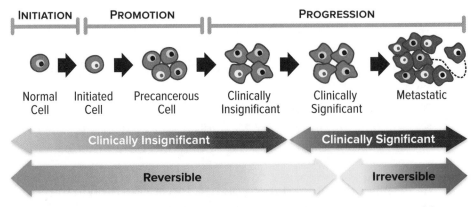

Figure Intro 1.1 visually displays how plastic the process of developing prostate cancer is. Bottom line: Prostate cancer is treatable, and in some cases reversible, if caught early enough.

**DEBUNKING MYTHS**

## PROSTATE CANCER IS IRREVERSIBLE

*Perhaps the most important information in* **Figure Intro 1.1** *(above), is that prostate cancer is* **REVERSIBLE,** *especially in its early stages.*

*Thankfully, new scientific research about active surveillance and its affect on prostate cancer has demonstrated that an anti-cancer lifestyle can actually reverse prostate cancer. It all depends upon where a man is on the spectrum of disease (see figure above) plus several other factors.*

*For many people, including some doctors, the idea that prostate cancer is reversible remains controversial.*

*The location of the line between reversible and irreversible prostate cancer varies from man to man. In general, we consider low-risk, low-volume prostate cancer to be reversible with active surveillance. Other risk factors such as the patient's age, overall health, pelvic health, and any previous pelvic surgeries are also part of the equation.*

*Also, it's important to realize that there's a big difference between "reversible" and "treatable." Prostate cancer that is not "reversible" may be very "treatable," with a high treatment success rate and minimal complications.*

**INFLAMMATION**

| | Problems | Solutions |
|---|---|---|
| **Inflammation** | 1. Immune System | 1. Treat infections & prostatitis |
| | 2. Diet | 2. Eat a low-glycemic (low-sugar) diet |
| | 3. Toxic Substances | 3. See **Page 264** |
| | 4. Inactivity | 4. Exercise 30 minutes a day |
| | 5. Structure | 5. See **Page 262** |
| | 6. Stress | 6. Start a stress reduction program |
| | 7. Hormones | 7. Have your hormone levels and ratios checked by a certified functional medicine doctor |
| | 8. Prostate | 8. Begin our 7-point program |

Figure 10.1 outlines the causes and solutions for inflammation — which is the root cause of many kinds of prostate disease — including cancer.

## INFLAMMATION IS THE ORIGIN OF VIRTUALLY ALL CHRONIC DISEASE.

Regaining your health after any kind of cancer diagnosis is all about reducing Inflammation and reversing its negative effects your body. This is no simple task.

***Why?** Because inflammation occurs on every level of your body: whole body, organ systems, tissues, your cells — even your DNA*. At some level, diseases like obesity, heart disease, stroke, diabetes, and prostate cancer are all manifestations of inflammation.

The causes of inflammation are everywhere. The sources include the food we eat (high-glycemic diet), the stagnant way we work (sitting for hours), the stress we carry around (increased cortisol), our misaligned bodies, and our over-worked immune systems ... to the toxic materials we ingest in the food we eat, the water we drink, and the air we breathe.

The point of this chapter is to make you aware of how a poor diet, inactivity, high stress, malfunctioning immune system, out-of-balance hormone levels, postural problems, and the presence of toxic substances in your body all work together to create prostate disease (cancer).

Once you are aware of what the problems are, then you can make a plan to fix them, which is what the **Chapter 10 Toolbox** is all about.

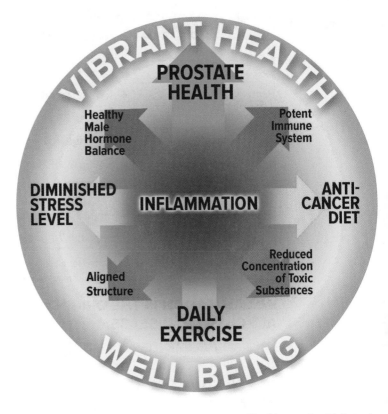

Figure 10.2 illustrates how the seven interconnected health areas (health factors) mentioned in this chapter can work together to restore your overall health and the health of your prostate.

If you want to regain your health, you're going to have to make some changes — and change is scary. It runs counter to our desire for the comfort of what's familiar.

To help you take make the right changes, we offer you our seven-point plan to rid your body of inflammation and allow your body's natural vitality to shine through.

**Figure 10.2** (above) reverses the direction of the seven health factors listed in **Figure 10.0** (from promoting prostate cancer to reviving prostate health). These two figures point out how these seven interconnected areas can either be your enemies (**Figure 10.0**) or your friends (**Figure 10.2**).

Even if you have been undermining your health for decades, **Chapter 10** will give you the tools to rejuvenate and revitalize your life. It's all about awareness.

**DIET**

| | Problems | Solutions |
|---|---|---|
| **DIET** | 1. Insulin/sugar problems & toxic chemicals in food | 1. Eat mostly organic vegetables (especially cruciferous vegetables) and low-glycemic fruit |
| | 2. High-glycemic diet | 2. Low-glycemic diet |
| | 3. Growth hormone/antibiotics in food | 3. Eat animal protein that is free of all hormones and antibiotics |
| | 4. Processed foods and trans fats | 4. Restore the balance between omega 3 & omega 6 fatty acids |
| | 5. Grains | 5. Limit grains and breads |
| | 6. Poor quality oils | 6. Use more olive and coconut oil |
| | 7. Alcohol, sweetened sodas, and caffeine consumption | 7. Limit alcohol, sodas, and caffeine |

**Figure 10.3** lists why eating a "Western Diet" has such a strong impact on inflammation, disease, cancer in general, and specifically prostate cancer.

Your diet is *the* fastest, easiest, and most powerful tool you have to improve your health. It is also the one thing you have complete control over. Unless you live in prison or are on a forced meal plan, you have complete control over what goes into your mouth.

Worldwide, the "Western Diet" is the single biggest cause of chronic disease. It is a recipe for inflammation with its processed foods, calories from sweeteners and simple carbs, oils that have been artificially modified, and meat that is awash in antibiotics and growth hormones.

To learn more about how your diet (and the other six wellness factors mentioned in this chapter) interact with your body, we encourage you to go to the **Chapter 10 Toolbox** and explore the basic tools there.

### WHEN IT COMES TO YOUR DIET, WHAT YOU DON'T EAT IS MORE IMPORTANT THAN WHAT YOU EAT. HERE ARE THE TOP 5 FOODS YOU SHOULD AVOID TO REDUCE YOUR LEVEL OF INFLAMMATION:

**1. Cut Out All Forms of Sugar** (**Ch 10** Digging Deeper)
Sugar is a toxin. Why would you want to eat a toxin? (Because it tastes so sweet, obviously.)

Sugar and its metabolic equivalents (sweeteners) come in many forms: agave syrup, brown sugar, brown rice syrup, cane juice, fruit juice concentrate, high fructose corn syrup, honey, maple syrup, molasses, sucanat, turbinado … the list goes on.

One look at the labels of your favorite foods will shock you about how much sugar is in them. All sweeteners flood your body with sugar, which boosts the production of insulin (a pro-inflammatory hormone). Insulin causes your body to store calories as fat and increases inflammation throughout your body. Just the taste of something sweet releases insulin.

If you want to lose weight, heal from cancer (and several other diseases), maintain your mental edge, and generally feel better, *cut out sweeteners.* As painful as this advice may sound, it's that simple.

## 2. Avoid Simple Carbs

Breads, pastas, cookies, crackers, popcorn, snack foods, breakfast cereals, granola, waffles, pancakes, candy, "energy' bars … even white potatoes are metabolized by your body the same way sugar is. They all boost insulin production, tell your body to store fat, and promote inflammation at every level.

## 3. Say "Goodbye" to Grains

Grains generally cause the same sugar rush, insulin spike, fat storage, and inflammation as simple carbs.

This response is true for "whole grains" and gluten-free grains. If you're going to eat grains, however, go with gluten-free whole grains. They are easier to digest and contain more nutrients.

## 4. Don't Eat Dairy

Consider this: Humans are the only animals that continue to drink milk after we have been weaned from our mothers. We are also the only animals to regularly drink the milk of another animal (cows and goats, mostly).

Several European studies have show that men who eat 2-3 servings of dairy products per day are up to eight times more likely to develop prostate cancer.

## 5. Just Say "No" to Alcohol

Sugar is a toxin. Alcohol is a poison. Why would you want to poison your body when you're trying to heal from prostate cancer? That makes no sense.

In 1988, the World Health Organization classified alcohol as a Group 1 carcinogen. Regular heavy alcohol consumption increases the risk for seven different types of cancer, including prostate, breast, colorectal, oral, and liver.

**NOTE**

*Before you begin any new diet, it's a good idea to get tested to see if you are allergic to certain foods. Food allergies/sensitivities create inflammation, so food allergy testing is a good place to start.*

### HERE ARE OUR BIG 3 FOODS YOU SHOULD EAT TO REPLACE THE OTHER 5 YOU JUST CUT OUT:

1. **Eat Lots of Organic Vegetables and Some Organic Low-Glycemic Fruit**

   Your goal is to make your diet 60-75 percent organic, non-starchy vegetables and low-glycemic fruit. Think of 60-75 percent as five cups (helpings) of fresh vegetables and fruit per day (4 cups of vegetables and 1 of fruit, such as berries).

   Include lots of cruciferous vegetables: broccoli, cauliflower, Brussels sprouts, kale, cabbage, bok choy, ... and many others. These vegetables contain compounds that kill cancer cells — so do berries!

   Onions and garlic not only improve the taste of food, they have cancer-fighting properties as well.

   **Warning:** The pesticides, herbicides, and fungicides in conventionally grown fruits and vegetables are poisons. No amount of rinsing will wash these poisons off — they are embedded in the body of the plant.

   **Warning:** The long-term results of feeding GMO (Genetically Modified Organism) food to lab animals are frightening. Avoid them wherever possible. Ask your grocer if your vegetables and fruit contain GMOs. If they don't know, don't buy it.

2. **Healthy Fats Are Your Friends**

   A diet rich in animal fats and trans fats is one of the clearest dietary links to prostate cancer. These unhealthy fats clog the tiny arteries throughout your body and promote heart attacks, strokes, and erectile dysfunction. Healthy fats, such as **avocados, seeds & nuts,** however, are important in the production of hormones, memory, supple skin, and younger-looking hair.

**Healthy Fats:** Olive oil, coconut oil, and clarified butter.

**Unhealthy Fats:** Margarine, trans-fats, cotton seed oil, soy oil, and safflower oil.

**So-So Fats:** Sesame oil, canola oil, and peanut oil.

3. **Clean, Lean Animal Protein Cooked at Low Temperatures is OK**

Several new studies show a connection between eating meat and developing cancer — specifically red meat, processed meat, and prostate cancer. Here's the information we think men concerned about prostate cancer need to know:

- If you eat animal protein, eat grass-fed, organic meat (or wild game/fish). The antibiotics, nitrates, and hormones in conventionally raised meats are linked to the rise of "super bugs," heart disease, and cancer.

- Avoid meat cooked at high temperatures (pan-seared, grilled, charred, deep fried, or blackened). Cooking at high temperatures creates compounds in the meat that promote prostate cancer.

- Cooking meat at high temperatures also makes the proteins and fats more difficult to digest.

- Avoid processed meats, luncheon meats, smoked meats, jerky, pastrami, bacon ... basically any meat that has been treated with anything. They are extremely unhealthy for your heart and your prostate.

- All the problems associated with eating meat are multiplied by eating a lot of it. Instead of feasting on 1/2lb. burgers or 16 oz. steaks, eat smaller portions of meat (no bigger than your wallet).

- Eat the leanest meats you can find. Animal fat is a sponge for toxic substances and carcinogens.

- Several studies connect eating red meat with prostate cancer. However, we are unaware of any studies showing the negative effects of eating slow-cooked, grass-fed, organic red meat. More research on eating this kind of red meat would be very valuable.

**INACTIVITY**

| | Problems | Solutions |
|---|---|---|
| **INACTIVITY** | 1. Chronic inflammation, pain, and habitual stress | 1-3. Move your body: Stand up every hour, walk around, do chores, stay active |
| | 2. Accumulation of toxic substances in excess body fat leads to being both overweight and unhealthy | 1-3. Build your strength, endurance, and flexibility slowly over time. Exercise daily but avoid overtraining. |
| | 3. Lack of exercise leads to stagnant circulation, fatigue, depression, and a diminished desire to move your body | 1-3. Combine slow/steady exercise with resistance training and interval training, which improves circulation and removes toxic substances |

**Figure 10.4** points to why exercise is essential for a healthy body (and prostate), and inactivity is an evil habit that ruins your health and robs you of your energy.

## EXERCISE IS A FEAST THAT NOURISHES THE BODY, ENLIVENS THE MIND, AND FREES THE SPIRIT.

If something is good for your heart, it's probably good for your prostate, too.

The human body was designed to walk from place to place to gather food, sprint full speed when chasing after prey animals (or being chased by predators), and doing short bursts of all-out exercise (tree climbing, rock climbing, and fighting) — all followed by rest.

The value of this variety of daily exercise is most visible in its absence. In our increasingly sedentary culture many of us sit for 8-10 hours a day. The absence of daily physical activity is especially alarming considering that almost 70 percent people in the United States are overweight.

So, how do you incorporate exercise into your daily life?

**NOTE**

*First and foremost: Always consult with your primary care physician, a physical therapist, or knowledgeable personal trainer before you embark on a new exercise regime. Talk with people who have a thorough understanding of any limitations you have, as well as proper exercise technique and the use of exercise equipment.*

It's important to realize that there is no single kind of exercise that is best for everyone. To get the most out of the time you spend exercising, it's about integrating different kinds of exercise to train smarter — not harder.

Also keep in mind that you have to play the ball where it lies. **If walking around the block is all your body can handle at first, that's fine.** Persistence is the key. The longer you stay with a comprehensive exercise program, the more you will be able to increase your endurance, vitality, and cardiovascular health.

## WE RECOMMEND A FOUR-PRONGED APPROACH:

### 1. Breathe hard for at least 30 minutes every day.

Do something every day that makes you breathe so hard that it is difficult to hold a conversation. You may have to get up a half an hour earlier or skip some other activity that is NOT helping you improve your health. Don't stop if you miss a day. Daily exercise is the goal, but 3-4 times per week is a huge improvement over sitting on the sofa seven days a week.

### 2. Resistance training is key to rebuilding your health.

When it comes to reducing inflammation, the value of pushing, pulling, lifting, and releasing some sort of resistance cannot be overemphasized.

It doesn't matter if you are using your body weight or some kind of equipment that provides resistance (a weight machine or free weights). Stressing your core muscles (the ones responsible for alignment and posture) and your skeletal muscles (the ones that move your body) helps you build strength, muscular endurance, balance; maintain healthy hormone levels; get a good night's sleep; and generally feel better about life.

Group classes help take the drudgery out of resistance training. Try Pilates, TRX, kettle balls, or any number of group fitness classes that use resistance.

If classes don't work for you, then start a resistance training program by doing push-ups and core strength exercises on the floor during TV commercials.

Weight lifting (using weight machines or free weights) is an exceptional way to boost strength, tone your body, improve circulation, and reduce inflammation, all of which can have a positive impact on your prostate.

The way you workout is also important. Without going into detail here, as a prostate cancer patient, your goal is to maximize the hormonal, circulatory, and health benefits of your workouts without pushing your body to the point where you hurt yourself or you are too sore to exercise the following day.

**No medals given for bravery. If you're hurt, you can't exercise; if you're too sore, you don't want to.**

*Rome was not built in a day. Neither was your temple. It's normal to jump into a new exercise program, especially after a health scare. The importance of a solid foundation cannot be overestimated. Go slow. Don't over do it. Remember: Your goal is to heal.*

3. **High-intensity exercise achieves the same results in a fraction of the time.**

   What is high-intensity exercise? Think of it as short bursts of going as fast as you can without hurting yourself. For some people that's a 50 percent effort; for others, it's closer to 100 percent. This "flat out for 30 seconds" kind of exercise mimics what our ancestors did while hunting or avoiding being hunted.

   We recommend 30 seconds of high-intensity exercise followed by 90 seconds to recover your breath and bring your heart rate back down. (You won't recover all the way, but your breathing and heart rate will come back down.) Eight of these cycles (30 seconds of "all out" effort followed by 90 seconds of "active recovery") is ideal. In 16 minutes, you will achieve similar results to jogging for two hours.

*You will probably have to build up to eight cycles. One cycle may be all you can do the first time — no problem. Simply add a cycle as you can until you get to eight.*

If it's been a while since you exercised or if you are obese, 30 seconds of high-intensity exercise might be just walking at a brisk pace, and your 90 seconds of recovery would be slowing down to a stroll. If you're already in good shape, you could do this 30/90 seconds pattern while walking, running, swimming, cycling, hiking, on a rowing machine, and so on.

This kind of interval training, does wonders for your heart, boosts your male hormone production, and improves your overall health.

Be careful: We recommend you start with one high-intensity workout session per week and build slowly to a maximum of three. Interval training can do wonders for your body, but if done incorrectly, it's also an easy way to injure yourself.

Substitute one 16-minute high-intensity workout for one "breathe hard every day for 30-minutes" workout. This way, you vary your exercise patterns, which takes the drudgery out of working out.

4. **Keep Your Spine Supple. (Also see "STRUC-TURE" later in this chapter.)**

## Healthy Pelvis — Happy Prostate

If your lower spine and pelvis are in good alignment and free from chronic pain, chances are the muscles and connective tissue in your pelvic floor will be strong yet supple. This kind of supple lower spine and pelvis allows for healthy blood and lymph circulation in and around the prostate gland, which promotes health and reduces inflammation.

There are several ways to improve how supple your lower back and pelvis are:

### EXERCISES

- **Core strengthening**: Postural muscles
- **Flexibility training:** Yoga and stretching
- **Pilates & Gyrotonics:** Strengthens and opens the spine through its full range of motion

### Hands-on Therapies

- Physical Therapy
- Osteopathic/Chiropractic manipulation
- Acupuncture
- Rolfing/Structural Integration
- Muscle Activation Technique
- Neurokinetic Therapy
- Craniosacral Therapy

If you are unfamiliar with these exercises or hands-on therapies, we recommend a simple Google search for which ones are available in your area.

**NOTE**

*The biggest challenge with any new exercise program is avoiding injuries. That's why it is important to intentionally underachieve for the first couple of months.*

As a prostate cancer survivor, it is far better to regain your health and fitness at a slightly slower pace than it is to get injured and not be able to receive the benefits of exercise and activities.

Yoga, hiking, swimming, weight lifting, Pilates, riding your bike ... are all wonderful activities that feel great and help your body heal. Just remember to take it easy for a while — there's no finish line here.

**STRESS**

| | Problems | Solutions |
|---|---|---|
| **STRESS** | 1. A prostate cancer diagnosis | 1. The "right fit" prostate cancer treatment plan |
| | 2. Fears about money and your close relationships | 2. Seek sound financial advice and open up to the people closest to you |
| | 3. Work-related issues | 3. Talk with co-workers and supervisors (if you can) |
| | 4. Feeling overwhelmed | 4. Daily deep breathing practice promotes feeling calm |
| | 5. Too much cortisol and adrenaline in your system | 5. Daily exercise, limit stimulants, prayer/meditation |

**Figure 10.5** outlines five common causes of chronic stress for prostate cancer patients. Whatever your stress level was before your diagnosis, expect it to skyrocket after a diagnosis. The challenge is learning how to cope with this new level of stress (on top of the old one) so you can move forward with your healing process.

**Stress comes in many forms:**

- Health problems (like a prostate cancer diagnosis)
- Money issues
- Grief/Death of a loved one
- Losing a job
- Difficult relationships
- Challenges at work
- Taking care of aging parents or a high-needs child
- Getting married
- Getting divorced
- Living in uncertainty or fear
- Traumatic events (and the PTSD that follows)
- ... the list goes on

The connection between stress and cancer is well documented. It is our observation that many people who "get" cancer often go through an especially stressful period a year or two before they are diagnosed.

The net effect of chronic stress is that it stretches the body's immune system beyond its ability maintain your well being. In the absence of a robust immune system, the unhealthy processes going on inside our bodies gain the upper hand, and that's when we get sick.

Any kind of cancer diagnosis multiplies the level of stress you were experiencing before the diagnosis, which only makes matters worse.

Think of it this way, if your stress level contributed to developing cancer — then the additional stress of being diagnosed with cancer just rocketed your previous stress level into the stratosphere.

It is difficult to tease apart the sources of your stress because many of them involve other people or situations that are outside of your control. Instead of trying to bend the river, we recommend that you use these eight strategies to move with the current — not against it.

**EIGHT PROVEN STRATEGIES FOR COPING WITH STRESS:**

1. **Daily Exercise:** It's cheap, easy, and unless it is too painful to move your body for 30 minutes every day, every aspect of your life will benefit from exercise — especially your stress level.

2. **Connect with the People Who Love You:** You cannot put a price tag on the support you receive from the people (and animals) who love you. Surround yourself with these people and let them care for you in their own way. The support of spouses, partners, family, friends, pets, and your community helps create an environment where healing is possible.

3. **Eat Good Food:** Your body thrives on good nutrition. The simple act of nourishing your body cuts down on the insulin level in your body. Find a way to work cruciferous vegetables, fish and lean chicken, organic fruit, and healthy fats into your comfort foods.

   For example, oven-roasted Brussels sprouts, cauliflower, broccoli, with a few cloves of garlic and a dash of olive oil and balsamic vinegar on top is delicious (add a little pulled chicken or a can of tuna and you have a complete meal). Likewise, replace your nightly bowl of ice cream with the same bowl of sliced fruit and berries — and a handful of chopped almonds on top. Delicious!

4. **Prayer/Meditation:** If you are a prayerful person, then now would be the time to pray. If you're not, you can achieve a similar level of peace simply by sitting in a chair with your eyes closed while gently noticing the rise and fall of your breath. Two 20-minute sessions of prayer or meditation each day, can significantly shift your stress level and completely turn your life around. If one 20-minute session is all you can fit in, then that's a great start!

5. **Chi (Qi) Gong:** This ancient Chinese martial art combines the joy of exercise with the calm of meditation. Chi Gong uses breathing techniques, physical postures, precise motions, and focused intention (meditation) to help move the universal life energy (Chi) throughout your body.

   Chi Gong practice (which looks like its more well known cousin: Tai Chi) is part moving meditation and part slow-flowing movement accompanied by rhythmic breathing and a deeply relaxed state of mind.

## 6. The Smile

This technique comes from Chi Gong and is perfect for people who don't have a lot of time to devote to prayer or meditation. All that's required is a quiet place and five minutes.

All you have to do is close you eyes and think of something that makes you truly happy. This is not "fake it until you make it." You need to feel your body, especially the muscles of your face, smile. Then, you send that smile to your prostate and pelvis.

The best time to practice "The Smile" is when you wake up or when you go to sleep.

## 7. Therapeutic Techniques

The following techniques deliver outstanding results for people who are experiencing debilitating stress or Post Traumatic Stress Disorder (PTSD).

A prostate cancer diagnosis can create what feels like being hit by never-ending waves of stress that bring old traumas and painful memories to the surface.

Although healing old issues and past traumas is always a good idea, sometimes the level of stress that comes up can feel overwhelming. That's when turning to a professional counselors trained in these techniques can be invaluable.

- **EMDR** (Eye Movement Desensitization and Reprocessing)
- **Brainspotting**
- **Emotional Freedom Technique**
- **Neuromodulation Technique**

The results of these therapies border on the miraculous, including reports of people healing from decades of stress and PTSD in as few as 5-10 sessions.

Patients frequently report that years of nagging thoughts and the endless replaying of painful images simply stop.

Patients often describe this sudden shift, like they dropped their old emotional baggage by the side of the road and just walked away.

### 8. Heart Math

Heart Math is an app (computer, mobile phone, and tablet) that uses simple bio-feedback techniques, tools, and technologies to help minimize the effects of stress and anxiety. If you are familiar with smart phone and computer apps and you only have a few minutes during the day to work on stress reduction, then Heart Math is a smart use of your time.

The HeartMath Inner Balance app and sensor work by replacing "the same old" negative responses to stress with feelings of confidence and ease. Heart-Math works by boosting the parasympathetic nervous system (the nervous system that calms the body) while decreasing the sympathetic nervous system (the system that gets you ready fight, run, or hide).

HeartMath improves focus, listening skills, and sleep — while decreasing anxiety, fatigue, and depression. Several studies have show that HeartMath enhances overall health, psychological health, and quality of life.

## IMMUNE SYSTEM

| Problems | Solutions |
|---|---|
| 1. Immune diseases/disorders (your body attacks itself) | 1. Consult a Functional Medicine doctor and test for depleted immune sys. |
| 2. Hidden Infections | 2. Test & treat for infections |
| 3. Allergies | 3. Test for food and environmental allergies |
| 4. Inflammation | 4. Low-glycemic diet |
| 5. Hormone Imbalances | 5. Test for hormone imbalances and treat them |

Figure 10.6 outlines some of the major ways that can prevent your immune system from healing your body of prostate cancer.

Your immune system performs a complex balancing act between destroying invading organisms (bacteria, viruses, and other pathogens), perceived threats (foods, pollen, molds, yeasts, and so on), and preventing your own defense systems from going too far and attacking your body, which can lead to auto-immune diseases.

An emergency room is another apt analogy about your immune system. Like an ER, your immune system takes care of what it perceives to be biggest problems first. The more health issues you have, the fewer resources your immune system has to devote to each one.

If your immune system is already depleted because of multiple allergies, infections, and lots of chronic inflammation, then it doesn't have the reserves required to fight off a new problem (like prostate cancer).

If you have prostate cancer, at some point in your recent past, your immune system was too busy taking care of other ongoing (chronic) problems to rise to the occasion when your cancer was still in its infancy.

**Here's the take-home message about your immune system:** In order to heal from prostate cancer, you have to start treating your body like a temple and taking care of your immune system so it can take care of you. Start by feeding your body what it needs (vegetables instead of sweet/starchy comfort foods), avoiding potential allergens (dietary or environmental), exercising daily, treating any chronic infections or diseases, starting a daily stress-reduction program, and having your hormones tested to see if your body is functioning well.

## HORMONES

| | Problems | Solutions |
|---|---|---|
| **HORMONES** | 1. Unhealthy testosterone-to-estrogen ratio (not enough testosterone or too much estrogen) | 1, 2. Test hormone levels & treat any imbalances |
| | 2. Low levels of free or total testosterone | |
| | 3. Immune system dysfunction | 3. Find a good Functional Medicine doctor |
| | 4. Metabolic issues | 4. Get lean: Body fat produces estrogen |
| | 5. Water stored in plastic bottles that leach estrogens | 5, 6. Block environmental estrogens & avoid "estrogenic" foods |
| | 6. Diet rich in soy and/or beer | |
| | 7. Difficulty falling asleep or difficulty staying asleep | 7. Find a good Functional Medicine doctor |

**Figure 10.7** gives a "tip of the iceberg" overview of how healthy hormone levels and ratios are essential to a healthy prostate. We recommend that you ask your doctor about your male hormone levels and a program to optimize them.

Healthy hormone levels are essential for good prostate health and function. Hormones like testosterone, estrogen, DHT, and DHEA all play an interconnected role in the health of your prostate.

Contrary to outdated medical information that was once considered the bedrock truth about prostate cancer and prostate health, normal testosterone levels do NOT contribute to a man's risk of developing prostate cancer.

In fact, men with low testosterone levels (Low T) are at a greater risk of developing prostate cancer. Recent medical studies continue to show that low testosterone:

- Does NOT protect men from prostate cancer
- INCREASES the risk of developing prostate cancer
- INCREASES the risk of developing the most aggressive kinds of prostate cancer (high-risk)

For more on testosterone and prostate cancer, see the Chapter 7 **Digging Deeper Section**. As with Low T, high levels of estrogen or a low testosterone-to-estrogen ratio can increase the risk of developing prostate cancer.

The three simplest ways to lower your estrogen levels (and raise your testosterone-to-estrogen ratio) are to

1. Get lean

2. Eliminate foods that contain estrogen and estrogen-like (estrogenic) compounds

3. Stop drinking water from plastic bottles.

Body fat also produces a type of estrogen. If you reduce your amount of body fat, you will reduce your estrogen levels too. Cutting out soy products (soy milk, tofu, tempeh, soy protein, and miso) and hops (beer) will shift your estrogen-to-testosterone ratio. Plastic bottles contain as many as 30 estrogen and estrogen-like compounds that leech into the water. Start drinking water from glass bottles instead.

We also recommend that you see a functional medical doctor and have your blood tested for these hormones:

- Testosterone (free and total)
- DHT
- DHEA
- Estrogen

**STRUCTURE**

| | Problems | Solutions |
|---|---|---|
| **STRUCTURE** | 1. Sacral or lower back injuries and/or surgeries | 1-6. Physical therapy, osteopathic manipulation, chiropractic, massage therapy, acupuncture, and MAT/NKT. (See **Page 263**) |
| | 2. Loose ligaments in lower back and/or pelvis | |
| | 3. Pelvic floor dysfunction | |
| | 4. Pudendal nerve entrapment | 1-6. Injection therapy such as PRP (Platelet Rich Plasma), stem cells, and Prolotherapy |
| | 5. Poor posture | |
| | 6. Organ and gland dysfunction within the bowl of the pelvis | |

**Figure 10.8** illustrates the impact that lower back and pelvic problems can have on prostate disease and prostate cancer. If you have prostate cancer/issues and anatomical problems in your lower back or pelvis, consider consulting one of the practitioners listed on **Page 263**.

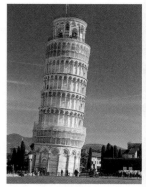

Your pelvic floor is an inter-woven web of muscles and connective tissues that form a hammock that keeps your intestines, urinary tract, and other internal organs in place. The best example we can think of to help you understand the importance of a healthy pelvic floor is the Leaning Tower of Pisa.

This famous leaning tower, where Galileo is said to have dropped two cannonballs to study the effect of mass on the speed of falling objects, doesn't lean because the tower is tilted. *It leans because the foundation is sinking on one side of the tower more than it is on the other.*

Think of your pelvic floor like the foundation beneath the Tower of Pisa. If the foundation of your pelvis is injured, tilted, too tight, too loose, or too tight in some areas and loose in others, then (like the part of the tower that is above ground) the organs inside your pelvis are at a greater risk of all sorts of structural complications.

Although pelvic floor problems are responsible for these complications, the real culprit usually lies in the structural integrity of the lower back and ligaments that connect

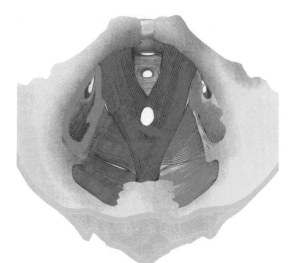

**Figure 10.9** Illustrates a birds eye view of a healthy pelvic floor — web of interconnected tissue that supports all the organs and glands of pelvis and lower abdomen — including the prostate.

the spine to the pelvis (iliolumbar ligaments) and hold the pelvis together (sacroiliac ligaments).

Spinal injuries, herniated discs, broken vertebrae or pelvic bones, spinal stenosis (diminished disc space), spinal surgeries, and other conditions can also interfere with the nerves that go to the pelvic floor and organs inside the "bowl" of your pelvis. (See **Figure 10.9**.)

Pelvic floor problems can affect everything from circulation, muscular strength, urinary function, digestion, inflammation, and infections ... to your ability to have and maintain an erection. In other words, the health of your lower back, pelvis, and pelvic floor have a huge impact on the health of your prostate.

Unlike changing your diet, getting more exercise, or learning to meditate — resolving pelvic floor, lower back, and other pelvic issues requires help from a skilled professional trained in hands-on body therapies such as:

- Physical Therapy
- Chiropractic manipulation
- Osteopathic medicine
- Acupuncture
- Rolfing
- Touch for Health
- Muscle Activation Technique (MAT)
- Neurokinetic Therapy (NKT)

**TOXIC SUBSTANCES**

| | Problems | Solutions |
|---|---|---|
| **TOXIC SUBSTANCES** | 1. From sources outside your body: soap, shampoo, cleansers, disinfectants, harsh chemicals, pesticides, herbicides, fungicides, fertilizers, heavy metals, and chemicals used in warfare like Agent Orange. | 1. Remove all harsh chemicals from your home: cleansers, pesticides, herbicides, fungicides, and so on. |
| | 2. Manufactured inside your body: Toxic substances usually created by bacteria and other microbes that live inside your body. | 1, 2. Eat organic fruits and vegetables — or at least non-GMO food. |
| | 3. Cannot be excreted: Toxins/toxic substances that your body is unable to excrete through normal channels: liver, intestines, lungs, kidneys, and skin. | 1, 3. Work with a Functional Medicine Doctor to improve your body's ability to get rid of toxins through normal pathways of excretion. |
| | 4. Poorly functioning immune system and long-term allergies. | 1, 4 & 5. Seek professional medical help from the best specialists you can afford. |
| | 5. Organ problems: liver, kidneys, lungs, heart, intestines, or skin. | |

**Figure 10.10** outlines how toxic substances come in three categories based on their origin and whether your body can process them: 1. From outside your body, 2. Made by your body, 3. Cannot be excreted by your body.

"Toxins" is a word that gets tossed around a lot by people who use cleanses and fasts as a form of self-purification. In that context, "toxins" could mean anything from the chemicals in household cleansers and weed killers to the byproducts of having a second helping of dessert and drinking too much wine last weekend.

Please don't misunderstand us: There are hundreds of peer-reviewed scientific papers that support the medicinal benefits of cleanses and fasts — especially intermittent fasting (micro-fasts) that last 12-16 hours.

For the purposes of this discussion, however, we will use the term "toxic substances" to mean both "biological toxins" (biochemicals produced by plants, animals or microbes that include spider bites, poison ivy, and the bacteria that causes botulism) and "environmental toxins" (industrial chemicals and heavy metals), as well as synthetic chemicals (pesticides, herbicides, and fungicides).

To these two groups of toxins, we should also add the ingredients of certain pharmaceutical medications. These ingredients cause the health problems that you hear rattled off quickly at the end of TV commercials: "XYZ may cause headache, nausea, vomiting, diarrhea, and in some cases, patients who take XYZ may develop the following conditions..."

Essentially, we are talking about chemicals that your body was not designed to metabolize or excrete. These chemicals come from three sources:

1. Outside your body
   (environmental toxins/toxic substances)
2. Biochemical
   (substances manufactured within your body)
3. Chemicals that cannot be excreted (usually toxins/ toxic substances that came from outside your body)

Because your body (mostly your lungs, liver, kidneys, intestines, and skin) has difficulty getting rid of these chemicals, these substances become trapped in your tissues, wreaking havoc on the DNA, cellular, organ, and whole-body levels.

As your body works overtime to get rid of these chemicals, the extra load weakens your organs (and immune system) and prevents them from performing their normal functions of cleansing and detoxifying the body.

So what can you do (short of moving to a deserted island) to eliminate your exposure to these toxic substances?

**Here are a few simple ideas:**

- Purchase organic and non-GMO food
- Dispose of all household cleaners that contain ingredients you cannot pronounce, and replace them with natural soap, baking soda, vinegar, and citrus solvents.
- Dispose of all herbicides, pesticides, and fungicides in your garage, in the basement, attic, or under the kitchen sink.
- Purchase bottled water in glass bottles or install a home water filtration system.

# THE PROSTATE CANCER PERFECT STORM

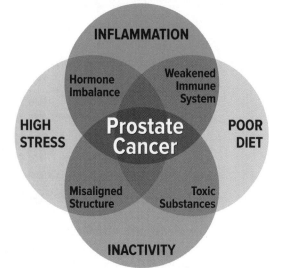

**Figure 10.11** displays the "Perfect Storm" of the seven health factors that create inflammation and increase the risk of prostate cancer. Obviously, factors like age, family history, other illnesses, and ethnicity also play a role in this diagram.

**INFLAMMATION MANAGEMENT SUMMARY**

Getting rid of inflammation is a complex process that requires more information than we can possibly present in a single chapter of a book. Here is a quick list of the top eight action steps we recommend (one for each health factor listed in this chapter — plus inflammation).

**1. Inflammation:** Treat prostatitis, BPH, and PIN.

**2. Diet:** Read food labels and reduce your consumption of all sweeteners, trans fats, and processed foods.

**3. Inactivity:** Walk, run, ride a bike, swim, hike, go to the gym, but raise your heart rate for 30 minutes every day.

**4. Stress:** Spend 20 minutes a day practicing stress reduction: prayer, meditation, Chi Gong, or Heart Math.

**5. Immune System:** Get treatment for all chronic allergies, lingering infections, and autoimmune disorders.

**6. Hormones:** Avoid all estrogens, estrogenic foods & beverages (soy & hops), and pseudo-estrogens in food storage containers (plastic bags and bottles).

**7. Structure:** Get evaluated for "pelvic floor dysfunction" by a physical therapist or other knowledgeable therapist.

**8. Toxic Substances:** Eat organic food & drink finely filtered water (not just water from a charcoal filter).

# Doctor Story
## DR. PHRANQ TAMBURRI, NMD

Naturopathic Medicine

Longevity Medical

Phoenix, Arizona

*I'm not in the business of telling people what to do. I am in the business of asking questions, listening, evaluating answers, and making suggestions based on those answers.*

*I built my practice around four questions:*

**1. What's the chance of you having clinically significant prostate cancer that is confined inside the gland and will be found at the same location in multiple prostate biopsies?**

*To answer that question, we usually have a long conversation about how we all have cancer in our bodies, Gleason scores, the number of prostate cancer cells replicating, the spectrum of PSA tests, Doppler MRI, digital rectal exams, which leads to the money question...*

**2. What's the chance that your prostate cancer will kill you in the next 5 years?**

*If your cancer is not metastatic, at what point will it cross the line and escape your prostate: 10 years, 20 years ... longer? In other words, what is your cancer's "metabolic momentum"? Predicting metabolic momentum is an amalgam of Gleason score, family & medical history, biopsy, PSA, and several other tests.*

**3. What else is adding to your PSA?**

*We need to know what we're treating. Besides prostate cancer, the #1 reason for a high PSA is prostatitis; the #2 reason is BPH. Most men have two or more going on at the same time.*

**4. How do we track your cancer over time?**

*Prostate cancer is like a polar bear: It can be a ferocious papa bear or a cute little cub. If we are trying to treat the bear and it's on an iceberg (BPH) in the middle of a blizzard (prostatitis), we've got to get the bear on land and stop the storm before we can treat it. If a patient has all three going on and his PSA falls, which one of the three improved?*

## LOOKING AHEAD

**CHAPTER 1:** You or your doctor is concerned about your prostate — We provide you with **Prostate 101**: where it lives, what it does, plus relevant statistics.

**CHAPTER 2:** Your doctor told you to **schedule a prostate biopsy** — We give you a **Prostate Biopsy Assessment Tool** to see if you actually need one, and what to expect if you do.

**CHAPTER 3:** You have a prostate biopsy — We explain the steps you need to take, whether you have a **negative biopsy or a positive biopsy**.

**CHAPTER 4:** You have a **positive prostate biopsy** — We provide you with a **Prostate Cancer Assessment Tool** to help you understand which kind of cancer you have.

**CHAPTER 5:** You need to select a prostate cancer treatment — We provide you with a summary of the most common types of treatment based on your **cancer risk type** (low-risk, moderate-risk, and high-risk).

**CHAPTER 6:** You have **low-risk, low-volume prostate cancer** and need to learn more about emerging treatments — We provide you with a summary of these treatments to help you understand the differences between focal, minimally invasive, alternative, whole gland, and traditional treatments.

**CHAPTER 7:** You have prostate cancer that is more advanced than low-risk, low-volume and need to know more about **whole-gland treatments** (both stand-alone traditional and combination treatments) — We provide you with a summary of these treatments.

**CHAPTER 8:** You want to know the **success and complication rates** for each type of treatment and for each cancer risk type (low-risk, moderate-risk, and high-risk) — We provide you with unbiased information to support your decision-making process.

**CHAPTER 9:** You feel **overwhelmed** by the news of a positive prostate biopsy — We give you the tools to surf this tidal wave of emotion and overcome the feeling of panic that almost always accompanies a positive biopsy report.

**CHAPTER 10:** You want to **use your cancer diagnosis as a springboard to better health** — We help you address your wellness goals with a proven plan that covers inflammation, diet, inactivity, stress, immune system, hormone optimization, structure, and removing toxic substances.

**WHAT'S NEXT?**

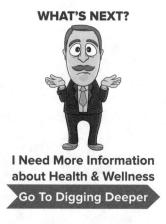

**I Need More Information about Health & Wellness**

Go To Digging Deeper

# WELCOME TO THE TOOLBOX
# CHAPTER 10 **TOOLBOX**

THIS TOOLBOX IS DESIGNED TO HELP YOU APPLY THE
SEVEN HEALTH FACTORS THAT IMPACT INFLAMMATION
AND THE RISK OF HAVING PROSTATE CANCER. THE
GOAL HERE IS TO HELP YOU REGAIN YOUR OVERALL
HEALTH AND THE HEALTH OF YOUR PROSTATE:

1. **Diet**

2. **Inactivity**

3. **Stress**

4. **Immune System**

5. **Hormones**

6. **Structure**

7. **Toxic Substances**

**The Chapter 10 Toolbox** gives you the opportunity to put the information presented in this chapter to work for you right away.

The beauty of the seven health areas listed above is that they will benefit anyone, but they are designed for men who have been recently diagnosed with prostate cancer or concerned about its prevention.

Regardless of your diagnosis, the kind of cancer you have, your age, or which type of treatment you select, you can apply the information about these seven health areas immediately and begin to receive their benefits.

Will they cure your cancer? That depends upon your age, which kind of cancer you have, how much, where it is in your prostate, and a host of other factors.

If you look at **Figure 10.12** on **Page 271**, you'll see two empty spaces at the end of each section: "pick two causes listed above" and "pick two treatments listed above."

These spaces allow you to choose two of the bullet points listed in each health area and begin working on them. Some of the actions are simple: "Move your body: Stand up every hour, walk around, do chores, stay active." Other actions are more complicated: "Eat mostly organic vegetables" or "test hormones levels & treat any imbalances."

T O O L B O X

As with all things in this book, begin at a pace that works for you. If shifting your diet and exercise habits is all you can handle, start there.

On **Page 266** we also included our top 8 actions steps we recommend for each health area.

**Remember:** It's more important to get started and stay on your path than it is to procrastinate about picking the perfect actions. So, let's get started.

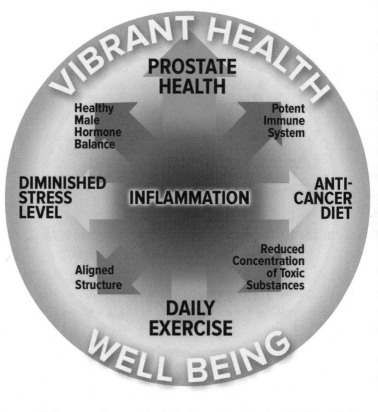

**Figure 10.2** reverses the seven health factors that we introduced in **Figure 10.0** at the beginning of the chapter. As you can see, if you reverse the direction of these arrows (health factors) from pointing towards disease to pointing towards health and well being, you reverse the course of your condition — from the inside out.

| | PROBLEMS | SOLUTIONS |
|---|---|---|
| **INFLAMMATION** | 1. Immune System | 1. Treat infections & prostatitis |
| | 2. Diet | 2. Eat a low-glycemic (low-sugar) diet |
| | 3. Toxic Substances | 3. See **Page 264** |
| | 4. Inactivity | 4. Exercise 30 minutes a day |
| | 5. Structure | 5. See **Page 262** |
| | 6. Stress | 6. Start a stress reduction program |
| | 7. Hormones | 7. Have your hormone levels and ratios checked by a certified functional medicine doctor |
| | 8. Prostate | 8. Begin our 7-point program |
| | **PICK TWO PROBLEMS LISTED ABOVE.** | **PICK TWO SOLUTIONS LISTED ABOVE.** |
| **DIET** | 1. Insulin/sugar problems & toxic chemicals in food | 1. Eat mostly organic vegetables (especially cruciferous vegetables) and organic fruit |
| | 2. High-glycemic diet | 2. Low-glycemic diet |
| | 3. Growth hormone/antibiotics in food | 3. Eat animal protein that is free of all hormones and antibiotics |
| | 4. Processed foods and trans fats | 4. Restore the balance between omega 3 & omega 6 fatty acids |
| | 5. Grains | 5. Limit grains and breads |
| | 6. Poor quality oils | 6. Use more olive and coconut oil |
| | 7. Alcohol, sweetened sodas, and caffeine consumption | 7. Limit alcohol, sodas, and caffeine |
| | **PICK TWO PROBLEMS LISTED ABOVE.** | **PICK TWO SOLUTIONS LISTED ABOVE.** |

**Figure 10.12** gives you the opportunity to use the seven health factors from Chapter 10 and select four aspects of each heading that you would like to use as a springboard to improve your health. We invite you to use the space below each heading to write down two "problems" you would like to work on, as well as two "solutions" you would like to implement.

**TOOLBOX**

| | PROBLEMS | SOLUTIONS |
|---|---|---|
| **INACTIVITY** | 1. Chronic inflammation, pain, and habitual stress | 1-3. Move your body: Stand up every hour, walk around, do chores, stay active |
| | 2. Accumulation of toxic substances in excess body fat leads to being both overweight and unhealthy | 1-3. Build your strength, endurance, and flexibility slowly over time. Exercise daily but avoid overtraining. |
| | 3. Lack of exercise leads to stagnant circulation, fatigue, depression, and a diminished desire to move your body | 1-3. Combine slow/steady exercise with resistance training and interval training, which improves circulation and removes toxic substances |
| | **PICK TWO PROBLEMS LISTED ABOVE.** | **PICK TWO SOLUTIONS LISTED ABOVE.** |
| **STRESS** | 1. A prostate cancer diagnosis | 1. The "right fit" prostate cancer treatment plan |
| | 2. Fears about money and your close relationships | 2. Seek sound financial support and open up to the people closest to you |
| | 3. Work-related issues | 3. Talk with co-workers and supervisors (if you can) |
| | 4. Feeling overwhelmed | 4. Daily deep breathing practice promotes feeling calm |
| | 5. Too much cortisol and adrenaline in your system | 5. Daily exercise, limit stimulants, prayer/meditation |
| | **PICK TWO PROBLEMS LISTED ABOVE.** | **PICK TWO SOLUTIONS LISTED ABOVE.** |
| **IMMUNE SYSTEM** | 1. Immune diseases/disorder (your body attacks itself) | 1. Consult a Functional Medicine doctor and test for depleted immune system |
| | 2. Hidden Infections | 2. Test & treat for infections |
| | 3. Allergies | 3. Test for food and environmental allergies |
| | 4. Inflammation | 4. Low-glycemic diet |
| | 5. Hormone Imbalances | 5. Test for hormone imbalances and treat them |
| | **PICK TWO PROBLEMS LISTED ABOVE.** | **PICK TWO SOLUTIONS LISTED ABOVE.** |

| | PROBLEMS | SOLUTIONS |
|---|---|---|
| **HORMONES** | 1. Unhealthy testosterone-to-estrogen ratio (not enough testosterone or too much estrogen) | 1, 2. Test hormone levels & treat any imbalances |
| | 2. Low levels of free or total testosterone | |
| | 3. Immune system dysfunction | 3.    Find a good Functional Medicine doctor |
| | 4. Metabolic issues | 4.    Get lean: Body fat produces estrogen |
| | 5. Water stored in plastic bottles that leach estrogens | 5, 6. Block environmental estrogens & avoid "estrogenic" foods |
| | 6. Diet rich in soy and/or beer | |
| | 7.  Difficulty falling asleep or difficulty staying asleep | 7.    Find a good Functional Medicine doctor |
| | **PICK TWO PROBLEMS LISTED ABOVE.** | **PICK TWO SOLUTIONS LISTED ABOVE.** |
| | • | |
| **STRUCTURE** | 1.  Sacral or low back injuries and/or surgeries | 1-6. Physical therapy, osteopathic manipulation, chiropractic, massage therapy, acupuncture, and MAT/NKT (See **Page 263**) |
| | 2. Loose ligaments in lower back and/or pelvis | |
| | 3. Pelvic floor dysfunction | 1-6. Injection therapy such as PRP (Platelet Rich Plasma), stem cells, and Prolotherapy |
| | 4. Pudendal nerve entrapment | |
| | 5. Poor posture | |
| | 6. Organ and gland dysfunction within the bowl of the pelvis | |
| | **PICK TWO PROBLEMS LISTED ABOVE.** | **PICK TWO SOLUTIONS LISTED ABOVE.** |

TOOLBOX

| | PROBLEMS | SOLUTIONS |
|---|---|---|
| **TOXIC SUBSTANCES** | 1. From sources outside your body: soaps, shampoos, cleansers, disinfectants, harsh chemicals, pesticides, herbicides, fungicides, fertilizers, heavy metals, and chemicals used in warfare like Agent Orange | 1. Remove all harsh chemicals from your home: pesticides, herbicides, fungicides, and so on.<br>1. Replace household cleaners with simple solutions like vinegar, baking soda, citrus solvents, and soap. |
| | 2. Manufactured inside your body: Toxic substances usually manufactured by bacteria and other microbes that live inside your body | 1, 2. Eat organic fruits and vegetables — or at least non-GMO food. |
| | 3. Cannot be excreted: Toxins/toxic substances that your body is unable to excrete through normal channels: liver, intestines, lungs, kidneys, and skin. | 1, 3. Work with a Functional Medicine Doctor to improve your body's ability to get rid of toxins through normal pathways of excretion. |
| | 4. Poorly functioning immune system and long-term allergies. | 1, 4 & 5. Seek professional medical help from the best specialists you can afford to see. |
| | 5. Organ problems: liver, kidneys, lungs, heart, intestines, or skin. | |
| | **PICK TWO PROBLEMS LISTED ABOVE.** | **PICK TWO SOLUTIONS LISTED ABOVE.** |
| | | |

## WHAT IS FUNCTIONAL MEDICINE?

*According to the Institute for Functional Medicine, "Functional Medicine addresses the underlying causes of disease, using a systems-oriented approach and engaging both patient and practitioner in a therapeutic partnership. It is an evolution in the practice of medicine that better addresses the healthcare needs of the 21st century."*

### HOW IS FUNCTIONAL MEDICINE DIFFERENT?
*Functional Medicine integrates the latest scientific information with lifestyle and environmental factors to create a new medical system that allows healthcare professionals to better understand what each patient needs.*

### WHERE TO FIND A FUNCTIONAL MEDICAL DOCTOR IN YOUR AREA
*For more information about Functional Medicine and Functional Medical doctors in your area, we invite you to visit the following websites:*

*http://www.abihm.org*
*http://www.abihm.org/search-doctors*
*https://www.functionalmedicine.org*

TOOLBOX

# GUIDE TO EATING OUT

## Restaurants

1. Say, "No thank you" to the bread or chips and salsa that automatically arrive on your table. These high-glycemic carbs are metabolized just like sugar. You are essentially "packing on the pounds" before your meal arrives.

2. Start your meal with a small salad. Salads usually arrive first and take the edge off your hunger, and your meal has a healthy start.

3. Consider ordering several side dishes or something from the "a la Carte" menu. That way, you can *get your vegetables* and still feel satisfied.

4. Avoid "all you can eat" buffet-style restaurants. They promote overeating.

5. Skip dessert. You will feel lighter, look thinner, and have fewer health issues.

## Parties

1. Eat a healthy mini-meal before you go. Include some veggies, protein, and healthy fats. Try a simple spring-mix salad with some chicken or canned tuna, sprinkle in a few seeds or nuts, and add half an avocado. It takes under 10 minutes to prepare.

2. Bring a couple of bottles of sparkling water.

3. Alcoholic beverages are the kings of "empty calories." Alcohol is metabolized into fat in your liver, and alcohol is a carcinogen. Best to avoid it. If you drink alcohol, alternate between alcoholic beverages and sparkling water.

4. Arrive a little late. You'll spend less time "grazing" the finger food.

5. Bring a healthy side dish or appetizer. That way, you have a go-to item — instead of nachos, pizza, Buffalo chicken wings, or seven-layer dip.

## At Work

1. Bring your own lunch. This practice will save you $5-10/day, and give you more control over what you eat. You also won't find yourself staring at a vending machine at 3:30, trying to decide between a Snickers bar or bag of Cheetos.

2. Eat less bread. You'll lose weight and lower your insulin production. Make yourself an open-faced sandwich. If you eat out, order a lettuce or tortilla wrap.

3. Avoid sweetened energy drinks. If you feel run down, have an unsweetened cup of coffee or tea. If your job allows, go for a 10-minute walk instead.

4. Bring your own bottled water (unless your work provides it). Avoid the estrogen by drinking water from glass bottles whenever possible.

5. Avoid crashing and burning by keeping a ready supply of healthy snacks in your desk, locker, or car: nuts, seeds, low-glycemic fruit, and bottled water.

TOOLBOX

**NOTES:**

TOOLBOX

# SPECIAL SECTION

# Spouse
# Stories

# SILENT HEROES

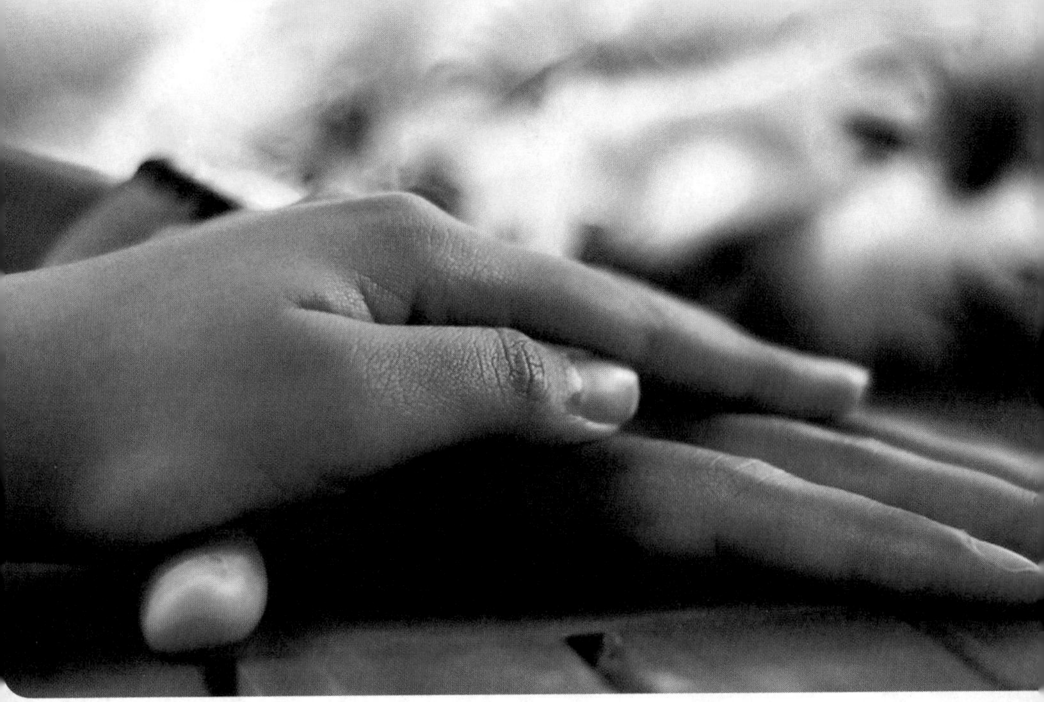

Stalwart

Intuitive

Loving

Empathetic

Nurturing

Tireless

*... In a word "Heroes."*

That's what we call the spouses, partners, family members, and friends of men who develop prostate cancer. These are the people who pick up the slack, take the notes, ask doctors the hard questions, hold the hands, speak up, help make the big decisions (and the little ones), cook the meals, carry the extra load, care for everyone else, create diversions, listen and listen and listen some more, but most of all ... "stand by their man." These selfless acts of love and devotion are what allows prostate cancer patients to breathe a little easier, make the best possible treatment decision, then get on with the business of living.

# NO CANCER DIAGNOSIS IS EASY ... BUT THESE PEOPLE MAKE IT EASIER

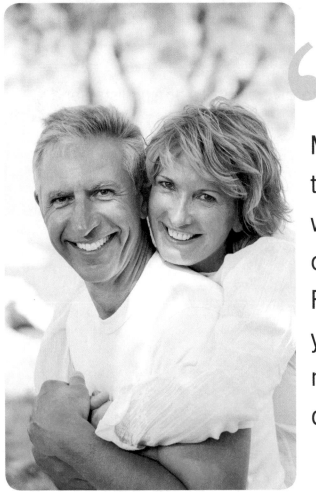

> My main message to partners of men with prostate cancer is simple: Focus on how much you love them — no matter what you're doing..."

## Marriage lowers the risk of dying from cancer

*Married men and women have a 20 percent better chance of surviving cancer than single people.*

*Researchers at the Dana-Farber Cancer Institute and Brigham and Women's Hospital in Boston analyzed data from 734,800 cancer patients. They found that men had a 23 percent higher chance of beating cancer if they were married.*

# CHRIS

Here are a few things I learned from supporting and loving my husband, Richard, during his time with prostate cancer.

It's OK to feel afraid, and there's less of an objective reason to feel afraid than you think. Prostate cancer, when properly treated, has a low remission rate.

**Two memories come to mind:**

1.   **Fear is part of the process:** After the diagnosis, I'd wake up feeling good, then a wave of fear would hit me like a bucket of cold water.

2.   **Intense emotions are natural:** Right after the surgery, the surgeon called and said this was a tricky surgery (and he had done thousands) but he thought he got it all. My insides melted with relief when I heard that.

The particulars of your situation matter, so take the time to get information. For example, Richard's second biopsy changed his stage to from low-risk to moderate-risk.

Lingering pelvic pain from that biopsy meant his insides were literally "glued together" from inflammation. After much research, and a bit of happenstance, we learned that surgery was the best option for Richard.

Also, we received great help from an incredible peer support system that I found online and one very knowledgeable prostate cancer mentor. The men and women in the support system were generous with their time and wisdom. I laugh now when I think about the number of men I've talked to about their private parts. Privacy goes out the window with prostate cancer. I think that's a good thing.

Finally, sex matters. Get some good books about sex after prostate cancer. Make the most out of what you have. I talked with men who had good sex but no erections. If you have any problems at all, I suggest you see a good sex therapist sooner than later. Our sex therapist's message to me was straight forward: Right now, you're responsible for making things work. Don't judge. Be open and just focus on loving.

My main message to partners of men with prostate cancer is simple: Focus on how much you love them — no matter what you're doing — whether you're feeling scared, doing research, meeting with doctors, going through treatment, having sex, or just drinking a cup of tea together at breakfast.

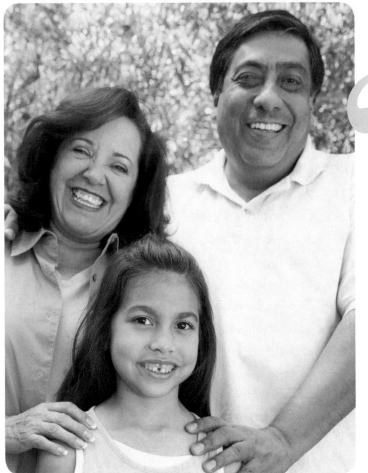

"We were told that surgery was our only option."

In 50 percent of the cancers studied by the researchers at the Dana-Farber Cancer Institute and Brigham and Women's Hospital, having a spouse was more beneficial than chemotherapy.

# REATHA

Here's my experience after we found out that my husband, Steve, had prostate cancer.

After the first biopsy, we were told the cancer was so small that the recommendation was to just watch it for a year and see what happened. After a year passed, another biopsy was done. This time, the cancer was more aggressive than they previously thought, so surgery was scheduled to remove Steve's prostate.

We were told that surgery was our only option.

Shortly after we scheduled the surgery, we began researching all the potential side effects from surgery. We were both very dissatisfied when we learned about the possible problems in terms of quality of life, and what that would mean for Steve and for us as a couple.

A few weeks before the surgery, Steve met a man who had been diagnosed with prostrate cancer several years ago. The man explained that he too had been scheduled for surgery when he heard of an alternative treatment called Cyberknife.

He explained that this type of treatment could be done over a period of a few days with little or no side effects, and that he was very happy with the results!

We looked into Cyberknife, scheduled an appointment, and had the procedure done in less than a month. Almost two years later, and Steve has had no side effects other than the occasional trouble urinating (treated with Flomax). Best of all: Steve's last PSA test was excellent with no sign of cancer.

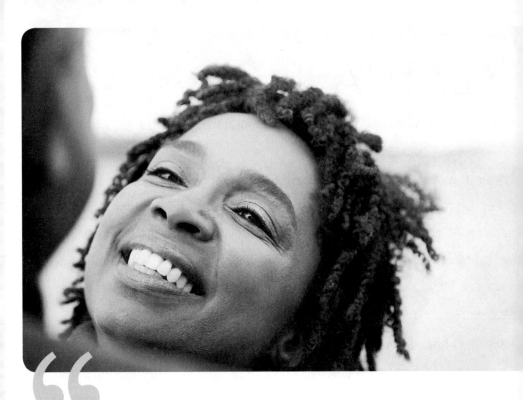

"He never said how afraid he was that he might be very sick or even die, but those feelings had taken over and he was now really beside himself."

*In the United States, the lifetime divorce rate is approximately 50 percent; for chronically ill people, the rate is closer to 75 percent.*

# SANDY

### The Agenda

After visiting a few different prostate cancer specialists, we were headed to Porter Hospital to talk with yet another one.

We had already met with a general practitioner, who referred us to a surgeon (who advised us to have surgery), a consultant (who laid out several different approaches), and we were now going to see a radiologist.

My husband, who grew up with the adage "You are nothing without your health," was trying to remain calm as we were overwhelmed with all this information. Sometimes, however, he panicked and felt completely out of control.

As he drove to the hospital for this appointment, he began searching the car for his agenda. After driving erratically for several miles, he finally pulled over and became convinced he had left it on the roof of the car when we left home. He became extremely upset, believing that he had lost it.

He insisted that I drop him off at the hospital, go back the same way we came and look for it on the road all the way back home. I told him we'd look for it after the appointment, but he absolutely could not accept that. He was in full panic mode. His fear, need for control, and anxiety were all focused onto the agenda and his need to find it. He never said how afraid he was or that he might be very sick or even die, but those feelings had taken over and he was now really beside himself.

I left him at the doctor's office and drove home where I found the agenda on the kitchen counter. I returned to the radiologist's office just as they were finishing, and I drove us home.

We had several more very tense weeks before the final decision was made to have surgery (radical prostatectomy). It was very successful, and many years later he is still cancer free.

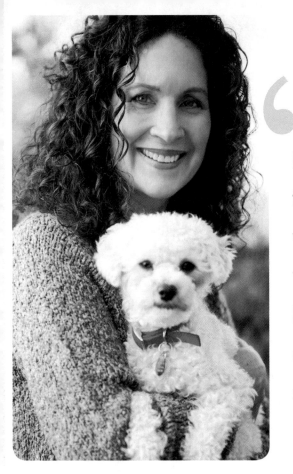

"I had barely started to mourn my mom when I was suddenly faced with what felt like insurmountable challenges. My life was starting to unravel."

*Dr. Michael J. Glantz of the University of Utah Huntsman Cancer Institute and colleagues from three other institutions collected data on 515 patients who received a diagnoses of a brain tumor or multiple sclerosis from 2001 through 2006.*

*Women in the study who were diagnosed with either of these diseases were seven times more likely to become separated or divorced than men with similar health problems.*

*When the men in this study became seriously ill, only 3 percent got separated or divorced. Among women, however, the separation/divorce rate was close to 21 percent.*

# ANA

My husband was diagnosed with prostate cancer a couple of months after my mother passed away.

I had barely started to mourn my mom when I was suddenly faced with what felt like insurmountable challenges. My life was starting to unravel.

The way I saw it, I had to two choices: crumple into nothingness or make myself stronger than ever.

The first choice was out of the question; it felt selfish and irresponsible. The two people I loved the most needed me: My father (who was suffering from Alzheimer's disease) had to be protected and cared for, and now, my husband needed my help and care too.

My time for grieving would have to wait for those few moments a week when I was alone. I didn't want to burden my ailing father or my newly diagnosed husband with my grief, my fears, or my concerns.

My saving grace was our doctor, who also happened to be an expert in prostate cancer. She immediately helped us weigh our options and literally took my husband and me under her wing. It was an immense relief and a blessing. Suddenly, we weren't alone.

More than that, I wasn't alone. I didn't have to do it all myself. Our doctor helped us through a maze of questions, doubts, and fears. Her wealth of knowledge was the balm for my anxiety.

I'll never forget the day she put it all into perspective for me. She said that in a couple of years, this nightmare would be behind us — a memory. She added that my husband was better off having this kind of prostate cancer than he would be with a permanent condition like diabetes.

This prostate cancer experience taught me so much about myself and about my husband. I discovered his resilience, his moral strength and his profound love for me. I found my resolve, determination, and faith to be stronger than I ever knew I could be. And love, there was always so much love all the way around.

My husband's treatment began with brachytherapy (radioactive seed implantation), which was followed with several weeks of radiation therapy. The irony is, shortly after my husband finished his treatments, my father passed away.

" Lesson #1: Never neglect the details, not even the tiny ones. That's when my husband's fight for life, really began."

*According to a 2004 article in the* Southern Medical Journal, *a study by Duke University Medical Center revealed that "nearly 90 percent [of patients] reported using religion to some degree to cope, and more than 40 percent indicated that it was the most important factor that kept them going."*

# KAY

It's been sixteen years since we've had cancer (my husband had prostate cancer). I try to appreciate how precious each and every day is — and not take my husband for granted. Many of our marital conflicts over the years have been a result of the stress and uncertainty of this disease and where it might lead us.

I have always been good at taking care of the little details. But somehow I neglected to ask my husband's primary care physician what his PSA numbers were. We were repeatedly told they were normal, but we never knew the actual numbers. The doctor knew my husband had received prostate cancer treatment (brachytherapy), but for reasons I'll never understand, he neglected to mention my husband's creeping PSA — until it was 6!

I was speechless! How can this be? We took care of this problem years ago. They must have missed some areas. Then my husband's doctor tried to blame us for my husband's rising PSA. He also gave us NO hope for the future.

Lesson #1: Never neglect the details, not even the tiny ones. That's when my husband's fight for life, really began.

My husband has never liked going to the doctor, he doesn't like prescription medications, and he can't stand being told not to eat or drink this or that. With this disease, however, he has had to make some changes. I made myself in charge all his appointments, prescriptions, and supplements.

We have kept our faith strong through all the ups and downs. Also, we never pass up the opportunity to remind friends and relatives (especially our son) about how important it is to have yearly PSA tests whenever we can. But for now, I'm happy for the life we have together. Every night I glance over at my husband while he sleeps, and thank God for the opportunity for more time together, and how grateful I am that he's still with me.

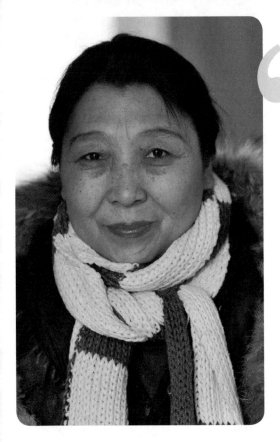

" I would advise spouses to be respectful of how your husband chooses to deal with their diagnosis (publicly or privately), and to always insist on getting a second opinion before rushing into treatment. Lastly, tell your spouse how much he means to you. Hugs are great medicine."

*As 2013 study published in* The Journal of Clinical Oncology *found that married patients were less likely to have metastatic disease when they are diagnosed, more likely to receive definitive therapy, and less likely to die as a result of their cancer.*

# JOAN

My husband, Jeff, was diagnosed with prostate cancer by accident.

After an unexpected layoff, Jeff scheduled a physical before our benefits expired. He was told to call the doctor back, and we were both in disbelief after hearing the dreaded "C" word. He had no symptoms, felt great, was active — and only 49 years old.

I was glad I was able to go with him to his appointments to provide emotional support — and learn the facts firsthand. It was a very emotional and crazy time, with so much information to absorb. I felt much better when we learned that his cancer was detected early, so it was very treatable. I could help relay this information to our children and family members, since they were also affected by the news.

The experience of being diagnosed and going through all the tests was especially scary for Jeff. Prostate cancer took his father very quickly.

Our first appointment was with a surgeon, who said Jeff was a perfect candidate for surgery. Jeff wanted to rush into surgery and get the cancer removed as soon as possible, so we scheduled surgery right away. Luckily, the doctor had to cancel the surgery. That cancellation opened the door for a second opinion with a urologist oncologist who recommended brachytherapy (radioactive seed implants).

After taking the time to research all the facts, Jeff felt most comfortable with brachytherapy, so that's the treatment we chose.

Many men don't want to talk with their spouse, family members, or other people close to them. I was glad Jeff was the opposite. He wanted to talk about his diagnosis and let other men know how important it was to get tested. Just by being open, Jeff received a huge outpouring of support, and he learned that many other men he knew had also gone through prostate cancer treatment.

I would advise spouses to be respectful of how your husband chooses to deal with their diagnosis (publicly or privately), and to always insist on getting a second opinion before rushing into treatment. Lastly, tell your spouse how much he means to you. Hugs are great medicine.

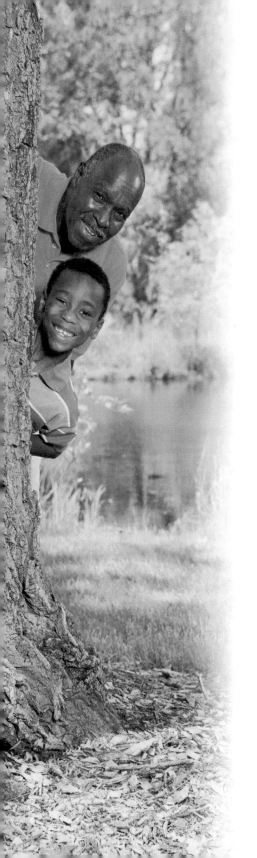

LOVE

MARRIAGE

ENHANCE

HEALTH

AND

HEALING

# Five Outstanding Resources for Spouses and Partners

### 1. American Cancer Society
*http://www.cancer.org/treatment/treatmentsandsideeffects/ emotionalsideeffects/copingwithcancerineverydaylife/ a-message-of-hope-for-spouses-families-friends*

### 2. Cancer Care
*http://www.cancercare.org/support_groups/ 77-caregiver_support_group_spouses_partners*

### 3. Us Too
- *http://www.ustoo.org/Spouses-Partners-Family*
- *http://www.ustoo.org/Us-Too-International*

### 4. You Are Not Alone Now
*http://www.yananow.org/ProstateCancerWomen.shtml*

### 5. Prostate Cancer Foundation
*http://www.pcf.org/site/c.leJRIROrEpH/b.5856543/k.6599/ Finding_a_Support_Group.htm*

# YOUR THOUGHTS

# Digging Deeper

# INTRODUCTION

**The following discussion of PSA screening was included here to help you understand how valuable PSA is to diagnosing and treating prostate cancer.**

- The Great American PSA Controversy

# The Great American PSA Controversy

The effectiveness of PSA blood tests is inarguable.

This statement is confirmed by a 2002 study of 2,042 prostate cancer patients at the Walter Reed Army Medical Center between 1988 and 1998. In this study, the percentage of men who were initially diagnosed with metastatic prostate cancer (disease that had already spread outside the prostate) decreased from 17 percent between 1988 - 1990 to 4 percent from 1996 - 1998. The percentage of patients who, on initial evaluation, had prostate cancer that extended through the prostate capsule or into adjacent structures fell from 15 to 6 percent over the same period.

According to *Advanced Urology*, due to the wide-spread use of PSA testing since the mid 1990s, fewer men are dying of prostate cancer. For example, 90 percent of all prostate cancers now are discovered before they spread outside the prostate. Thanks to this early detection advantage, the five-year survival rate is nearly 100 percent.

By helping diagnose more men when prostate cancers is in an early stage, PSA testing allows patients to consult with their physicians about the full spectrum of treatment options — everything from active surveillance to surgery. Without early detection, however, many of these options are off the table because the cancer is too advanced.

Here's a little data to support that claim: Between 2008-2012, 21.4 out of 100,000 U.S. men died from prostate cancer, compared to 39.2 per 100,000 men in 1992, just before PSA testing became widespread. That's an **83 percent improvement!**

In 2012, the U.S. Preventive Services Task Force (USPSTF) recommended *against* prostate-specific antigen (PSA) screening for prostate cancer. The USPSTF claims "There is moderate or high certainty that the service has no net benefit or that the harms outweigh the benefits."

We have one simple question: **Why?**

For a thorough answer to that question, we direct you to the USPSTF's website: (*http://www.uspreventiveservicestaskforce.org/page/document/recommendationstatementfinal/prostate-cancer-screening*). Before you go there, we recommend you consider the following information:

- Early cancer detection and treatment, due in part to PSA testing, is the primary reason the death rate from prostate cancer has fallen in recent years.

- If your PSA total is higher than 2.0 ng/ml, additional tests (4Kscore Test, PCA3, and SelectMDx) combined with preventative lifestyle measures are highly encouraged.
- Eighty-five percent of men who have prostate cancer also have a PSA above 4.0 ng/ml.
- Twenty-five percent of men who have a PSA between 4.0 and 10.0 ng/ml and a normal DRE have prostate cancer.
- If your PSA is more than 10.0 ng/ml, you have a 50-75 percent risk of prostate cancer, depending upon your DRE.
- If your PSA free is below 10 percent, there is a 56 percent risk of prostate cancer.
- Not everyone with an elevated PSA has prostate cancer, and not everyone with a normal PSA is cancer free either.
- PSA rises with non-cancerous BPH (benign prostatic hyperplasia), a condition many men have as they get older.
- PSA increases with prostatitis, an infection/inflammation of the prostate.
- Your PSA goes up slowly as you age, even with no prostate complications.
- Ejaculation can cause a temporary rise in PSA. For this reason, most practitioners recommend abstaining from ejaculation for a full 48 hours before being tested.
- Medications such as Proscar and Avodart falsely lower PSA levels. If you are taking these medications, let your doctors know so they can adjust for them.
- Riding a bicycle also increases your PSA numbers. Avoid cycling for 48 hours before a PSA test.

## PSA Screening: Our Position

Our position is that a thorough medical history followed by a digital rectal exam (DRE), plus a PSA free and PSA total blood tests is the best way to *begin* an evaluation of a man's prostate.

There are two major types of PSA screening (PSA total and PSA free) and two types of calculations based on PSA total (PSA velocity and PSA density). Each of these four PSA numbers provide doctors and patients with different pieces of the prostate puzzle. If you had all four of these PSA numbers, you would have a much better understanding about the health of your prostate.

We also believe that the best use of PSA screening is in combination with newer, more advanced tests for prostate cancer such as Select MDx, 4Ks-core Test, and PCA3. The combination of all these tests provides doctors with a more accurate and comprehensive picture about what's going on inside a patient's prostate. (For more information on these and others tests please go to **Chapter 2** and the **Chapter 2 Toolbox.** )

## Check Engine Light Analogy

We invite you to think about PSA screening as you would a dashboard "check engine" light. If you drive a newer model car, you will notice all sorts of different warning lights when you first start your car. Still, none of these warning lights tell you exactly what is causing the problem: a blown head gasket, a coolant system leak, a fouled spark plug, a frayed belt, a faulty sensor ... and so on.

What these "check engine" lights do tell you is that something is wrong, and you need to get some professional help.

The same is true for a basic PSA screening (PSA total). It does NOT tell you the source of the problem; it only tells you that there is one — something is causing an abnormal amount of PSA to leak out of your prostate. Combining PSA total with PSA free, PSA velocity, and PSA density (which requires an image of your prostate) can help pinpoint the problem, as well as rule out certain conditions.

For example, an elevated PSA could be caused by an enlarged prostate (BPH), prostatitis, and several other conditions. Without additional testing, there's no way of knowing whether prostate cancer is causing of the rise in PSA.

## So Why All the Controversy about PSA Screening?

From our perspective, discouraging men from having routine (annual) PSA screening after 50 is like throwing the baby out with the bath water.

Yes, in the past, PSA testing was overused by urologists in a rush to have patients undergo a prostate biopsy. The thinking used to be that the earliest hint of prostate cancer meant the patient needed a radical prostatectomy (surgery) ASAP. Catch the cancer early, remove the prostate, and the patient has better chance of living a full life.

The problem with this simplistic narrative is that treatment complications can be worse than living with a minute amount of prostate cancer that will never develop into an aggressive form of the disease.

In some cases, the long-term negative psychological effects of permanent impotence and incontinence can be more devastating than the knowledge of living with a minute amount of low-risk prostate cancer.

In other words, the treatment can be worse than the disease. For many urologists, that's a bitter pill to swallow.

## The United States Preventative Services Task Force (USPSTF)

Since 2008, the USPSTF has been on a mission to discourage primary care physicians from providing PSA tests for their patients. Their findings indicate that the benefits of PSA screening are outweighed by the risk of harm associated with the additional procedures recommended after an elevated PSA screening.

We agree with the USPSTF that prostate cancer surgery (radical prostatectomy) and many types of external beam radiation are "overkill" in cases where men have of low-risk, low-volume prostate cancer. Men with this kind of cancer are better candidates for either active surveillance or some of the emerging (focal) treatments we discuss in **Chapter 6.**

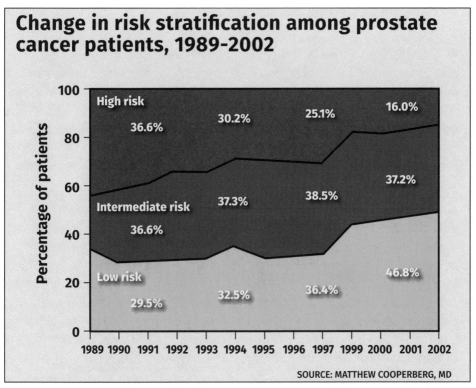

**Figure DD Intro 1.0** illustrates the dramatic decrease in the identification of high-risk patients after the use of PSA testing became widespread (middle 1990s). Also, note the significant increase in the number of low-risk patients after the middle 1990s.

However, throwing PSA screening "under the bus" just because it effectively identifies many cases of low-risk, low-volume prostate cancer (as well as many cases of high-risk, high-volume prostate cancer) would be like punishing your children for eating all the food on their plates because it could lead to obesity.

It is our opinion that the USPSTF position misses the mark and their recommendations ignore the value of combining PSA screening with newer diagnostic tests.

But don't just take our word. Let's go to the source.

## PSA Screening: The USPSTF Position

The following paragraphs were taken directly from the USPSTF website (*http://www.uspreventiveservicestaskforce.org/Page/Document/UpdateSummaryFinal/prostate-cancer-screening*).

We have woven this narrative together using direct quotes from the USPSTF website. The only alteration to the text is that we have inserted ellipsis (...) to indicate a break in the narrative. We apologize if the transitions between paragraphs is a little choppy.

> ❝ *(PSA)-based screening programs have been advocated as a possible means to reduce the mortality rate, as the test can detect asymptomatic, early-stage tumors. Beginning in the 1990s, utilization of the PSA test became widespread in U.S. clinical practice; data from nationally representative surveys and community primary care clinics consistently show that the majority of American men aged 50 years and older receive regular PSA tests...*

> ❝ *In 2008, the U.S. Preventive Services Task Force (USPSTF) recommended against screening for prostate cancer in men aged 75 years and older. It concluded that the evidence was insufficient to assess the balance of benefits and harms of screening for prostate cancer in men younger than age 75 years, due to a lack of evidence that screening reduced mortality. The subsequent publication of initial mortality results from two large, randomized controlled trials of prostate cancer screening (the* U.S. Prostate, Lung, Colorectal, and Ovarian Cancer Screening Trial *and the* European Randomized Study of Screening for Prostate Cancer *prompted the USPSTF to request an updated systematic evidence review of direct evidence on the benefits and harms of PSA-based screening for prostate cancer. The USPSTF commissioned a separate report examining the benefits and*

*harms of treatment for localized prostate cancer, given that the over-all outcomes of early detection are intrinsically tied to the subsequent use of therapies...*

** *Until we have a better test and better treatment options, based on a comprehensive review of the science, the USPSTF recommends that men not get the PSA test to screen for prostate cancer. Whether or not to be screened is a decision each man should make once he understands the facts and based on his own values and preferences. The USPSTF encourages you to learn more, and if you have questions to have a conversation with your nurse or doctor ...*

*To learn more about the benefits and harms of prostate cancer screening, see the USPSTF fact sheet (PDF File, 293 KB; PDF Help) read more below, or read the full USPSTF evidence reviews, which may be found on the Task Force's Web site at http://www.uspreventiveservicestaskforce.org/prostatecancerscreening.*

** *Five randomized controlled trials (two fair- and three poor-quality) and two meta-analyses evaluating the impact of PSA-based screening on prostate cancer mortality were identified. A report describing results from a single center participating in one of the fair-quality trials was also identified. Of the two highest-quality trials, the* U.S. Prostate, Lung, Colorectal, and Ovarian Cancer Screening Trial *found no statistically significant effect of PSA-based screening on prostate cancer mortality after 10 years...*

** *The* European Randomized Study of Screening for Prostate Cancer *also found no statistically significant effect in all enrolled men (ages 50–74 years) after a median followup (sic) of 9 years but reported a 0.07% absolute risk reduction in a prespecified (sic) subgroup of men aged 55 to 69 years...*

** *Neither meta-analysis indicated a reduction in prostate cancer mortality with the use of PSA-based screening. When a benefit was found, PSA-based screening resulted in an estimated 48 additional men being treated for each prostate cancer death that was averted. Twelve percent to 13% of screened men had false-positive results after 3 to 4 screening rounds, and clinically important infections, bleeding, or urinary retention occurred after 0.5%–1.0% of prostate biopsies...*

** *PSA-based screening is associated with the detection of additional cases of prostate cancer, but small to no reduction in prostate cancer-specific mortality...*

> **❝** *For additional information, we recommend you consult the United States Preventative Services Task Force website:* http://www.us preventiveservicestaskforce.org/Page/Document/UpdateSummaryFinal/ prostate-cancer-screening.

## Our Analysis of the USPSTF's Position

**USPSTF:** "It [a USPSTF report} bases its recommendations on the evidence of both the benefits and harms of the service and an assessment of the balance. The USPSTF does not consider the costs of providing a service in this assessment."

**The Authors:** Excluding the cost of a PSA test sounds noble, but according to Healthcare Bluebook.com (*https://healthcarebluebook.com/*) a fair price for PSA screening is only $58. Compared to other prostate tests and procedures, that's a drop in the bucket:

- MRI of the prostate (with contrast): $1,152
- Standard (TRUS) prostate biopsy: $2,627
- Surgical removal of the prostate: $16,179

**USPSTF:** There is adequate evidence that false-positive PSA test results are associated with negative psychological effects, including persistent worry about prostate cancer. Men who have a false-positive test result are more likely to have additional testing, including 1 or more biopsies, in the following year than those who have a negative test result. Over 10 years, approximately 15% to 20% of men will have a PSA test result that triggers a biopsy, depending on the PSA threshold and testing interval used.

**The Authors:** Any elevated PSA test is cause for concern for any man who has one — the check engine light is on. Any urologist worth their salt will explain to their patient these simple percentages based on PSA (assuming a normal digital rectal exam):

- If PSA 2-4, 15% probability of having a positive prostate biopsy
- If PSA 4-10, 25% probability of having a positive prostate biopsy
- If PSA >10, 50% probability of having a positive prostate biopsy

Likewise, a good urologist will mention that an enlarged prostate (BPH) and prostatitis (prostate infection) can also cause an elevated PSA test. These two "mimickers" need to be ruled out with additional tests before proceeding on to imaging or a prostate biopsy.

**USPSTF:** New evidence from a randomized trial of treatment of screen-detected cancer indicates that roughly one third of men who have a prostate biopsy experience pain, fever, bleeding, infection, transient urinary difficulties, or other issues requiring clinician follow-up that the men consider a "moderate or major problem"; approximately 1% require hospitalization.

**The Authors:** We couldn't agree more. That's why we highly encourage any man who receives a higher than normal PSA test or abnormal digital rectal exam to follow up with additional blood and urine biomarker tests like PSA free, PCA3, SelectMDx, and 4Kscore Test, as well as image tests like MRI or CAT scans — before having a prostate biopsy.

There are three good reasons to have these tests and images done first:

### 1. "First, do no harm."

Hippocrates, the father of Western Medicine, taught this simple philosophy to his students almost 2,500 years ago.

### 2. Price

Prostate biopsies are more expensive as all other diagnostic prostate tests and scans *combined*.

### 3. False Positives & False Negatives

A elevated PSA test result that is caused by something other than prostate cancer can lead to a unnecessary prostate biopsy. A false negative prostate biopsy (one that missed some hidden cancer) leads a man to believe that he doesn't have cancer when he actually does.

Both of these results can create problems for the patient — for different reasons. The first one frightens men that they might have prostate cancer, when they actually don't. The second gives them false hope that they don't have cancer, when in fact, they do.

Which group would you rather be in?

**USPSTF:** Although the precise, long-term effect of PSA screening on prostate cancer specific mortality remains uncertain, existing studies adequately demonstrate that the reduction in prostate cancer mortality after 10 to 14 years is, at most, very small, even for men in what seems to be the optimal age range of 55 to 69 years. There is no apparent reduction in all-cause mortality. In contrast, the harms associated with the diagnosis and treatment of screen-detected cancer are common, occur early, often persist, and include a small but real risk for premature death.

**The Authors:** The above statement is in direct contradiction to the overwhelming majority of the data on the impact of PSA testing on prostate cancer survivorship. We are curious to hear how the USPSTF reconciles the above statement with the 83 percent reduction in prostate cancer mortality between 1992 and 2008-2012.

**USPSTF:** Many more men in a screened population will experience the harms of screening and treatment of screen-detected disease than will experience the benefit. The inevitability of overdiagnosis and overtreatment of prostate cancer as a result of screening means that many men will experience the adverse effects of diagnosis and treatment of a disease that would have remained asymptomatic throughout their lives. Assessing the balance of benefits and harms requires weighing a moderate to high probability of early and persistent harm from treatment against the very low probability of preventing a death from prostate cancer in the long term.

The USPSTF concludes that there is moderate certainty that the benefits of PSA-based screening for prostate cancer do not outweigh the harms.

**The Authors:** Ask any practicing urologist whether the benefits of PSA testing (screening) outweighs the risks, and 99 out of 100 will reply with an emphatic, *"Yes!"*

Will most of these same doctors also admit that in the past the American medical establishment overtreated men with low-risk, low-volume prostate cancer?

*Yes.*

Did this practice lead to complications from prostate biopsies and traditional treatments that caused unnecessary harm?

*Yes.*

Did the rise in PSA testing catch more men with low-volume, low-risk prostate cancer when the treatment success rates are highest, the number of treatment options are the greatest, and the treatment complication rates are the lowest?

*Without question.*

The USPSTF is essentially saying the same thing as we are in this book. The big difference between our points of view is that PSA testing is still a valid and important first step in detecting prostate cancer.

PSA testing, however, is not the only step, but it remains a good first step. The next steps include other biomarker tests (4kscore Test, PCA3, SelectMDx, and others) and prostate imaging (MRI & CAT scans).

The other major difference between our point of view and the USPSTF's is that emerging treatments (See **Chapters 5 & 6**) have much lower complication rates than traditional treatments — therefore, fewer "harms."

So who is the USPSTF punishing by discouraging men from having regular PSA screenings: doctors who encourage their patients with an elevated PSA to have a prostate biopsy without first taking advantage of other biomarker and imaging tests — or men who continue to have undiagnosed prostate cancer because they were told to skip having a PSA test by their primary care physician?

Obviously, there is a middle path between those two extremes, and thanks to all the other lab tests and scans mentioned in **Chapter 2**, PSA screening isn't the only prostate cancer detection tool available.

**Bottom Line:** PSA screening remains a valuable (and in some cases a life-saving) prostate cancer detection tool.

# Digging Deeper
## CHAPTER 1

**This Digging Deeper Section includes the following tools and resources to help you understand more about prostate cancer longevity and death rates:**

- Prostate Cancer Longevity
- Cancer Death Rates in the United States

# Cancer Longevity: The Henrietta Lacks Story

Normal cell death (apoptosis) does not occur in prostate cancer cells. That's a big part of the problem in curing cancer — the cells refuse to die. Under the right laboratory conditions, cancer cells can live for decades.

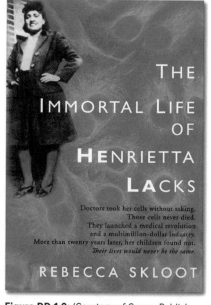

The longevity of cancer cells has been well documented. To summarize 50 years of scientific study: cancer cells live longer than normal cells. In some cases, much, much longer.

Most other cells in the body have a predictable life expectancy: a cell divides (usually several times), it matures, and then it dies. Some cells, like colon cells, only live a few days; while, neuron cells in your cerebral cortex can last a lifetime.

**Figure DD 1.0**: (Courtesy of Crown Publishing Group) The cover of Rebecca Skloot's best-selling book about Henrietta Lacks.

The longevity of cancer cells is more like that of a neuron; under the right conditions, they can live indefinitely.

The "immortality" of cancer cells is a big part of what makes eradicating cancer more of a challenge than curing the common cold.

Perhaps the most interesting example of the longevity of cancer is Henrietta Lacks.

In the *New York Times* bestseller, *The Immortal Life of Henrietta Lacks,* author Rebecca Skloot explores Ms. Lacks' story, all the different research that involved her cancer cells, and how her family never knew — and was never compensated. The book was named the 2010 "Book of the Year" by more than 60 media outlets.

As compelling as the story of Ms. Lacks and her cancer cells is, we only mention it here, to illustrate how difficult it is to kill certain cancer cells.

The "immortal" quality Ms. Lacks' cervical cancer cells made these cells invaluable to cancer researchers the world over. They have even been used in experiments performed in space.

The following book summary was taken from Rebecca Skloot's website (*http://rebeccaskloot.com/the-immortal-life/*):

> *Her name was Henrietta Lacks, but scientists know her as HeLa. She was a poor black tobacco farmer whose cells—taken without her knowledge in 1951—became one of the most important tools in medicine, vital for developing the polio vaccine, cloning, gene mapping, in vitro fertilization, and more. Henrietta's cells have been bought and sold by the billions, yet she remains virtually unknown, and her family can't afford health insurance.*
>
> *Soon to be made into an HBO movie by Oprah Winfrey and Alan Ball, this New York Times bestseller takes readers on an extraordinary journey, from the "colored" ward of Johns Hopkins Hospital in the 1950s to stark white laboratories with freezers filled with HeLa cells, from Henrietta's small, dying hometown of Clover, Virginia, to East Baltimore today, where her children and grandchildren live and struggle with the legacy of her cells.* **The Immortal Life of Henrietta Lacks** *tells a riveting story of the collision between ethics, race, and medicine; of scientific discovery and faith healing; and of a daughter consumed with questions about the mother she never knew. It's a story inextricably connected to the dark history of experimentation on African Americans, the birth of bioethics, and the legal battles over whether we control the stuff we're made of.*

## Prostate Cancer Statistics

In **Chapter 1**, we introduced you to some basic prostate cancer statistics. We believe it's important to understand the big picture and see where you fit in the spectrum of other men with prostate cancer.

We also know how easy it is to get lost in the numbers — kind of like missing the forest for the trees. When things get scary (as with a prostate cancer diagnosis), it's normal to shift your attention to things that are tangible (like numbers), instead of feeling swept away by a raging sea of emotions.

If you find yourself stuck on numbers and percentages, here are a few thoughts about statistics that are designed to help you remain grounded, function as normally as possible (given the circumstances), and stay sane.

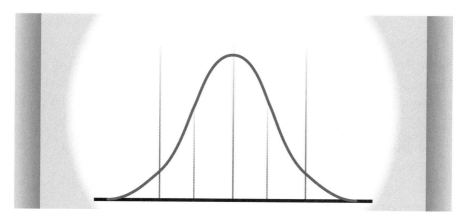

**Figure DD 1.1** illustrates a standard bell curve.

## 1. You Are More than a Statistic

No matter what kind of prostate cancer you have (low-risk, high-risk, low-volume, high-volume, Gleason 3 + 3, Gleason 4 + 3, and so on), you have a kind of cancer that will respond differently to treatment than another man with exactly the same numbers. In other words, you are biologically unique, so is your immune system. Some people's immune systems are better at fighting bacterial infections; others are better at killing cancer. Regardless of the strengths and weaknesses of your immune system, it's important to know that you are a complex biological being that is greater than sum of your parts. You are NOT a statistic.

## 2. Statistics Only Apply to Groups

If you look a standard bell curve (see **Figure DD 1.1** above), the first thing you notice is the shape. It looks like a bell (hence the name) or perhaps the outline of a hill.

What this curve represents is lots of different data points that collectively create this shape. There are more data points underneath the highest part of the bell curve and fewer data points at the ends.

So what does this information tell us about your prostate cancer?

That depends on what's being measured. For example, if you are looking at a graph that measures 15-year survival rate, you want to be at far right end of the bell curve (the men that live the longest). If the bell curve measures how much cancer was found in a prostate biopsy, you want to be at the far left end of the curve (as little cancer as possible).

Regardless of what's being measured, you are not a statistic. Statistics only apply to groups of data points, or for the purposes of this discussion, groups of men — specifically, groups of men who have prostate cancer.

Are you a group of men? No. So how does any of this statistical information that describes a group of men apply directly to you? Good question.

Statistical data (information) may reflect your condition perfectly, or the information may only be most applicable to a certain subset of men who have prostate cancer — and you don't belong to that group.

Even if you do belong to a certain subset of men with prostate cancer, the take home message is that what applies to your group of men in general, may or may not apply specifically to you.

As we mentioned on the previous page, your body's ability to fight this disease and heal may be superior to other men who have cancer numbers that are similar to yours. Likewise, your immune system's ability to combat this disease may be lower than men who have cancer numbers similar to yours.

Regardless of where you fall on any curve (collection of data points), you are more than a number. Your body's ability to respond to treatment depends on a constellation of health factors (some you have control over, others you do not). All you can do is improve your overall health (and therefore the health of your prostate) and find the best possible medical team to treat the kind of cancer you have.

Everything else rests in much bigger hands.

## Where Do You Fit in a Prostate Cancer Timeline?

The good news is that you are living in an age of declining cancer death rates. As you can see from **Figures DD 1.2 and 1.3** below, the only cancer death rates that have increased in the past 25 years are pancreatic cancer (men and women) and liver cancer (men).

The average 5-year survival rate for pancreatic cancer in both men and women is only four percent. The average 5-year survival rate for liver cancer in men and women is only slightly better: 17 percent.

Thanks to early detection and more effective treatments, prostate cancer is not as deadly as it once was. For example, both the number of men who develop prostate cancer and the numbers of men who die from the disease have been dropping steadily since 1995. As you can see from **Figure DD 1.2,** other major cancers (lung, colon, and stomach) also display similar curves.

The bad news, however, is that cancer is more prevalent than every before. The American Cancer Society estimates that approximately 1 in 2 men living in North America will develop some form of cancer during their lifetime. For women, the estimate is closer to 1 in 3. For prostate cancer, the numbers are closer to 1 in 7 (14%).

What does that information tell us? It means that every other man you meet on the street is likely to develop cancer sometime in their lives! The same is true for every third woman. Those are staggering numbers.

When it comes to developing cancer, 1-7 are better odds than 1-2 or 1-3, but 14 percent of men is still way too high.

Let's take a look behind the statistics at other information that points to an improving situation for men who have been diagnosed with prostate cancer.

1. The next generation of blood biomarker, epigenetic, and genomic testing give doctors new tools that can accurately predict the kind of prostate cancer a man has. Advancements like MRI Fusion prostate biopsies also help locate exactly where the cancer is (see **Chapter 2**).

2. If your cancer is contained within your prostate, there is a very good chance of a cure (see **Chapter 8**).

3. New treatments are available that have minimal complication rates, which means that men can reasonably expect to maintain their ability to have an erection and NOT leak urine (see **Chapter 8**).

4. Lifestyle factors are powerful medicine (see **Chapters 8 & 10**).

5. In the next 10 years, breakthroughs in immunotherapy will dramatically improve doctors' ability to treat prostate cancer (and other cancers).

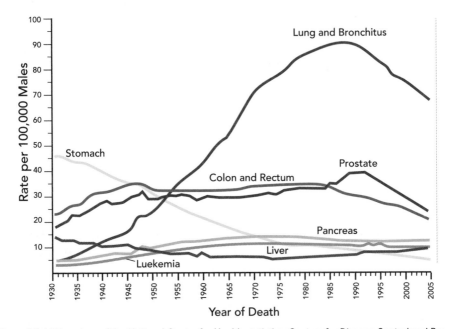

**Figure DD 1.2** (courtesy of the National Center for Health statistics, Centers for Disease Control and Prevention), illustrates the cancer death rates for *men* in the United States from 1930 through 2005. As you can see, prostate cancer death rates spiked in the U.S. between 1990-1995 and has been on the decline ever since.

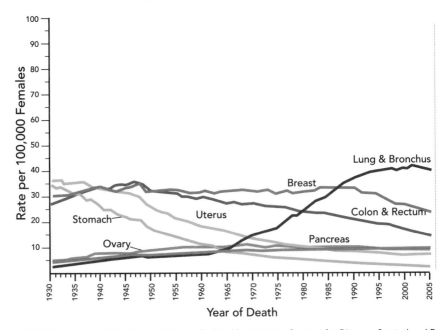

**Figure DD 1.3** (courtesy of the National Center for Health statistics, Centers for Disease Control and Prevention), illustrates the cancer death rates for *women* in the United States from 1930 through 2005. As you can see, breast cancer death rates in the U.S. have been falling steadily since about 1990.

# Digging Deeper
## CHAPTER 2

This Digging Deeper Section includes the following tools and resources to help you gain a better understanding of how genetics, biomarkers, and complications fit into your decision to have a prostate biopsy:

- How family history and genetics play into your prostate cancer equation.
- Why do African-American men have the highest rate of prostate cancer?
- What biomarkers can reveal about the health of your prostate.
- What you need to know about prostate biopsy complications.

# Family History (Genetics)

According to Dr. David Crawford of the University of Colorado Medical Center, "Cancer is a collection of genetic changes. The longer it sticks around, the harder it is to treat."

Your risk of developing prostate cancer more than doubles if your father or brother has the disease. Your risk is higher if you have a brother with prostate cancer. The risk of developing prostate cancer is also much higher for men with several relatives who have developed the disease, especially if they are diagnosed under the age of 50.

Genetic mutations in specific genes also increase the chances of developing prostate cancer. Scientists have located several genes that appear to raise the risk of inheriting at least one type of prostate cancer. For example, there are strong indications that inherited mutations in the MRS1, RNASEL, ELACS, BRCA1 and BRCA2 genes increase the risk of prostate cancer. The BRCA1 and BRCA2 genes also carry an increased risk for breast and ovarian cancer running in some families.

According to Cancer.org, inherited DNA mutations in certain genes may account for 5 to 10 percent of all prostate cancer.

In a study by Seller et al. of 41,827 women with breast cancer, the researchers found that 11.4 percent of the women had a father or brother with prostate cancer, 15.2 percent had a mother or sister with breast cancer, and 2 percent had a family history of both breast cancer and prostate cancer.

In follow-up studies, the risk of women developing breast cancer after the initial survey rose to 42 percent if there was a family history of breast cancer. The risk jumped to 71 percent when there was a family history of both kinds of cancer.

Clearly, these cancer rates are much higher than the general population and suggest a strong genetic link between breast and prostate cancers. Information on diet, lifestyle, and environmental factors (exposure to toxic substances) would have been helpful to see which had a bigger impact: lifestyle-induced epigenetic DNA modifications or inherited genetic mutations — but that's a different study.

## Gene Changes

Every time a cell prepares to divide, it copies its DNA. Sometimes errors occur during the copying process, which alters the new cell by either a genetic mutation (change in the cell's DNA) or an epigenetic modification (a change in DNA expression).

Prostate cancer is caused by both mutations or modifications of a prostate cell's DNA. Scientists have made great progress in understanding how certain changes in DNA can make normal prostate cells become cancerous.

The genes within our DNA control when cells grow, divide, and die. "Oncogenes" help cells grow, divide, and stay alive as long as possible. "Tumor Suppressor Genes" slow down cell division, repair DNA errors, and cause cells to die at the appropriate time (apoptosis). Stimulating oncogenes or blocking tumor suppressor are two ways to help cancer find a foothold.

This process may be driven by DNA changes (mutations). Mutations can either be inherited from a parent or can be acquired during a person's lifetime.

**Several mutated genes have been linked to a man's inherited tendency to develop prostate cancer:**

**RNASEL (formerly HPC1):** The normal function of this tumor suppressor gene is to help cells die when something goes wrong. Inherited mutations in this gene may allow abnormal cells to live longer than they should, which can lead to an increased risk of prostate cancer.

**BRCA1 and BRCA2:** These tumor suppressor genes normally help repair mistakes in a cell's DNA (or cause the cell to die if the mistake can't be fixed). Inherited mutations in these genes more commonly cause breast and ovarian cancer in women; however, inherited BRCA gene changes also account for a small number of prostate cancers in men.

**DNA mismatch repair genes (such as MSH2 and MLH1):** These genes normally help fix mistakes (mismatches) in DNA that are made when a cell is preparing to divide. Men with inherited mutations in these genes have a condition known as Lynch Syndrome (also known as hereditary non-polyposis colorectal cancer, or HNPCC), which puts these men at an increased risk of developing colorectal, prostate, and other cancers.

As you can see, several inherited gene mutations can raise prostate cancer risk, but these mutations only account for a low percentage of cases.

Recently, research has found a connection between some common gene variations and a higher risk of developing prostate cancer. Studies to confirm these connections are needed to see if testing for these gene variants would help predict an increased risk for prostate cancer.

It is important to keep in mind that the majority of DNA mutations and modifications linked to prostate cancer occur over the course of a man's lifetime — not because of an inherited genetic malfunction.

# More on BRCA1 & BRCA2 Mutations

BRCA1 and BRCA2 are human genes that produce tumor suppressor proteins. These proteins help repair damaged DNA and, therefore, play a role in ensuring the stability of the cell's genetic material. When either of these genes are mutated or altered in such a way that their protein production either stops or ceases to function properly, any new DNA damage may not be repaired correctly. As a result, cells are more likely to develop additional genetic alterations that can lead to cancer.

Men with BRCA1 or BRCA2 mutations have a higher risk of prostate cancer. Furthermore, these cancers are more likely to develop at a younger age in men with a BRCA mutation. Men with these mutations do, however, have a lower chance overall of developing cancer than women with a same mutations. Also, men with BRCA2 mutations, and to a lesser extent BRCA1 mutations, are at increased risk of breast cancer.

A detrimental BRCA1 or BRCA2 mutation can be inherited from a person's mother or father. Each child of a parent who carries a mutation in one copy of these genes has a 50 percent chance of inheriting the mutation. BRCA1 and BRCA2 mutations are usually dominant, meaning that the mutation is expressed, even if a person's other copy of the gene is normal.

Because harmful BRCA1 and BRCA2 gene mutations are relatively rare in the general population, most experts agree that mutation testing of individuals who do not have cancer should be performed only when the person's individual or family history suggests the possible presence of a harmful mutation in BRCA1 or BRCA2.

People of Ashkenazi Jewish descent have a higher prevalence of BRCA1 and BRCA2 mutations than the general U.S. population. Other ethnic and geographic populations around the world, such as the Norwegian, Dutch, and Icelandic peoples, also have a higher prevalence of specific BRCA1 and BRCA2 mutations.

Men from families with a history of breast and ovarian cancer should consider testing for a BRCA gene mutation particularly if any of the breast cancers occurred before age 50 (in either female or male relatives). Men with breast cancer themselves are highly likely to have a BRCA mutation and should consider testing. Men who have prostate cancer and a family history of breast cancer should also think about testing..

DNA (from a blood or saliva sample) is all that's needed for mutation testing. The sample is sent to a laboratory for analysis. It usually takes about a month to get the test results.

A positive test result indicates that a person has inherited a known harmful mutation in the BRCA1 or BRCA2 gene; therefore, this person has an increased risk of developing certain cancers. However, a positive test result cannot tell whether or when an individual will actually develop cancer. For example, some women who inherit a potentially cancer causing BRCA1 or BRCA2 mutation will never develop breast or ovarian cancer.

## Enhanced Screening

There can be benefits to genetic testing, regardless of whether a person receives a positive or a negative result.

The potential benefits of a true negative result include a sense of relief regarding the future risk of cancer, learning that one's children are at less of a risk of inheriting the family's cancer susceptibility, and the possibility that special checkups, tests, or preventive surgeries may not be needed.

A positive test result may also bring relief by resolving uncertainty regarding future cancer risk and allow people to make informed decisions about their future — including taking steps to reduce their cancer risk. In addition, people who have a positive test result can choose to participate in medical research that could, in the long run, help reduce deaths from hereditary prostate, breast, and ovarian cancers.

# Why Do African American Men Have the Highest Rate of Prostate Cancer ?

The sad truth is the incidence of prostate cancer and the prostate cancer death rate for African American men is higher than any other racial or ethnic group.

According to the Surveillance, Epidemiology & End Results (SEER) program of the National Cancer Institute, between 2009-2013, the prostate cancer incidence rate for the general population was 129.4/100,000. For African Americans, the incidence rate was 203.5/100,000 for the same period. Between 2008-2012, The American Cancer Society reports that the death rate from prostate cancer for the general population was 21.4/100,000. For African Americans, the death rate was 47.2/100,000 for the same period.

The fact that the prostate cancer death rate for African-American men is more than twice that of other American men points to a host of issues: medical, biological, genetic, socio-economic, and racial disparities.

Access to quality health care, availability of follow-up care, affordable health insurance, and lifestyle factors (living in urban "food deserts," diets high in saturated fats and low in fresh vegetables, and obesity) all have a hand in this unfortunate situation.

We know some of the factors involved in African-American men developing and dying from prostate cancer because the disease is not as prevalent in England as it is in North America. The PROCESS study found that prostate cancer incidence for black men living two major British cities (London and Bristol) between 1997 and 2001 was 166/100,000. The CDC's data for the prostate cancer incidence rate for African Americans in 2001 was 234.1/100,000 — a 41 percent difference.

According to a 2009 study, *Prostate Cancer Disparities in Black Men of African Descent,* "The growing literature on the disproportionate burden of prostate cancer among other Black men of West African ancestry follows the path of the Transatlantic Slave Trade. To better understand and address the global prostate cancer disparities seen in Black men of West African ancestry, future studies should explore the genetic and environmental risk factors for prostate cancer among this group."

These racial disparities apply, even when other factors are the same or accounted for. For example, in 2009, the Southwest Oncology Group (SWOG) published a study on the racial disparities in prostate cancer death rates. This study observed 1,843 white and black men with prostate cancer who had the same disease stage, identical treatments, and follow up care. Even when socio-economic factors were taken into account, the SWOG study found that African American men in this study were 21 percent more likely to die from prostate cancer than their white counterparts.

Racial and ethnic backgrounds, however, do not doom men to die from prostate cancer or make them immune to the disease. For example, Japanese men have some of the lowest rates of prostate cancer diagnosis and mortality in the world. However, men born in Japan who immigrate to Hawaii have prostate cancer rates that fall in between Japanese men living in Japan and white American men living in Hawaii, which suggests that dietary and environmental factors play important roles in the development and progression of prostate cancer.

Because of a higher incidence of prostate cancer and prostate cancer mortality in African-American men, we recommend that African-American men begin having regular digital rectal exams and PSA screenings at age 40.

# What Biomarkers Can Reveal about the Health of Your Prostate

Biomarkers are measurable indicators of some biological process, condition, or general state of health. Because testing for biomarkers is generally non-invasive (or less invasive than more traditional tests), they can provide important information about a specific disease (like prostate cancer) as well as information about a person's overall health (information that would come from blood or urine tests at an annual physical).

Because of their less invasive nature, biomarkers play an increasingly important role in prostate cancer diagnosis, monitoring, and treatment. Coupling biomarkers with MRI and CT scans gives doctors a more accurate picture of prostate health and helps pinpoint areas of disease.

Because the complications from prostate biopsies increase in frequency and severity with each additional biopsy, the development of reliable, non-invasive tests that accurately report whether a man is likely to have (or not have) prostate cancer (and if so, what kind of cancer) is an important step in replacing the prostate biopsy as the diagnostic "gold standard."

In addition, biomarkers provide physicians with better guidelines about when to biopsy (or re-biopsy). Biomarkers also help minimize false negative biopsies (and therefore re-biopsies), which ultimately lowers the number and severity of complications that a patient experiences, so biomarkers are also an ally in the battle against diagnostic "harms."

Below and on the next page, we discuss where biomarkers come from and why doctors use them at specific points in the diagnostic process.

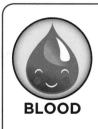

**BLOOD**

**PSA free, PSA total, PSA density, and PSA velocity** are the most commonly used blood biomarkers to detect prostate cancer.

The **4Kscore Test** combines four prostate-specific biomarkers (**PSA free, PSA total, PSA intact, & hK2**) with clinical information to provide men with an accurate assessment of their risk for aggressive prostate cancer.

**Figure DD 2.0** (which continues on the following page) provides a general overview of the three most common types biomarkers to evaluate a man's risk of having prostate cancer — or which kind of cancer he has if other tests confirm the presence of cancer.
Numerous biomarkers are in clinical trials or have recently come on the market. We have not mentioned them here until their effectiveness has been more thoroughly researched and documented.

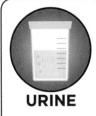

**URINE**

**PCA 3** is a unique strand of non-coding RNA that occurs at elevated levels in more than 90% of prostate cancer tissues; however, does not occur at elevated levels in normal or enlarged prostate tissue samples.

**SelectMDx** uses reverse transcription PCR (RT-PCR) to measure mRNA levels of the DLX1 and HOXC6 biomarkers. Higher expressions of DLX1 and HOXC6 mRNA are associated with an increased probability for high-grade prostate cancer (Gleason Score ≥ 7).

**TMPRSS2-ERG** is a urine biomarker that is frequently associated with significant prostate cancer. **TMPRSS2-ERG** can be used in combination with PSA density and prostate biopsy information to rank how aggressive a patient's prostate cancer aggressive is.

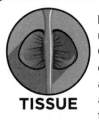

**TISSUE**

**PTEN** is a tumor suppressor gene involved in cell cycle regulation. The absence of **PTEN** gene is associated with higher Gleason scores, increased risk of cancer progression, and cancer recurrence after treatment. It is also associated with advanced localized cancer, and metastatic disease. The **PTEN** assay is a prognostic fluorescence in situ hybridization (FISH) test typically ordered in conjunction with a prostate biopsy. For patients with a cancer diagnosis, the PTEN assay may help determine the rate of progression; therefore, the most appropriate form of treatment.

**ConfirmMDx** is an epigenetic marker for methylation that has a 90% negative predictive value for up to 30 months after a prostate biopsy. A recent study by Dr. David Crawford evaluated the accuracy of this test on 138 patients who had a negative **ConfirmMDx** result. Only 6 of the 138 patients (4%) had a second prostate biopsy.

**Prolaris** is a genomic test that uses a panel of 46 genes that further investigates a low-risk prostate cancer diagnosis to determine whether the diagnosis is accurate — as opposed more aggressive prostate cancer masquerading as low-risk disease. **Prolaris** can also be used before treatment to ID patients who have high-risk prostate cancer, as well as after surgery to confirm the pre-operative diagnosis.

**Oncotype DX** is a genomic test that looks for the presence of 17 aggressive prostate cancer genes. It is used to confirm that low-risk and low-to-intermediate-risk prostate cancer found during a prostate biopsy does NOT include more aggressive disease.

**ProMark** is a biopsy-based prostate cancer test that uses immunofluorescent imaging analysis to quantify the expression of certain biomarkers and classify a patient's cancer. A recent clinical validation study demonstrated **ProMark** ability to differentiate between indolent from aggressive disease.

**Decipher** is a different type of genomic tool based on 22 RNA biomarkers that evaluates the risk of metastasis after a radical prostatectomy (surgery).

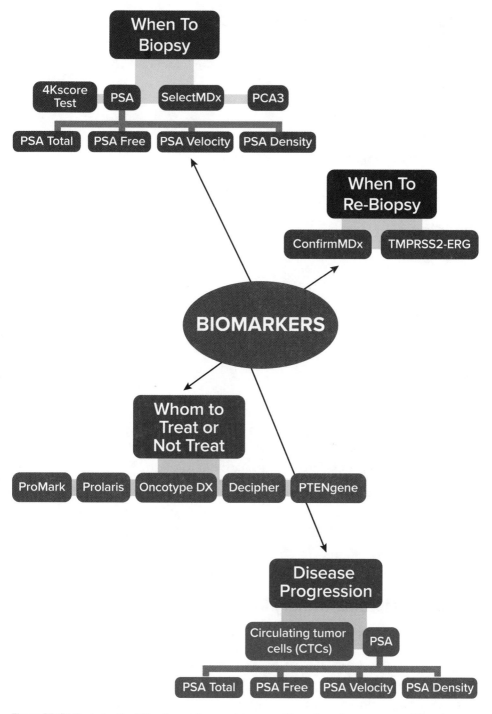

**Figure DD 2.1** illustrates the "When" regarding prostate cancer biomarkers: As you can see, different biomarkers are used at different times in the progression from diagnosis to biopsy (re-biopsy) to treatment. Note that the biomarkers change as the need for different information changes.

# Prostate Biopsy Complications

Prostate biopsy complications can be as minor as blood in your urine for a week to 10 days or as deadly as a bacterial infection like sepsis.

The major prostate biopsy complications include:

- Bleeding
- Pain
- Urinary symptoms/ Urinary retention
- Sexual dysfunction
- Infection

## Bleeding

Bleeding is the most frequently reported complication after biopsy, but it is usually minor and is resolved spontaneously. Significant bleeding, however, is rare (requiring hospitalization occurs in less than 1 percent of cases) but can be life-threatening.

## Pain

The use of anti-anxiety agents combined with periprostatic lidocaine injection appears to significantly reduce pain.

**Transrectal Biopsy:** If performed correctly, lidocaine injections into the prostate and surrounding tissues significantly reduces or eliminates the pain from the prostate biopsy needles being shot into the prostate. Without lidocaine, the procedure is too painful to tolerate.

**Transperineal Biopsy:** because perineal biopsies are significantly more painful than rectal biopsies, a periprostatic nerve block is frequently used with perineal biopsies to reduce pain without increasing complications.

Anti-anxiety medications are commonly used with both types of biopsies to help patients relax (specifically to relax the anal sphincter).

## Urinary Symptoms/Urinary Retention

An exacerbation of lower urinary tract symptoms may also occur after biopsy, particularly in men with an enlarged prostate, but urinary retention is infrequent. Prophylactic alpha-blockers in men with large or symptomatic prostates may be helpful. Although urinary symptoms are not uncommon after a prostate biopsy, these symptoms (pain and/or itching along the urinary tract, the need to urinate immediately, the need to urinate often, and the feeling of never being able to completely empty the bladder) usually resolve themselves within 48 hours after the biopsy. In some rare cases, these symptoms can drag on for months after the biopsy — or the symptoms may come and go intermittently.

## Erectile Dysfunction (ED)

Depending upon the age and health of the patient, difficulty having or maintaining an erection is common for 7-10 days after a prostate biopsy.

Men who have prostate cancer are more likely to have ED after a prostate biopsy than men who do not. The question remains whether the men who are diagnosed with prostate cancer and have ED are having an emotional or physiological reaction. Being told, "You have prostate cancer," is enough to pull the emotional rug out from under even the most confident and self-assured man.

## Mortality

All men undergoing a prostate biopsy should begin taking antimicrobial prophylaxis (oral or injectable antibiotics) 24 hours before the procedure, and should be educated on the signs and symptoms of significant bacterial infection. Patients should seek immediate medical care at the nearest emergency room if they experience any of these symptoms:

- Flu-like symptoms
- Fever and chills
- Muscle aches and pains
- Pressure between the legs
- Sharp pain or intense burning while urinating
- Difficulty or inability to urinate
- Overall weakness
- Feeling lightheaded
- Difficulty standing up straight
- Uncontrollable shivering

A systemic bacterial infection (sepsis) is the most significant complication of a prostate biopsy. Sepsis is caused by the biopsy needles passing through the rectum and picking up bacteria on their way to the prostate. If left untreated, sepsis is often fatal.

If you or a person in your care has recently had a prostate biopsy and experiences any of these symptoms, go to the nearest emergency room immediately! Septic shock is setting in, and time is of the essence.

Septic shock can cause multiple organ dysfunction syndrome (also called "multiple organ failure") and death. The mortality rate from septic shock is about 40 percent (and significantly greater if left untreated).

Sepsis is on the rise. Two decades ago, sepsis was reported in less than 1 percent of cases. Today, that number is 2-4 percent of cases depending upon the study. The rise of antibiotic-resistant bacteria, especially floro-quinolone-resistant bacteria, is believed to be the cause.

## Patient- and Procedure-Related Complications

Another way of think about prostate biopsy complications is to look at where they come from — the patient side or the procedure side.

As a consumer of healthcare, it is important to know what you have control over and what you do not. Even with the things you don't have control over (your doctor's skill level, the room where the biopsy takes place, how the procedure is performed), you do have control over which procedure is performed, when it is performed, and how many times.

The following check list gives patients a better idea of what causes prostate biopsy complications and how they can minimize their risk.

## Patient-Related Complications

If you answer "Yes" to any of the following questions, we strongly recommend you talk with your doctor before having a prostate biopsy:

- ◆ Do you have diabetes?
- ◆ Do you have an enlarged prostate (BPH)?
- ◆ Have you traveled outside the United States recently?
- ◆ Do you have a urinary tract infection or have you had one recently?
- ◆ Have you taken antibiotics, especially fluoroquinolones, recently?
- ◆ Have you been hospitalized recently?
- ◆ Are you a doctor or hospital employee?
- ◆ Have you had a positive urine culture recently?

## Procedure-Related Complications

The following factors increase your risk of complications from a prostate biopsy.

- ◆ A higher number of prostate biopsy needle cores (20 vs. 12)
- ◆ Repeat biopsies (Your risk of having complications goes up with each additional biopsy.)
- ◆ Transrectal biopsies and transperineal biopsies have different complication rates. For more information, see **Chapter 2**, Page 50.

| | BLEEDING |
|---|---|
| **Blood in Urine** | • A small amount of blood in the urine is common after prostate biopsy. This condition may last for several days and usually heals itself. Overall, less than 1% of cases of blood in the urine require hospitalization. |
| **Rectal Bleeding** | • Rosario et al. found that rectal bleeding was more common than previously reported (36.8%). Only 2.5% of rectal bleeding was found to be a major or moderate problem. However, when rectal bleeding is severe, it is a serious health threat that requires immediate medical attention. |
| **Blood in Ejaculate** | • Rosario et al. found that 92.6% of all men reported blood in their ejaculate during the 35 days after biopsy. <br> • Manoharan noted the decline of blood in ejaculate over time: 84% in week 1, 66% in week 2, and 32% after week 4. |
| **Anticoagulants** | • Prostate biopsies may be safe if the patient is taking aspirin, because the frequency of bleeding complications is low; however, the data about more powerful anticoagulants like Warfarin and Clopidogrel is less conclusive. <br> • Patients who take Warfarin require special consideration because of Warfarin's interaction with the antibiotics commonly used to prevent infection after a prostate biopsy. |

**Figure DD 2.2** discusses the four most common types of post-prostate biopsy bleeding issues and how common they are among men who have had a biopsy.

| | COMPLICATIONS |
|---|---|
| **Pain** | • Lidocaine injections (10–20 ml) in and around the prostate are safe, well tolerated, and significantly reduce pain compared to no anesthetic. <br> • The use of a periprostatic nerve block as prostate biopsy anesthesia significantly reduces the patient's perception of pain without increasing the complication rate. |
| **Lower urinary tract symptoms & urinary retention** | • The range of acute urinary retention after a biopsy ranges from 0.2 to 2%. Retention is usually transient and controlled by alpha-blockers <br> • Patients with preexisting urinary symptoms or who have large prostates should consider taking alpha-blockers shortly before, during, or after the biopsy to reduce the risk of urinary retention. <br> • Painful urination or difficulty urinating occurs in 6 to 25% of cases. |
| **Erectile dysfunction** | • A study of 85 men who underwent a single 12-core TRUS biopsy found no significant differences in pre- and post biopsy ability to get and maintain an erection. Men with biopsy-proven cancer, however, had significant changes in post biopsy erectile dysfunction compared to men without cancer — including deterioration of sexual desire, ability to achieve orgasm, intercourse satisfaction, and overall satisfaction. |

| | |
|---|---|
| **Infection** | • A Cochrane review showed that prophylactic antibiotics significantly reduces bacteriuria, bacteremia, fever, urinary tract infection (UTI), and hospitalization<br>• A recent international survey reported that 98.2% of men undergoing a biopsy in 84 countries received antimicrobial prophylaxis, with fluoro-quinolones being most commonly prescribed (92.5%)<br>• Although the reported duration of use varies widely, most studies show no significant benefit beyond 24 hours after the procedure.<br>• Types of infection include: bacteriuria, UTI, epididymitis, meningitis, vertebral osteomyelitis, sepsis, and septic shock.<br>• Recent studies have suggested an increase in microbial resistance to antibiotics, particularly fluoroquinolone.<br>• The most common pathogen is E. coli, which have high rates of resistance to fluoroquinolones as well as ampicillin and sulfamethoxazole -trimethoprim. |
| **Reducing infectious complications** | • Taylor et al. reported no significant decrease in the frequency of sepsis using a targeted approach, compared with other patients receiving standard prophylaxis (0% vs 2.6%; p = 0.12).<br>• To date, there are no randomized studies showing that targeted prophylaxis using rectal swabs results reduces infection and cost compared with standard or expanded prophylaxis.<br>• Strategies to reduce the risk of infection:<br>  ◆ Assessing risk factors for resistant bacteria (previous/recent antibiotics)<br>  ◆ Reducing the number of biopsy cores<br>  ◆ Ruling out prostatitis<br>  ◆ Avoiding unnecessary repeat biopsies<br>  ◆ Bathing the rectum with betadine solution right before the biopsy<br>  ◆ Better sterile protocols for ultrasound gel<br>  ◆ Use more biomarkers and MRI fusion biopsy for accuracy and decreasing the number of needle cores |
| **Mortality** | • Patients should be instructed to seek immediate medical attention for signs of a post-biopsy infection.<br>• An analysis of death after a prostate biopsy showed that the age of the patient and the number of previous biopsies both increased the possibility of dying.<br>• In Canada, Nam et al. reported a 0.09% 30-day mortality rate after biopsy.<br>• In US SEER–Medicare data, 55 men (0.31%) who underwent biopsy died within 30 days compared with the 1,474 controls (1.09%). |

**Figure DD 2.3** (beginning on previous page) provides information about possible complications from a prostate biopsy. Pain and urinary symptoms frequently resolve themselves within the first month after a biopsy. Most men do not experience a significant erectile dysfunction; however ED can take months to overcome. Infections from a prostate biopsy can be fatal. The rise of antibiotic-resistant bacteria has increased the risk of infection, causing urologists to pay attention to this potentially deadly problem.

Obviously, the goal is to have a "complication-free" prostate biopsy. Knowing which behaviors and health factors increase or decrease your changes of having complications allows you to make better decisions.

---

# Mark's Big Septic Scare

I developed sepsis after my third prostate biopsy.

To make a long story short, I went into septic shock four days after the biopsy. Thankfully, I had the sense to get out of bed in the middle of the night and drag myself to the emergency room of the nearest hospital.

Fortunately for me (but not for them), three men had recently died at that hospital from prostate-biopsy induced sepsis that led to multiple organ failure. Had it not been for a new sepsis protocol that the hospital had put in place a few weeks before I arrived at the ER, I might have been patient number four.

One of the ER doctors told me that I was 6-12 hours away from complete organ failure.

After a really rough night, I was admitted to the hospital the following morning and spent the next five days on the infectious disease floor. I felt sicker than I ever have in my life for the first couple of days, but gradually the antibiotics began winning the war against E. coli.

While I was in the hospital, I acquired C. diff. (A horrible bowel bacteria that keeps you tethered to the toilet for weeks.) So as the systemic bacterial infection was going away, a new bacterial infection in my intestines was trying to kill me.

The happy irony of this entire experience was receiving a phone call from my urologist's nurse. With joy in her voice, she told me that my prostate biopsy looked great: no cancer, no PIN, no inflammation. Great news indeed!

When I told her that her that I was in the hospital with sepsis from my biopsy, all she said was, "Oh, I'm so sorry." And then quickly got off the phone.

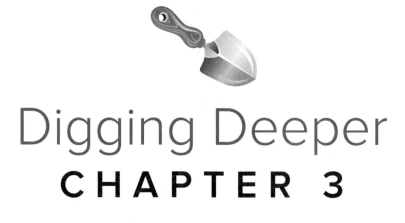

# Digging Deeper
## CHAPTER 3

This Digging Deeper Section includes the following tools and resources to help you better understand the results of your prostate biopsy:

- What's the difference between epigenetic tests like ConfirmMDx and genomic tests like Prolaris, Decipher, and Onco*type* DX?
- Throughout this book, when we talk about "prostate cancer," we are really saying "Acinar Adenocarcinoma." Actually, there are 6 other kinds of prostate cancer. Each of these cancers are unique, require their own treatment protocol, and represent about 1% of all prostate cancers.

# The Role of Epigenetics in Detecting "Hidden" Prostate Cancer

According to whatisepigenetics.com, "Epigenetics is the study of heritable changes in gene expression ... that do not involve changes to the underlying DNA sequence — a change in phenotype without a change in genotype — which in turn affects how cells read the genes. Epigenetic change is a regular and natural occurrence but can also be influenced by several factors including age, the environment/lifestyle, and disease state."

In other words, epigenetics involves changes within cells, tissues, organs, and organisms that occur due to modifications in the *expression* of certain genes — without alterations or mutations to the DNA of the genes themselves.

Epigenetics may explain differences between identical twins or why children who were born after one of their parents made a significant lifestyle change (drank more, ate more, smoked more — or the opposite) behave differently than their older siblings who were born before these changes occurred.

**What do epigenetic changes mean for men with prostate cancer?**

Epigenetic testing offers doctors a new way to reduce the approximately 175,000 false negative prostate biopsies that occur in the United States every year. Tissue biomarker tests, like ConfirmMDx, look for evidence of prostate cancer cells in otherwise healthy prostate biopsy tissue samples.

Here's how: One way for prostate cancer to spread is by "turning off" tumor suppressor genes (genes that protect cells against cancer) in the DNA of healthy prostate cells. Tumor suppressor genes can be turned off by a molecular process known as "methylation."

DNA Methylation (also called "hypermethylation") is a biochemical sequence in which methyl groups (one carbon atom bonded to three hydrogen atoms — $CH_3$) attach themselves to various genes in a cell's DNA.

Adding methyl groups changes the appearance and structure of the tumor suppressor gene's DNA enough that it prevents the gene from transcribing its instructions to the cell. The same genes are still there; however, the change in the gene's appearance and structure renders it inactive.

An easy way to visualize methylation is to put some tape over the key to your front door. The key remains the same, but it no longer opens the door. Another way to think about methylation is a string of fabric that prevents a zipper from working. The zipper is fine, but the string prevents the teeth of the zipper from meshing together.

Prostate cancer cells typically produce more methyl groups than healthy prostate cells. Epigenetic tests, like ConfirmMDx, look for abnormally high concentrations of methyl groups in prostate biopsy tissue samples. Higher methyl group concentrations (methylation) indicates the presence of prostate cancer, even if the biopsy is negative for cancer.

Why? Because molecular changes (methylation) can be detected earlier than cellular changes (PIN and prostate cancer). This is especially true of early stage prostate cancer when the size of the tumor is so small that finding it with a prostate biopsy needle requires great skill, advanced technology, and a little luck.

Epigenetic tests also help doctors focus future biopsies on the areas of the prostate with the highest methylation concentrations; therefore, the highest probability of harboring hidden cancer.

We would be remiss if we failed to mention that an absence of methyl groups ("hypomethylation") can also help cancer find a foothold in the DNA of certain genes. That, however, is a different process altogether.

## What's the Difference Between Epigenetic and Genomic Testing?

The basic difference between epigenetic testing and genomic testing involves what's being measured.

Epigenetic tests for prostate cancer measure certain biomarker molecules that are known to be involved in gene activation or gene silencing — like methyl groups. The presence or absence of these biomarkers can tell us a great deal about the health or disease of the these cells.

Genomic tests for prostate cancer look for the presence of larger sections of genetic material (genes) that are present in aggressive prostate cancer. If a genomic test is positive for this kind of genetic material, then the patient needs to have a definitive form of treatment.

## Genomic Testing Helps Doctors Accurately ID the Kind of Cancer

According to the World Health Organization, "genomics addresses all genes and their inter relationships in order to identify their combined influence on the growth and development of the organism."

Genomic tests like Decipher, Oncotype DX, and Prolaris give doctors the tools to separate true low-risk prostate cancer from more advanced cancers that may be masquerading as low-risk cancer. All three tests pick up where blood biomarkers, urine biomarkers, and prostate biopsy information leave off: PSA, 4Kscore Test, SelectMDx, PCA3, Gleason score, cancer stage, cancer type, percentage of positive needle cores, and so on.

Decipher, Oncotype DX, and Prolaris all measure the presence or absence of specific genetic material (either DNA or RNA). These genomic tests look for the presence of certain sequences of genetic material that occur in higher concentrations of aggressive high-risk prostate cancer but are absent (or present in much lower concentrations) in non-aggressive low-risk cancer.

To borrow from Prolaris' advertising message, the point of genomic tests is to help doctors separate the sheep (non-aggressive prostate cancers) from the wolves in sheep's clothing (aggressive prostate cancers).

If a patient's prostate biopsy indicates that he has low-risk cancer, but a genomic test detects the presence of genetic sequences from an aggressive form of prostate cancer, the genomic results reveal that the cancer is more aggressive than previously thought — a wolf in sheep's clothing.

Knowing which kind of cancer a man has is important for two reasons:

1. Genomic tests allow doctors to accurately match the type of treatment with the kind of cancer the patient has. The correct pairing of treatment and disease prevents doctors from undertreating the cancer; therefore, giving patients the best possible chance of a cure.

2. Although not as life threatening as undertreatment, overtreatment can also be a problem because of complications like impotence and incontinence, which can have a lifelong impact on a man's quality of life. The correct pairing of treatment type with the kind of cancer a man has helps prevent overtreatment and its attendant complications.

**Figure DD 3.0** (on the following page) provides a few basic characteristics of the seven different kinds of prostate cancer and which types of treatment are most (or least) effective for each. Please note that treatment options for the most common kind of prostate cancer (Acinar Adenocarcinoma) are the focus of **Chapters 5-8.** The other six cancers in **Figure DD 3.0** do not respond to treatment the same way that Acinar Adenocarcinoma does.

# The Seven Types of Prostate Cancer

| Types | Characteristics | Treatments |
|---|---|---|
| Acinar Adeno-carcinoma | • 95% of all prostate cancers.<br>• Starts from gland cells within the prostate. | • Standard treatments are discussed in Chapters 5-8. |
| Ductal Adeno-carcinoma | • Starts in the cells that line the ducts (tubes) of the prostate gland.<br>• Often grows and spreads faster than acinar adenocacinoma. | • Less sensitive to hormone therapy than acinar adenocarcinoma. |
| Urothelial/ Transitional Cell | • Often starts in the bladder and spreads to the prostate.<br>• Can also start in the cells that line the urethra. | • Surgery to remove your prostate and bladder.<br>• On occasion, adjuvant chemotherapy is given. |
| Squamous Cell | • Starts with the flat cells covering the prostate gland.<br>• Often grows and spreads faster than acinar adenocacinoma. | • Often diagnosed in an advanced stage.<br>• Treatments for acinar adenocarcinoma do not work as well for this type of prostate cancer. |
| Carcinoid | • It start from cells of the neuro-endocrine system.<br>• Slow growing —patients may be asymptomatic for years.<br>• Very rare. | • Monitoring recommend of slower-growing cancers.<br>• Surgery recommended for faster-growing localized cancers.<br>• Chemotherapy effective for advanced cancers. |
| Small Cell | • This is a type of neuroendo-crine tumor and is made up of small round cells.<br>• PSA not helpful for diagnosis or follow up.<br>• Fast growing, difficult to detect, often diagnosed in advanced stages. | • Hormone therapy does not work.<br>• Chemotherapy developed for small cell carcinoma of the lung is often effective.<br>• Radiation is effective as either primary or secondary treatment. |
| Sarcomas | • Sarcomas start from muscle cells.<br>• Often grows quickly.<br>• Occurs mainly between 35-60. | • Radical prostatectomy.<br>• Adjuvant radiation and chemotherapy may be required, depending on the extent of the disease. |

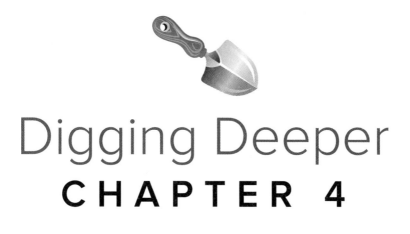

# Digging Deeper
## CHAPTER 4

This Digging Deeper Section includes the following tools and resources to help you understand the results of your prostate biopsy and how to interpret these results:

- Prostate Cancer Calculators
- MRI-Fusion Biopsy

# Prostate Cancer Calculators

Prostate cancer calculators can be helpful in providing information about the kind of cancer a man has, as well as the type of treatments that would be appropriate for that kind of cancer.

It's important to realize that no calculator, computer program, or algorithm can replace the interaction between an insightful doctor and an informed patient.

Why?

Because any single health factor can outweigh all the others. For example, if a man has low-risk, low-volume prostate cancer, but the tumor is located against the capsule of the prostate (outside edge), the situation is much more dire than if the same tumor was located in the middle of the prostate.

To help patients become more informed, we have included the following links to three prostate cancer calculators. We encourage you to explore each one by plugging your numbers into each one and see if the results are consistent — or where they vary.

This information makes for great conversations with your doctor(s) when it comes time to make a decision about which treatment option is best for you.

> Note: There are several prostate calculators designed for doctors and medical researchers, but after exploring each of them, they are cumbersome and require greater understanding of prostate cancer than most patients have.
>
> 1. *http://www.prostatecalculator.org/*
>
> 2. *http://deb.uthscsa.edu/URORiskCalc/Pages/calcs.jsp*
>
> 3. *http://www.thecalculator.co/health/Gleason-Score-for-Prostate-Cancer-Calculator-714.html*

# MRI Fusion Prostate Biopsy

There are two types of pelvic MRI:

1. **The Standard external MRI:** This type of MRI is useful in detecting the presence of prostate cancer in the surrounding tissues of the prostate (seminal vesicles, lymph nodes, rectum, bladder and bony structures in the pelvis).

2. **The Trans-rectal MRI:** This kind of MRI is used mainly to examine the prostate itself.

Over the past decade, better quality MRIs (stronger magnets) and multi-parametric enhancements (diffusion-weighted imaging and dynamic contrast studies) have improved image quality and helped distinguish between normal tissues and cancer, as well as between lower- and higher-risk prostate cancer.

In addition, using modalities such as spectroscopy, which can measure the amount of Choline and Citrate present in the prostate tissue, helps doctors tell the difference between BPH and prostate cancer.

A major challenge for urologists has been the 30-35 percent accuracy of random TRUS biopsies. In the past, this lack of accuracy has led to the need for follow-up biopsies, which increases the risk of complications.

Improvements in MRI technology and the ability to transfer the MRI image to a transrectal ultrasound has created a new generation of targeted prostate biopsies: MRI-TRUS fusion (also called "MRI-Fusion").

The MRI-fusion uses the MRI, which is performed, interpreted and stored in the device by a radiologist. This three-dimensional reconstruction of the prostate is then fused with real-time ultrasound, allowing the target(s) to be seen on the screen of the ultrasound machine. The biopsies are then performed trans-rectally aiming for the targets displayed on the ultrasound screen.

This technology offers a way to pinpoint, sample, and track suspected cancers with greater precision and improved detection rates (75-80% versus 30-35%). The image fusion process combines relevant information from MRI and ultrasound into a single image, which provides more information than either image alone.

As with a TRUS biopsy, MRI-Fusion biopsies can be done in an office setting and combine the knowledge of an expert radiologist with the expertise of a urologist.

## Who Benefits Most from MRI-Fusion Technology

It would be easy to argue that all men who have a prostate biopsy would benefit from this new technology; however, there are two clinical scenarios that benefit the most:

1. Men in active surveillance
2. Men who have had a prior negative biopsy but continue to have elevated PSA levels.

Men on active surveillance already have prostate cancer that has been identified by a prostate biopsy (presumably low-risk, low-volume cancer). The previous biopsies indicate the areas of the prostate that contain cancer. An MRI-fusion biopsy can guide the biopsy needles to within 1.2 mm of their target, so doctors can revisit areas from the previous biopsy with a level of accuracy that cannot be achieved with a TRUS biopsy.

The second group poses a significant challenge for urologists because (until recently) repeat TRUS biopsies were the only real alternative available — and the complications from prostate biopsies go up with each additional biopsy.

In addition, these patients may have cancer in areas that are not routinely biopsied, such as the anterior prostate or close to the urethra. If a patient has an aggressive form of cancer in an unusual location, the disease might progress long before a diagnosis could be made.

Because MRI-Fusion biopsies provide a more accurate image of the prostate, it allows doctors to spot previously "unseen" cancers and save lives — while minimizing the need for repeat biopsies and their attendant complications.

New biomarker technologies can also help previously biopsied patients gather more information about the health of their prostate. The epigenetic test ConfirmMDx has a of 98 percent negative predictive value when performed on prostate biopsy tissue samples.

If negative, it can help avoid a unnecessary re-biopsy. If positive, it can direct doctors to specific areas of the prostate that are more likely to harbor hidden cancer; therefore, improving the chances of finding the cancer.

Blood- and urine-based biomarkers such as 4Kscore Test, PCA3, and SelectMDx can also provide important information for men on active surveillance and men with an elevated PSA and negative prostate biopsy results.

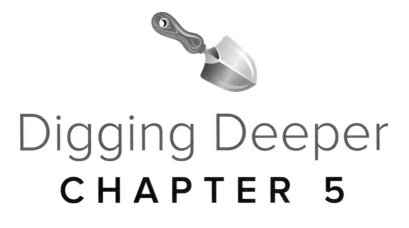

# Digging Deeper
## CHAPTER 5

This Digging Deeper Section includes the following tools and resources to help you better understand your prostate cancer diagnosis and begin to evaluate your treatment options based on the kind of cancer you have:

- Doctor Selection Tips
- Watchful Waiting vs. Active Surveillance
- A Deeper Look at Active Surveillance

# Doctor Selection Tips

*Even though the Declaration of Independence states that: "All men are created equal" — all doctors are not. For this reason, we strongly recommend that you consult with local prostate cancer support group(s) and meet with prostate cancer survivors who live in your area to find out which doctors and hospitals deliver the best results and the highest level of care.*

## KISSING A FEW FROGS

*When it comes to finding the right doctor, you may have to kiss a few frogs (so to speak) before you find your prince. That's normal and to be expected.*

*Men with low-risk, low-volume prostate cancer should get a second, third, or even fourth opinion before making a final decision.*

*Seek professional opinions from doctors who specialize in different kinds of medicine. For example, if your first doctor is a surgeon (urologist), we recommend you get a second opinion from a doctor who specializes in a different type of treatment — radiation, cryotherapy, or some other form of treatment.*

*Men with high-risk, high-volume prostate cancer do NOT have the luxury of a third or fourth opinion. With a high-risk diagnosis, time is of the essence.*

## FINDING THE RIGHT DOCTOR IS CRUCIAL

**Here's what to look for:**

*1. The doctor's skill, knowledge, and experience (use the Internet, talk to local prostate cancer survivors, seek out operating room nurses)*

*2. His/Her treatment success rates (5-, 10-, 20-years after treatment)*

*3. What are the complications of the recommended treatment?*

*4. Compare this doctor's complication rates with other doctors in your area*

*5. Do you feel comfortable about putting your prostate, your future sex life, and your ability to have a normal lifestyle in this doctor's hands?*

*6. Did this doctor take the time to answer your questions in a satisfactory way?*

## TRUST YOUR GUT

*As silly as it sounds, listening to your "intuition" is extremely important at a time like this. Your "gut" doesn't second guess itself; your mind, however, flip-flops all the time. Now is the time to listen to your survival instincts.*

*The last thing you want is regrets. You want to look back in ten years and say, "I would make that same decision in a heartbeat."*

| Watchful Waiting | Active Surveillance |
|---|---|
| • WW is generally suitable for men with other significant health issues. | • Works best for low-risk, low-volume patients. |
| • Commonly used when life expectancy is 5 years or less. | • Involves close monitoring and regular follow-up with the following tests and scans: PSA free, total, velocity and density; PCA 3 or SelectMDX, 4Kscore Test, MRI scans, and prostate biopsies. |
| • Usually does NOT involve prostate cancer follow-up appointments or curative treatment. | |
| • Treatment is palliative (focused on relieving pain and alleviating symptoms). | • Active surveillance may lead to definitive treatment if cancer progresses based on the numbers from any of the above tests. |

**Figure DD 5.0** displays the key differences between Watchful Waiting and Active Surveillance. Although these two treatments were once considered to be the same, there are striking differences between the two. The biggest difference is that Watchful Waiting is usually an end of life "lack of treatment" choice. Active Surveillance, on the other hand, involves significant lifestyle changes that can have dramatic affects on a man's overall health; therefore, his prostate health as well.

# Watchful Waiting vs. Active Surveillance

At one time, watchful waiting and active surveillance were considered the same type of treatment — more or less a "wait and see" approach to early stage prostate cancer. Today, watchful waiting is essentially a form of non-treatment. It is usually reserved for men who are too old/unhealthy to undergo treatment or have another pressing health problem that is a greater concern. Active surveillance, on the other hand, involves significant lifestyle changes. These lifestyle changes are discussed in greater detail in **Chapter 10**.

There are probably as many different kinds of active surveillance programs as there are practitioners advocating them. In other words, different doctors focus on different behaviors that they believe can help their patients regain their overall health and the health of their prostate.

Obviously, active surveillance programs vary between patients, as no two men are the same. That said, most active surveillance programs focus on these common lifestyle areas:

1. Diet
2. Nutritional supplements
3. Daily exercise
4. Stress management

5. Getting more/better quality sleep

6. Improved immune system function

7. Balancing hormones

8. Correcting structural problems

9. Removing toxic substances from your body and your environment

10. Prayer, meditation, and mindfulness

When evaluating patients for active surveillance, doctors frequently look at two factors:

1. The kind of prostate cancer a man has

2. How willing is he to comply with the program.

Men with low-risk, low-grade, low-volume prostate cancer are the best candidates for active surveillance because their cancer is less likely to spread or pose a threat to their health.

In 1995, pathologist Dr. Jonathan Epstein, M.D. developed clinical criteria to help determine which men with Stage T1c prostate cancer were good candidates for active surveillance, and which men should consider more aggressive treatment. (See below).

Since 1995, the revolution in biomarker testing (blood, urine, prostate biopsy tissue samples — both epigenetic and genomic) has expanded the range of active surveillance beyond just men with type T1c cancer.

## Men with Stage T1c cancer are a good candidate for active surveillance if:

- ◆ It is found in only one or two biopsy needle cores, AND
- ◆ It makes up less than half of each needle core, AND
- ◆ The Gleason score is 6 or lower, AND
- ◆ PSA Density is in the 0.1 – 0.15 range, AND
- ◆ Free PSA is greater than 15 percent

## Men with Stage T1c cancer are a good candidate for more aggressive treatment if:

- ◆ It is found in three or more biopsy needle cores, OR
- ◆ It is present in greater than half of any one biopsy needle core, OR
- ◆ The Gleason score is 7 or higher, OR
- ◆ PSA Density is greater tan the 0.1 – 0.15 range, OR
- ◆ Free PSA is less than 15 percent

# A Deeper Look at Active Surveillance

Low-risk prostate cancer patients with low-volume disease are the best candidates for active surveillance. Patients with higher Gleason scores who have intermediate-to-high-volume disease are not good candidates for active surveillance because they are more likely to die from prostate cancer without definitive treatment.

The above statement is supported by data obtained from the PIVOT study, which compared radical prostatectomy to watchful waiting among 731 men with localized prostate cancer. In this study, men in the intermediate- to high-risk category who underwent a radical prostatectomy were less likely to die from prostate cancer than were the men in the watchful-waiting group.

Even though low-risk, low-volume patients are the best candidates for active surveillance, a small percentage of these men will see their cancer progress, sometimes to metastatic disease.

There is also the question of how to classify and treat patients in the "intermediate disease" category who have low-volume disease, because many of their cancers behave like low-risk cancer. It is this group that may benefit most from genomic testing to determine the true nature of their cancer and how to best to treat it.

Genomic testing of prostate biopsy tissue (Oncotype DX, Prolaris and Decipher) have proven helpful in identifying which low- to intermediate-risk patients have been properly diagnosed and which ones have more significant prostate cancer. Although these tests use different screening protocols, they all have the ability to recognize aggressive cancers that have a higher risk of becoming metastatic.

These tests measure the level of genes involved in tumor proliferation (how fast cancer cells divide) and assess tumor aggressiveness. This type of testing adds valuable information to standard prostate cancer tests like Gleason Score, PSA, cancer staging, number of positive needle cores, and other pathological characteristics. Genomic testing also reduces the number of unnecessary treatments and follow-up biopsies.

As more men take advantage of genomic testing (to identify cancers that are or will become more aggressive) and epigenetic testing (to uncover hidden cancers earlier than before), there is every reason to believe that the number of active surveillance treatment failures will decrease.

In addition, second opinions on pathology specimens can also be helpful in the assignment of proper Gleason scores; therefore the placement of patients into the right risk category.

Another important, and often overlooked, parameter is the age of the patient. The Scandinavian Prostate Cancer Group Study 4 (SPCG-4) studied the survival rate of patients who had localized prostate cancer. The study compared men who underwent radical prostatectomy versus men who choose watchful waiting. The patients who underwent radical prostatectomy were less likely to develop metastatic disease and die from prostate cancer than men in the watchful waiting group.

These findings were only statistically significant for men younger than 65 years. Thus suggesting that patients in the low-risk category who are older than 65 do not receive any longevity benefit from surgical removal of the prostate. They will, however, incur a higher incidence of impotence and incontinence; therefore, decreasing their overall quality of life.

## Active Surveillance Protocols

Active surveillance protocols vary greatly, and a lack of universally accepted standards needs to be reached to help ensure that each active surveillance patient receives the best possible treatment.

To complicate matters, many major academic institutions in the United States have their own active surveillance standards regarding the patients they accept, treatment protocols, and follow-up procedures. In addition, the treatments and lifestyle modifications used in active surveillance programs vary from doctor to doctor (and patient to patient).

On the one hand, new research on active surveillance is being done all over the world, which is great. On the other hand, the lack of active surveillance standards makes it difficult to make apples-to-apples comparisons of the data and results from all these different studies.

As new blood, urine, and tissue biomarker tests such as 4Kscore Test, PCA3, SelectMDx, Prolaris, Oncotype DX, and Decipher become commonly applied standards for codifying cancer, logic dictates that a clearer picture will emerge regarding who is/is not a good candidate for active surveillance.

The 10 lifestyle modifications listed earlier in this section are only points of departure for what should be a highly tailored treatment plan that is individualized for each patient. Whether a particular protocol is the right one for any, most, or all active surveillance patients will require a great deal of additional study.

The Canary PASS Study is an example of the kind of multi-institutional prospective study that could be adapted to provide the kind of information needed to help create more universal standards about which patients are the right ones for an active surveillance protocol.

The Canary PASS Study evaluated watchful waiting outcomes for patients with clinically localized prostate cancer. The study enrolled 907 patients. Each patient received a PSA screening every 3 months, a DRE every 6 months, and re-biopsy (minimum of 10 cores each time) at 6, 12, 24, 48 and 72 months after diagnosis.

The Canary PASS Study defined disease progression if Gleason score increased and tumor volume increased greater than 34 percent . Most men remained in watchful waiting for 5 years without adverse reclassification. From this group, however, 24 percent of patients were reclassified to a higher risk category. Of the 907 patients, 172 participants underwent treatment. Of those 172 men, 55 chose treatment despite not having any evidence of clinical progression.

The fact that 55 patients opted for treatment without any clinical evidence of progression speaks volumes about the anxiety of having any amount of cancer and the possibility of its progression.

In addition, the Canary PASS Study concluded that clinical characteristics alone do not completely distinguish indolent cancers from more significant ones. This data suggest the need for genomic testing, better imaging studies, and possibly more accurate biopsy techniques (such as MRI-fusion biopsy). Unfortunately, studies using these newer techniques have yet to be published.

It is also important to note that the Canary PASS Study did not differentiate between watchful waiting and active surveillance patients. In other words, some of these patients may have made health-affirming "active" lifestyle changes, while other may have just gone about their lives as they had before they received a prostate cancer diagnosis.

## Improved Imaging for Active Surveillance Patients

Magnetic Resonance Imaging (MRI) provide much higher resolution images than CT scans or Trans-rectal Ultrasound (TRUS). Over the past decade the image quality of MRIs has improved to help distinguish between normal and cancer tissue and between lower- and higher-risk cancer.

When advanced MRI technology is used in a targeted MRI-ultrasound fusion biopsy, it has the ability to detect, locate, track, and sample areas suspected of harboring cancer with precision; therefore, helping active surveillance patients by recording the precise areas previously biopsied, and noting whether the cancer in these areas has progressed.

## What Happens When Active Surveillance Fails?

As mentioned on the previous page, there is a need for more universal follow-up standards for active surveillance patients, and an even greater need for a clear definition of disease progression.

That said, many institutions in the United States look for changes in the following areas as an indication that the patient's cancer is progressing and that definitive treatment is warranted:

- DRE
- PSA velocity
- PSA thresholds  (PSA greater than 10)
- Gleason Score
- Number of positive biopsies

Of all these parameters Gleason Score is the best predictor of progression and the most likely to trigger a definitive treatment.

In order to minimize the possibility of cancer progression, active surveillance patients and their physicians should take full advantage of all of the recent advances in blood and urine biomarkers, genomic testing, imaging, and MRI-fusion biopsies.

# Digging Deeper

## CHAPTER 6

This Digging Deeper Section includes additional information about the following therapies to help you understand the complex and evolving field of "Emerging" prostate cancer treatment.

- The evolution from whole-gland treatments to smaller, focused, targeted treatments

# The Evolution from Whole-gland Treatments to Smaller, Focused, Targeted Treatments

The trend towards smaller, focused, targeted therapies has been motivated by a similar rationale as to the push towards active surveillance:

- Minimize treatment complications
- Improve treatment outcomes
- Decrease the number of prostate cancer deaths

All three of these points are appealing to many prostate cancer patients who are looking for the most effective yet least invasive treatment — especially patients who are frightened by the possibility of lifelong quality of life issues like incontinence and impotence.

As we mentioned in **Chapter 6,** since "emerging" treatments for prostate cancer are relatively new, they do not have 25-year survival rate statistics to support their efficacy. This lack of supporting data naturally sparks the question: "How do I know if this treatment will work?" This question looms over any new type of treatment — especially any new type of cancer treatment.

Since prostate cancer kills approximately 26,000 men a year in the United States, the dilemma is real. Should you to go with a less-proven (focused) treatment that has a lower risk of complications or a more traditional (whole gland) treatment that carries a higher complication risk.

On one side of the scales are treatment success rates, on the other side are treatment complication rates. The choice ultimately boils down to risking a less invasive type of treatment with the possibility that cancer could come back (and potentially spread into the rest of the body) versus going with a more traditional treatment that has a longer track record but also has a higher risk of complications from treatment.

**Chapter 8** provides both quantitative and qualitative information designed to help men make this agonizing decision.

## From a medical perspective, we see this concern from two perspectives:

**1. Overtreatment (with all its attendant complications):** This is especially a concern for men with low-risk, low-volume disease who may be good candidates for focal treatment or active surveillance. The overtreatment group best describes candidates for focal treatment (also called "emerging" or "targeted" treatments).

**2. Undertreatment (with the risk of cancer returning and spreading):**
Because prostate cancer can be a deadly disease, men with more aggressive cancers are understandably more concerned with "getting all of the cancer" than they are about possible complications. That's not to say that complications and quality of life issues are not a important to men with more advanced cancer; they are just not the top of the concern list.

# Focal Treatment vs. Active Surveillance

The first question that doctors who regularly work with low-risk, low-volume prostate cancer patients ask themselves is whether this patient would be a better candidate for active surveillance or focal therapy.

The truth is that there is a significant amount of treatment overlap for many low-risk, low-volume patients — to the point where some practitioners consider the active surveillance/focal treatment group as one and the same.

So why treat men with low-risk, low-volume cancer with focal therapies if they are good candidates for active surveillance? The best answer is that some patients have so much anxiety about their disease that removing the small amount of cancer in their prostate will help them feel more confident and less stressed about their condition. With focal treatment, they are actively doing something to get rid of their cancer — and that is very important for both their physical and mental health.

Lastly, patient education is crucial and should involve clear information and guidelines for post-treatment follow up. Also, this post-treatment information should include making the patient aware of the possibility of recurrence or that a smaller lesion not previously seen could become apparent with time and require further treatment.

A good analogy is skin cancer, where removal of a lesion does not rule out the need for careful follow-up to prevent a recurrence or the growth of a new lesion elsewhere else on the body.

As with active surveillance patients, focal therapy patients should have regular follow-ups to make sure there are no signs that the cancer has returned. If the cancer does come back, these patients should be treated with a definitive whole-gland treatment (where the entire prostate is removed, frozen, or destroyed by radiation).

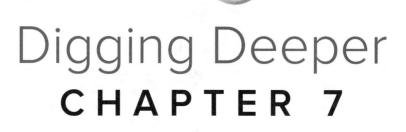

# Digging Deeper
## CHAPTER 7

This Digging Deeper Section includes information designed to help you better understand the relationship between testosterone and prostate cancer:

- How testosterone affects prostate cancer
- Intermittent Hormone Therapy

# Testosterone and PCA

Despite what you may have heard, testosterone does not cause prostate cancer!

If it did, the following three conditions would be true:

1. Twenty-year-old men, who have the highest testosterone levels, would also have the highest prostate cancer levels — but they have the lowest.
2. The prostate cancer rate would be highest for men with the highest testosterone levels — but after dozens of studies, no such connection can be found.
3. The most aggressive forms of prostate cancer would occur in men with the highest testosterone levels — but the opposite is true — the most aggressive forms of prostate cancer occur in men with the lowest levels of testosterone.

## What Does This Mean for Men with Prostate Cancer?

That 60 years of medical dogma that high testosterone levels cause prostate cancer is wrong.

Dr. Abraham Morgentaler and his colleagues at Harvard Medical School demonstrated that when testosterone levels are low, both healthy and cancerous prostate cells absorb testosterone like a sponge. However, once prostate cells reach a saturation point for testosterone at the low end of normal range for adult men, they stop absorbing testosterone.

## Testosterone & Prostate Cancer in a Nutshell

1. Men with LOW testosterone levels are:
   - NOT protected from prostate cancer
   - More likely to develop prostate cancer
   - More likely to have a higher grade and stage of prostate cancer
   - More likely to develop high-risk disease

2. Men with HIGH testosterone levels are NOT at a higher risk of developing prostate cancer

3. Men with prostate cancer do NOT have higher androgen levels than other men who do not have prostate cancer.

4. Normal testosterone levels do NOT have an impact on prostate cancer.

## What the Medical Research Says about Testosterone

■ In 21 long-term studies that looked at the relationship of testosterone to prostate development, the vast majority revealed no significant connection.

■ Data from 18 different studies, which combined 3,896 men with prostate cancer and 6,438 without prostate cancer, found NO connection between testosterone levels and prostate cancer.

■ In 19 controlled testosterone replacement therapy studies, the data showed no increase in PSA or prostate cancer, when compared to a placebo control group.

■ In 1,576 individual cases, there was NO connection found between testosterone and PSA.

■ Weekly intramuscular injections of testosterone (250 – 600 mg) that created abnormally high blood levels of testosterone (1138 – 2800 ng/ml) did NOT change either PSA or prostate volume.

# Intermittent Hormone Therapy

To understand the evolution from continuous hormone therapy to intermittent hormone therapy, we need to understand the reasons behind this move, and why it is so important. We also need to know how blocking the production and uptake of testosterone affects men and their bodies.

Today, it is widely accepted that an intermittent androgen blockade offers many patients the best way to maximize the therapeutic benefits against prostate cancer and minimize the side effects of a hormone (testosterone) blockade.

With intermittent hormone therapy, patients use the medications that block testosterone production for six to twelve months. A low PSA level is maintained during this time, and research indicates that the tumor burden is significantly reduced. (Most protocols call for at least three months of undetectable PSA levels.).

During the next period, the patient stops taking the medication that blocks testosterone production until the PSA rises to a predetermined level. (This level varies and depends upon the doctor, the patient, the patient's age, and overall health status).

Some patients refer to this period as a "drug holiday" because testosterone frequently returns to pre-treatment levels, which reverses many of the side effects that occurred during testosterone deprivation. This "holiday" often helps men recover their sexual function, improve their level energy and ability to exercise, regain their mental clarity, and restore their quality of life.

Once the PSA levels rise to that predetermined level, the medication(s) that blocks testosterone production and uptake are restarted.

## How Effective Is Intermittent Hormone Therapy?

To answer that question, we must first state the goals of intermittent hormone therapy:

1. Improve prostate cancer survival rate over continuous therapy — or at least maintain the same longevity as continuous therapy.

2. Reduce the negative side effects of a hormone (testosterone) blockade.

In 2015, Dr. Sindy Mangan, MD et al. published a review and meta-analysis of 10,510 references that included 22 articles and 15 trials (6,856 patients) that were published between 2000 and 2013. The study was titled, *Intermittent vs Continuous Androgen Deprivation Therapy for Prostate Cancer: A Systematic Review and Meta-analysis.*

## There were three critical observations from this study:

**1. Longevity:** No significant difference in overall survival occurred between patients on intermittent or continuous therapy.

**2. Quality of Life:** A minor improvement was reported in quality of life with intermittent therapy. Most trials observed an improvement in physical and sexual functioning with intermittent therapy.

**2a. Erections:** Intermittent therapy patients reported an improved level of sexual function. The quality of this finding, however, would be even more valuable had the level of sexual function been recorded before intermittent hormone therapy began. Did patients have a satisfying sex life before intermittent therapy?

**3. Hormone Resistance:** The use of intermittent therapy did not increase the time to hormone resistance (where the cancer is no longer responding to hormone therapy).

Intuitively, it makes sense that intermittent therapy would increase the time it takes to reach hormone resistance. In fact, two out of 4 studies in this meta-analysis did show that the time to reach hormone resistance increased with intermittent therapy; two other studies, however, did not.

## This study also poses some crucial questions regarding standardized protocols:

1. What is the ideal length of time for both the treatment and off-treatment (recovery) periods?

2. Traditionally, rising PSA total has been the signal to start or restart hormone therapy. The question remains, is PSA the best signal to begin the recovery periods and re-start hormone therapy? What if other biomarkers were combined to create a new formula for calculating when to begin and end hormone therapy recovery periods

2a. If PSA total is the best signal to start and restart hormone therapy, how high should the PSA total levels be allowed to go before therapy begins (or begins again) 10, 20, 50 ... 100 mg/nl?

## Other unanswered questions about the benefits of intermittent hormone therapy:

1. Does intermittent hormone therapy delay the development of hormone-resistant strains of prostate cancer; therefore, improving the longevity of the patient?

2. How does intermittent therapy affect bone health (reduce fractures, improve bone density)?

The longer patients stay on a testosterone blockade (hormone therapy), the greater the risk of side effects becoming irreversible and more pronounced. Hence, the push to find an alternative form of treatment.

## Side Effects

■ **Hot flashes and sweats:** Although they may improve gradually, some men have them throughout the entire hormone therapy. The National Institute for Health and Care Excellence (NICE) recommends medroxy-progesterone as the best treatment for hot flashes.

■ **Fatigue and weakness:** These symptoms are not uncommon, and regular and gentle exercise will help minimize them. Over exercising is the biggest error committed by patients with a recent cancer diagnosis, which can lead to more fatigue and weakness.

■ **Decreased bone density:** The stronger the bone, the less likely metastatic cancer cells are to take hold in them. Preemptive use of calcium and other minerals, vitamin $D_3$, and weight bearing exercise can strengthen the bone.

- **Decrease testicular size:** "Testicular shrinkage" is likely reversible if the hormone blockade is less than 1 year

- **Decreased libido and erections:** The majority of men who receive injections (luteinising hormone, LH, agonist and antagonist) report a lack of libido and inability to get an erection, while only half of the men on oral anti-androgens (Casodex) report these symptoms.

- **Male breast enlargement:** Breast swelling and tenderness is a particular problem with high dose Casodex. Taking Tamoxifen can help to reduce breast tenderness in about 6 out of 10 men. An alternative way to manage these side effects is a low dose of radiation to the breasts before treatment begins.

- **Weight gain and loss of muscle mass:** These side effects are common and may require calorie management and regular exercise. A low glycemic diet, rich in vegetables and fiber, with good quality protein and fats can be helpful.

- **Depression and memory impairment:** Although often manageable, cognitive challenges may be serious enough to require management by a mental health professional — and sometimes medication. Proper counseling and open discussions about these side effects before treatment begins can help buffer the mental-emotional effects of hormone therapy.

- **Risk of heart attack:** There is some evidence to suggest that men over age 65 who are on hormone therapy are at a higher risk of heart attack. Heart attacks are more likely if the patient already has a heart condition. In these cases, an evaluation by cardiology is imperative. In some cases, certain patients should avoid hormone therapy.

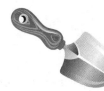

# Digging Deeper
## CHAPTER 8

This Digging Deeper Section includes a sample "action plan" to help you find the best treatment to match the kind of cancer you have:

- Creating a Successful Action Plan

# Creating a Successful Action Plan

We included this checklist to help you put together a prostate cancer action plan. This checklist walks you through all the steps in the treatment process that we have discussed up to now, and provides a organized format for all the medical information, numbers, results, opinions, and options.

Since **Chapter 8** is all about weighing the pros and cons of possible prostate cancer treatments and doctors, we thought it would be a good idea to give you a space for all this information.

Clearly, this is too much information to carry around in your head. It's also important to realize that each piece of medical information is weighted differently. For example, while a PSA free number is important, it is less important than the results of a genomic test.

Hopefully, this list gives you greater clarity and helps you make smart decisions.

## TESTS                                    (enter your information here)

### 1. Blood Biomarkers

    A. PSA total

    B. PSA free

    C. PSA density

    D. PSA velocity

    E. 4Kscore Test

### 2. Urine Biomarkers

    A. PCA3

    B. SelectMDx

## SCANS

### 1. Ultrasound

### 2. MRI

### 3. CAT

### 4. Bone Scan

## PROSTATE BIOPSY (enter your information here)

### 1. TRUS Biopsy

### 2. MRI-Guided Biopsy

### 3. MRI-Fusion Biopsy

## PROSTATE BIOPSY RESULTS

### 1. Negative

A. Epigenetic Test

i. ConfirmMDx

### 2. Positive

A. Cancer Stage

B. Gleason Score

C. PSA

D. Number of Positive Core Samples

E. Percent of Cancer in Biopsy

F. Genomic Tests

i. Oncotype DX

ii. Prolaris

iii. Decipher

### 3. Prostate Cancer Risk Assessment

A. Low-risk

B. Moderate-risk

C. High-risk

# MEDICAL APPOINTMENTS   (enter your information here)

## 1. First Opinion

    A. Name of Doctor

    B. Type of Doctor

    C. Doctor's Treatment Recommendation

    D. Doctor's Personal Success Rate

    E. Doctor's Personal Complication Rate

    F. What Do Former Patients Say?

    G. What Does Your Gut Say?

## 2. Second Opinion

    A. Name of Doctor

    B. Type of Doctor

    C. Doctor's Treatment Recommendation

    D. Doctor's Personal Success Rate

    E. Doctor's Personal Complication Rate

    F. What Do Former Patients Say?

    G. What Does Your Gut Say?

## 3. Third Opinion

    A. Name of Doctor

    B. Type of Doctor

    C. Doctor's Treatment Recommendation

    D. Doctor's Personal Success Rate

    E. Doctor's Personal Complication Rate

    F. What Do Former Patients Say?

    G. What Does Your Gut Say?

# TREATMENT OPTIONS
(enter your information here)

## 1. First Treatment Option

    A. Pros & Cons

    B. Success Rates vs. Complication Rates

    C. Which Complications Could You Live with?

    D. Which Complications Would Be Unbearable?

## 2. Second Treatment Option

    A. Pros & Cons

    B. Success Rates vs. Complication Rates

    C. Which Complications Could You Live with?

    D. Which Complications Would Be Unbearable?

## 3. Third Treatment Option

    A. Pros & Cons

    B. Success Rates vs. Complication Rates

    C. Which Complications Could You Live with?

    D. Which Complications Would Be Unbearable?

## 4. Fourth Treatment Option

    A. Pros & Cons

    B. Success Rates vs. Complication Rates

    C. Which Complications Could You Live with?

    D. Which Complications Would Be Unbearable?

# Digging Deeper
## CHAPTER 9

This Digging Deeper section includes the following tools and resources to help you cope with the emotional aspects of a prostate cancer diagnosis:

- Healthy Happy Strong List
- National Suicide Prevention Hotline
- Suicide Prevention
- Mark's Unsuccessful Suicide Story

# Healthy, Happy, Strong

Here's the list of activities that we recommend you do on a daily basis as you continue to surf the emotional tidal wave after a prostate cancer diagnosis. These activities are the ones that men report helped them reconnect with themselves after their diagnosis.

These activities can be done at any time, anywhere. Don't feel compelled to do all of them; however, we suggest you pick two or three and commit to doing one of them every day.

## A. Move Your Body

Daily exercise is one of the best things you can do to take care of your nervous system after being punched in the gut by a prostate cancer diagnosis. We recommend 30 minutes of exercise every day to start.

Note: If you haven't exercised for a while, go slowly at first and intentionally underachieve for the first couple of weeks, if not months. The last thing you want is the double whammy of injuring yourself in an attempt to improve your health.

If 30 minutes of exercise a day would be going from 0 to 60, then start with 10 minutes of exercise a day and add 10 more minutes a day by the end of each week. If you follow this program, you will be up to 30 minutes of exercise a day by the third week.

Whenever you start a new exercise regime, pay attention to what your body tells you. If your body hurts during or after exercise, we recommend that you try a different kind of exercise.

If you have the money to do so, now would be a good time to work with a personal trainer — both in terms of learning how to train smarter and for the daily motivation.

All exercise is helpful:

- Walking
- Hiking
- Running
- Cycling
- Swimming
- Weight lifting
- Skiing

- Ice skating
- Team sports (basketball, soccer, volleyball, baseball / softball, hockey ...)
- Group fitness
- Aerobics
- Dance

- Pilates
- Yoga
- Martial arts
- Interval training
- Golf
- Tennis

...You get the idea

The goal is to break a sweat, breathe harder, get your heart rate up, and feel like you pushed yourself slightly outside your comfort zone.

For most people, the sweet spot happens when you raise your heart rate to the point where it's challenging to hold a conversation. This level of exertion elevates your mood and boosts your body's production of the hormones and neurotransmitters that promote happiness.

## B. Music Therapy

Like James Brown said, "Get up offa that thing and dance 'till you feel better."

There are so many ways to brighten your world with music: sing in the shower, play an instrument, croon in your car, crank your favorite music until the neighbors come knocking, make a play list of your special songs and keep it on your smart phone so you can listen to it anytime, dance around the kitchen in your underwear, or get out of the house and go listen to some live music at a local venue.

Beethoven or Bruno Mars, it doesn't matter.

What's important is that you let the music soothe you, move you, get down and groove you.

## C. Creative Outlets

If you draw, paint, work with wood, sculpt, make origami animals, write songs, rebuild car engines, or create art out of found objects, NOW is the time to indulge your creative side. Like music and meditation, these outlets take your mind off of your diagnosis and give you time to do something that gives you a feeling of satisfaction — maybe even joy.

## D. Meditation

Meditation is powerful medicine; however, sitting meditation can be difficult to do when you're completely stressed out.

That's why we recommend any activity that takes you mind away from what's going on inside your body: walking in nature, fly fishing, motorcycle riding, gardening, wood working, cooking, repairing bicycles ... whatever your passion happens to be.

All it takes to do sitting meditation is a chair, a quiet space, and 20 minutes. You sit down in that quiet space and practice mindful breathing. What is "mindful breathing?" Good question.

In its simplest form, mindful breathing, is being aware of your breath without thought or judgment or any attempt to control it. You are simply following your breath in and out. There's no right or wrong; there's no destination, there's nothing to achieve.

When your thoughts wander away from your breath (as they will) you simply refocus your attention back to your next breath, and then the next, and so on. The mind chatter will come and go. Some days are better than others.

If you detach yourself from all the thoughts and worries that demand your immediate attention, soon you will find yourself resting in your breath.

Those few moments of stillness are priceless.

## E. Prayer

If you are a prayerful person, now is the ideal time to:

- Pray for your health and healing
- Ask other people to pray for you
- Invite groups of people to pray with you
- Request other people at your place of worship pray for you
- Have the leader of your religious community hold a healing vigil for you and invite whomever you like

If you are open to prayer, but it's not part of your daily life, a simple and honest prayer for help and healing opens the door to possibilities that you may not have considered.

---

### Health Outside the Box

Australian Veterinarian, Dr. Ian Gawler, was diagnosed with aggressive bone cancer. One of his legs was amputated and he was given conventional treatment, but the cancer continued to spread. His doctors gave him less than a month to live.

Feeling his life was coming to an end, Dr. Gawler began meditating three hours a day and switched to a strict plant-based diet. Within weeks, his bone deformities began to disappear. Within months, they were gone.

That was over 35 years ago. Today, Dr. Gawler is an internationally recognized authority on health and healing. He holds numerous retreats and seminars in his native Australia. (*http://www.iangawler.com*)

If you are opposed to prayer on principle, meditation (see above) offers many healing and calming benefits without bringing your beliefs into question.

## F. Get Out of the House

In moments of crisis, we all tend to close the blinds, hole up, and disconnect from the outside world. That's normal and perhaps healthy — for a while. After a week or two, that sort of isolation starts to become counter-productive.

We strongly recommend you get out of the house as often as you can, even if it's just to walk your dog, run errands, or go to your local market to buy some healthy food. Get out and mingle with people. Feel the fresh air on your skin. Share a smile with a stranger. You never know who you'll meet and what they will have to offer you.

## G. Get Out in Nature

You can't put a price tag on being in nature. It lifts your spirit and refreshes your senses.

A walk in the woods, through an open field, or along a shoreline reunites us with something primal.

If you're fortunate enough to live close to hiking trails, open space areas, or a body of water, add visiting them to your weekly to-do list. If you live in an urban area, try taking walks in a local park (assuming it's safe).

If you have a friend, family member, loved one, or beloved dog to accompany you, all the better.

Just being able to look up at the sky and watch the birds fly overhead is worth the effort it takes to get away from the traffic and congestion for a while.

For some men, fishing and hunting are what pulls them outdoors. If that's your story, plan a fishing or hunting trip soon.

# Suicide Statistics after Receiving a Prostate Cancer Diagnosis

Being told, "You have prostate cancer," often sets off a serious emotional crisis. The words "you" and "cancer" in the same sentence can trigger feelings of extreme anxiety, uncertainty, confusion, helplessness, and a fear of death.

In general, the more advanced the cancer, the greater the shock. However, this emotional response may have little to do with the size of the tumor, Gleason score, or how early it was detected. Any cancer diagnosis can kick up a hornet's nest of emotional issues that leave people feeling devastated and out of control.

For many men, a prostate cancer diagnosis is like staring down the barrel of their own mortality.

---

**National Suicide Prevention Hotline**

**1 (800) 273-8255**

**1 (800) 273-TALK**

*Counselors are available in English and Spanish (24/7/365)*

---

This form of psychological stress can cripple a man's self-esteem in a matter of minutes. Two hours before, he knew who he was and where he was going in life. And then Wham-O! Nothing makes sense. He doesn't know which way is up.

For some men, the level of stress, panic, and sadness is so severe that suicide looks like a perfectly reasonable option.

According to a 2005 study reported in the *American Journal of Geriatric Psychiatry,* researchers did a population-based review of men over 65 living in South Florida. The average annual incidence of suicide for these men was 55.3 per 100,000 people. For men with prostate cancer, however, the rate was 274.7 per 100,000 people. That's a **397 percent** increase in the suicide rate when compared to the general population.

There were almost five times as many suicides among men 65 and older who had prostate cancer than men the same age, living in the same area, who did NOT have prostate cancer.

Those numbers speak volumes about the need for addressing the emotional side of a prostate cancer diagnosis!

The same article also stated that 128 suicides were reported among 77,439 Swedish men with prostate cancer — 43 more suicides than were expected based on the suicide rate in the general population. Perhaps the most interesting finding of this study is that the suicide risk did not go up for men with early prostate cancer (T1c–T2), but it did increase for men with locally advanced disease, metastatic disease, and in those receiving androgen deprivation therapy.

## Suicide Rate Before PSA Testing

The suicide rate was even higher before PSA testing became the standard of care circa 1993.

A 2010 Harvard Medical School study examined the suicide rates among 342,000 men who had been diagnosed with prostate cancer from 1979 – 2004. The suicide rate among the men with prostate cancer was 40 percent higher in the year following their diagnosis, and 90 percent higher in the first three months after their diagnosis, than it was among men the same age who didn't have prostate cancer.

Harvard Medical School researchers also discovered that post-diagnosis suicide rates dropped dramatically after 1993. Presumably, this drop in the suicide rate occurred because PSA screening alerted men to the possible presence of prostate cancer before the disease became advanced, which lead to a less devastating diagnosis.

## What's the Take-Home Message?

Suicidal feelings should be taken seriously. If you have been diagnosed with prostate cancer and feel suicidal, know that you're not alone. These feelings happen to lots of men in your situation, including one of the authors of this book.

Don't mess around. If you're feeling suicidal, get help immediately!

Call the National Suicide Prevention Lifeline number: *1 (800) 273-8255.*

Trained counselors are available in English and Spanish: 24/7/365.

Finding a skilled professional counselor or therapist to help you get through the first couple of months after a diagnosis can be a crucial part of your recovery.

If you don't know of a good counselor or therapist in your community, ask your doctor or someone you trust. Do whatever you need to do in order to work through the suicidal feelings and other symptoms of being emotionally overwhelmed that often accompany a prostate cancer diagnosis.

**Remember:** Killing yourself because you have prostate cancer would be like joining cancer's team. We recommend that you embrace life instead.

## MARK'S UNSUCCESSFUL SUICIDE STORY

After I was diagnosed with prostate cancer (T1c, Gleason 6, PSA: 5.1), I had two physicians tell me that radical prostatectomy was my only option. Both doctors told me that they would do "a radical" if they were in my shoes, no questions asked.

But I asked a lot of questions. When I asked the first urologist I saw about the complications from the surgery, he told me that he was 90 percent sure that he would "keep me dry" (as in I wouldn't need to wear diapers) and about 70 percent sure that I could get an erection if I took Viagra. When I asked him about what my odds were of having an erection without Viagra, he told me that they were lower, but hedged about giving me a number, saying that there were some conflicting data from recent studies.

I was devastated. I was 46 years old. I was counting on having an active sex life for a long time! The thought of wearing diapers never even entered my mind.

The second urologist told me pretty much the same thing. At the end of the appointment, he did mentioned that there might be an experimental saturation brachytherapy technique that would work in my case, but there was no guarantee I wouldn't develop secondary cancers from the radiation.

The day after my second appointment, my house of cards caved in.

I got into a huge fight with my father, who had come out to Colorado to support me in my time of need. He was adamant that I have surgery, despite my reiterating, "that's my last option." So I sent him home.

By the end of that week, I had distanced myself from my girlfriend and her children and began planning how I was going to kill myself.

I decided to buy a handgun, drive up into the mountains, and blow my brains out.

The problem was I couldn't find a gun store. I went to a couple of sporting goods store, but they only sold air pistols. That made me feel even more pathetic — I couldn't even pull it together and buy a gun to kill myself!

I drove around in my Prius like a maniac for 10 minutes, which in retrospect must have looked really silly: burning rubber at green lights in a Prius. Really?

Slowly a thought sunk in: *Maybe I'm having a tough time killing myself because that's not what I'm supposed to do. Maybe there's a bigger purpose to my life that hasn't even scratched the surface of yet. Maybe there are doctors out there who can really help me, instead of just telling me about the procedure they do best. Maybe I don't have to have surgery and end up impotent and incontinent.*

Long story short — I didn't kill myself. I didn't have the surgery or radiation either. I took a different path: I embraced everything that I thought would improve my overall health and the health of my prostate (more on that in **Chapter 10** and the **Chapter 10 Toolbox**). Today, as far as anyone can tell, I am prostate cancer free, my PSA is normal, and I feel great.

If you're thinking about suicide after a prostate cancer diagnosis, I can tell you from person experience: "Don't do it." Your chances of living a long, health, sexually active life may be a lot better than you think.

# Digging Deeper
## CHAPTER 10

This Digging Deeper section provides you with a deeper understanding of how to use the seven health factors mentioned in Chapter 10 to help you heal your entire body — and the prostate it contains.

- The Bittersweet Truth about Sugar
- Glycemic Index & Glycemic Load
- The HELP Protocol

# The Bittersweet Truth about Sugar

By Dr. Emilia A. Ripoll, M.D.

If you've ever visited Dr. Joseph Mercola's website and viewed any of his articles on sugar, or seen Dr. Robert Lustig's *The Complete Skinny on Obesity* series on YouTube, then you already have a good understanding about how toxic sugar is and how America's addiction to it has hijacked our national health.

Both Mercola and Lustig focus on fructose being one of the main culprits behind the decline in the health of Americans and the rampant rise in diseases linked to obesity (heart disease, diabetes, hypertension, and cancer). I agree, and I would like to broaden the discussion to include simple carbohydrates such as sugar and other sweeteners.

It's not that carbohydrates are inherently bad. They're not. The real villain in the consumption of simple carbohydrates is the rise in blood sugar, which is followed by increased levels of the hormones insulin and leptin.

The aging and inflammatory effect on our bodies caused by elevated levels of insulin and leptin are both sad and preventable. As a physician, I feel compelled to inform my patients and friends how to avoid these pitfalls and enjoy fuller and healthier lives.

Let's take a look at five prevailing myths about sugar and see how debunking these myths liberates you from old unhealthy habits.

## Myth #1: A Calorie Is a Calorie

A calorie is NOT a calorie.

The antiquated "calories-in versus calories-out" model that treats all calories as equal is thoroughly dismantled and discredited by Gary Taubes in his best-selling book, *Why We Get Fat: And What to Do About It*. I highly recommend this book to anyone who is interested in health or has ever struggled with their weight.

As Taubes points out, different amounts of the fats, proteins, and carbohydrates may all contain the same number of calories, but these calories are not metabolized the same way in your body. This often misunderstood, yet extremely important, concept is the key to understanding why diet is so important to your health. As Lustig puts it, different foods may be "equi-caloric, but not equi-metabolic."

Most carbohydrates are metabolized with the help of insulin. Fructose, fruit sugar, is metabolized though a different pathway (more on that in a bit). I should add that insulin is also involved in protein metabolism, but it takes only 20 percent of the insulin that it would take to metabolize 4 oz. of sugar to metabolize 4 oz. of animal protein.

For example, let's use the simplest carbohydrate your likely to eat: refined sugar (sucrose). Sucrose is that wonderful white stuff that turns bitter coffee into sweet seduction. Sucrose is made up of two smaller sugar molecules: glucose and fructose. It is 50 percent glucose and 50 percent fructose.

With the help of insulin, glucose is metabolized by every cell in your body (bones, brain, and everything in between). This process begins even before the first molecule of glucose in your coffee hits your bloodstream.

Like Pavlov's dogs that drooled when they heard a bell, the mere anticipation of receiving sugar is enough to cause your pancreas to start producing insulin. Once the sweet receptors on your tongue signal that something yummy is on the way, insulin production shifts into gear.

This adaptation is essential to your health, as it is insulin's job is to move glucose out of your blood stream, where it can cause all sorts of problems (diabetes being the biggest), and into your cells where it is used right away or stored for later use.

Fructose follows a different pathway where it is metabolized only in the liver and stored directly as fat.

So eating sugar (glucose plus fructose) is a double whammy in the fat production and storage department. If you only take home one thing from this article, let it be this: The more simple carbohydrates you consume, the more fat your body stores.

For people trying to lose weight or maintain a healthy weight, cutting back on foods and beverages that contain sugar and other insulin-producing sweeteners is much smarter than restricting their consumption of proteins and fats (even though fats contain twice as many calories per volume as carbohydrates).

If you just said to yourself, *Wow, that's so simple.* You're right. It is simple... but it's not easy.

Why? Because sugar tastes really, really good. So do all of sugar's metabolic equivalents: evaporated cane juice, brown sugar, honey, high fructose corn syrup, agave syrup, maple syrup, brown rice syrup, molasses, and fruit juice concentrate. Food manufacturers have been taking advantage of this simple biological fact for decades, which is why sweeteners are so prevalent in processed foods.

I invite you to walk down any isle in any supermarket and start looking at the labels. Pay attention to the ingredients and "sugars," listed in grams. Both Mercola and Lustig recommend no more than 15 grams of fructose per day. Depending on the sweetener, fifteen grams of fructose means approximately 30 grams of total sugar, which is enough to shift some people out of fat burning mode and into fat storage mode.

For a real shocker, begin your exploration of product labels in the break-fast cereal isle.

## Myth #2: Natural Sweeteners are Healthier than Sugar

Life would be so much sweeter if this myth were true.

Sugar, evaporated cane juice, brown sugar, honey, maple syrup, molasses, and high fructose corn syrup all contain roughly equal amounts of glucose and fructose.

This may be a particularly difficult concept to get your mind around because we've been taught that honey and maple syrup are "natural" products, so they have to be better for you than high fructose corn syrup. Sadly, that's not the case. Evaporated cane juice is a natural product too — before it is further dehydrated and refined into table sugar.

Agave syrup has a low glycemic index (GI = 30, which is lower than apples), and its high fructose content makes it "sweeter" than sugar. In fact, agave can be upwards of 90 percent fructose (table sugar is 50 percent fructose). Because fructose is metabolized directly into fat in the liver, even with agave's low glycemic index, it still promotes fat storing instead of fat burning.

There are three natural sweeteners that don't contain fructose at all: brown rice syrup, stevia, and luo han guo. One of them is laden with arsenic, one is available in health food stores, and the other I've only seen on the Internet.

## Brown Rice Syrup

Brown rice syrup is a nutty, buttery tasting syrup created by cooking rice (usually white rice) with enzymes derived from barley sprouts and then decanting the excess water. Brown rice syrup's glycemic index is relatively low (25), but its composition is weighted heavily towards glucose; hence, it triggers an even larger insulin pulse than regular sugar.

Brown rice syrup's biggest health problem is NOT the insulin production it triggers but the arsenic it contains. Beginning in early 2012, the FDA reported large amounts of arsenic in two infant formulas whose main ingredient was brown rice syrup. These formulas had six times the recommended arsenic levels for drinking water (10 parts per billion). Subsequent reports have shown that some organic brown rice samples also contain alarmingly high levels of arsenic.

The high levels of arsenic in rice and rice products (brown rice syrup, rice cereals, rice cakes) are thought to come from rice fields that once grew cotton. According to the Federal Agency for Toxic Substances and Disease Registry, lead-arsenate pesticide residue continues to linger in soils where cotton was once grown, even though these chemicals were banned in the 1980s.

The smart thinking on brown rice syrup is to avoid it until this arsenic issue is resolved. Consumer Reports has lots of good information on arsenic in rice and other grains. For more information, I recommend you go online and read their articles.

## Stevia

Stevia is derived from the leaves of plants in the sunflower family that are native to semitropical and tropical areas of South and Central America. Stevia contains no sugars, no calories, has a glycemic index of zero, and is up to 300 times sweeter than sugar.

Some people don't like the taste of stevia; they find that stevia doesn't satisfy their sweet tooth. Fair enough. But it also won't make you fat or increase your chances of developing a host of inflammatory diseases related to elevated insulin and leptin exposure (obesity, diabetes, heart disease, cancer, and others).

From a health perspective, Stevia is one of the better sweeteners. Nevertheless, the pancreas' reaction to the stimulation of the sweet receptors on the tongue still causes an increase in insulin production — even if the anticipated glucose never arrives.

There were some studies in the 1980s that showed that daily Stevia use was linked to cancer of the penis in rats; however, the vast majority of subsequent studies contradict these early findings.

Since 2000, the World Health Organization, the European Food Safety Authority, and the FDA have all consider stevia as "generally recognized as safe" or GRAS.

# Luo Han Guo

Like stevia, sweeteners made from the luo han guo fruit (sometimes called Buddha fruit or monk fruit) are 300 times sweeter than sugar, contain zero calories, and have a glycemic index of zero. Luo han guo is a member of the gourd family and has been cultivated by Buddhist monks in southern China and northern Thailand since the 13th century; however, it did not appear in North America until the late 20th century.

Traditionally, luo han guo has been used in beverages designed to cool the body (hot weather, fever, hot flashes, and inflammation). In 2009, the FDA granted luo han guo GRAS status. No restrictions were placed on consuming the fruit or using its extracts as sweeteners.

As of the writing of this article, the only place I've been able to find luo han guo is online.

# Myth #3: Drinking Sugar Is OK

If you're feeling particularly adventurous, take a trip down the beverage isle of your local market and look at how many grams of "sugars" are in sodas, sweetened teas, energy drinks, and other beverages.

According to Lustig and other experts, drinking one 12 oz. can of Coke per day for a year (that's 10 extra teaspoons of sugar a day or roughly 30 pounds of sugar per year) will result in 15 additional pounds of fat — just from drinking one sugary soft drink every day.

Maybe former New York City mayor, Michael Bloomberg's crusade against soft drinks was right after all.

The simple truth is that drinking sugar is drinking sugar — no matter where the sugar comes from — Pepsi or organic apple juice. Both beverages contain the same amount of sugar per volume.

The only advantage to drinking juice is a moderate amount of vitamins and minerals. Also, if you drink apple or orange juice that contains a lot of fiber (pulp), the fiber will slow the rate of carbohydrate absorption in the small intestine, which minimally suppresses insulin production, and induces some measure of satiety. None of which happens when drinking a Pepsi.

Perhaps the biggest problem with drinking sugar is that the fructose in high fructose corn syrup (the sweetener used in most sodas and energy drinks) does not suppress the hunger hormone, ghrelin, which tells your brain that your stomach is full. This is how you can drink a 64-ounce Big Gulp of soda sweetened with high fructose corn syrup and still feel hungry 20 minutes later.

The other major hunger-suppression hormone, leptin, is produced by your fat cells, and works to signal your brain that your body either needs energy or does not need energy. Insufficient leptin levels signal your brain that your body is starving; an abundance of leptin tells your brain that your body feels sated.

As with insulin, if your body is exposed to too much leptin for too long, it becomes resistant to this hormone, and the once functional feedback system breaks down — and obesity, inflammation, and early aging ensue.

According to Lustig, when your body is awash in insulin from eating a high-sugar/high-carbohydrate diet, the insulin blocks the normal leptin signaling in your brain, so your brain thinks that your body is starving.

When this confusion happens, your fat cells release leptin, which would normally tell your brain that your body don't need any more food (energy); however, that normal leptin signaling process doesn't happen if your brain has been overridden by insulin or if your body/brain have become "leptin resistant."

According to Taubes, even though your leptin levels are high (which should trigger your brain to control hunger), your fat cells actually begin acting like a tumor, requesting more and more energy (sugar), until you are essentially eating to keep your fat cells satisfied to the detriment of the rest of your body.

Experts including Mercola, Lustig, and Taubes believe that the only way to break this cycle of insulin and leptin overload is through a low-sugar/low-carbohydrate diet that includes healthy fats (coconut oil, olive oil, avocados, nuts, and clarified butter) and moderate amounts of protein.

## Myth #4: Exercise is the Answer

Exercise is an important part of a healthy lifestyle; however, you cannot exercise your way to health if you are eating a high-sugar/high carbohydrate diet — even if you are exercising multiple hours a day to burn more calories than you take in.

The problem is not a lack of calories burned during exercise (or being weak willed or lazy). The problem is that a diet high in simple carbohydrates (sweeteners and starchy carbohydrates) signals your body to store fat. Once this "fat-storing mode" becomes your new normal, your body shifts towards storing the food you eat as fat (thanks to the high levels of the hormones insulin and leptin) and shifts away from giving your muscles and your reproductive·system the energy they need in order to maintain your overall health.

## Myth #5: What I Eat and Drink Only Affects Me

I understand this sentiment. The reality, however, is a different story.

The ripple effect of our dietary choices quickly goes far beyond the boundaries of our skin to include our families, our communities, our work force, our country, and even our planet.

According to the CDC, the global cost of treating metabolic syndrome (the symptoms of which include obesity, heart disease, type 2 diabetes, several types of cancer, hypertension, excessive fat in the blood, non-alcoholic fatty liver disease, polycystic ovarian syndrome, and dementia) accounts for 75 percent of all global health care expenses.

The CDC also estimates that the global cost of just treating type 2 diabetes is $150 billion per year.

Here's a little information from the CDC that brings this message home:

| Year | Global Sugar Consumption | Global Diabetes Rate |
|------|--------------------------|----------------------|
| 1985 | 98 million tons | 30 million people |
| 2010 | 160 million tons | 346 million people |

Within one generation, the global sugar consumption almost doubled. In that same time period, however, the diabetes rate increased more than 11 times. You don't have to be an epidemiologist to see that we have reached the tipping point.

## What Can You Do?

Here are five simple suggestions you can do to shift you diet away from sugar and other simple carbohydrates.

1.  Drink water instead of sodas, energy drinks, and fruit juice. This switch might feel like a punishment for the first couple of weeks, but soon you'll start to crave the clean, clear, quenching quality of water. I recommend you drink purified water that comes in glass bottles, because plastic bottles leach estrogen-like chemicals into the water.

2.  Read the label on any food that comes in a box, bag, bottle, or can. Select products for yourself and your family that contain the least amount of sweeteners and sugars. All this reading of labels may sound like it will turn a trip to the market into a prison sentence, but you will quickly learn to spot products that are "unsweetened." Actu-

376 PROSTATE CANCER: A NEW APPROACH TO TREATMENT AND HEALING

ally, "Spot the Sugar" is a fun game to play with your kids while you're shopping.

3. Visit your local health food store and pick up some stevia. You may find it satisfies your sweet tooth. And with zero calories and a glycemic index of zero, it is one of the, if not *the,* best sweetener.

4. Introduce salads and other green leafy vegetables into your diet plan. Eating five to seven servings of vegetables a day will have a dramatic effect on your health.

5. Replace traditional snack foods with seeds and nuts. Raw or dry roasted pumpkin seeds, almonds, walnuts, cashews, and pistachios make great between-meal snacks. They contain healthy oils that satisfy your appetite without raising your insulin level. Avoid "roasted" nuts because they are cooked in unhealthy omega-6 oils, which denature the proteins in the nuts.

---

## GLYCEMIC INDEX & GLYCEMIC LOAD

Glycemic index and glycemic load offer information about how foods affect blood sugar and insulin. The lower a food's glycemic index or glycemic load, the less it affects blood sugar and insulin levels.

**Glycemic Index**

A number associated with a particular type of food that indicates the food's effect on a person's blood glucose levels (also called "blood sugar levels"). A value of 100 represents the standard, an equivalent amount of pure glucose.[1] This number shows how much a person's blood sugar level increases after eating a particular type of food — an apple, slice of bread, roasted chicken breast, broccoli, and so on.

**Glycemic Load**

A number that estimates how much a particular type of food will raise a person's blood glucose level after eating it. One unit of "glycemic load" approximates the effect of consuming one gram of glucose. [1] Glycemic Load is calculated by multiplying the grams of carbohydrates available in a particular type of food by the food's Glycemic Index (see above), and then dividing by 100.

For more information about glycemic index and glycemic load, we encourage you to visit: *http://www.health.harvard.edu/healthy-eating/ glycemic_index_and_glycemic_load_for_100_foods*

1. Glycemic Research Institute

# The HELP Protocol

By Dr. Emilia A. Ripoll, M.D.

Use the information included here as a general guide. Each suggestion is designed to help you get started on your healing journey.

There's no guarantee that if you integrate one (or all) of these suggestions that your body will spontaneously heal itself; however, if you put these suggestions to work and stick with it, I can promise you that will start to feel healthier, happier, stronger, and more alive.

## Exercise and Lifestyle

Get outside, oxygenate your body, feel the sun on your skin and face, crank up your body's natural Vitamin D machinery. Just 30 minutes of brisk walking, six days a week can make a tremendous difference. Looking for something more strenuous? Try cycling, hiking, swimming, running, or tennis. If you can't exercise outdoors (it's too cold during the winter or you live in an unsafe neighborhood), join a gym, sign up for a CrossFit or Fitwall class, join a salsa or tango dance class, buy a mini-trampoline and jog on it while watching your favorite TV show, crank up the music and dance in your living room like no one's watching, work up a healthy sweat — it feels good.

## Move Your Pelvis

A healthy pelvis is the key to a happy body. Activities like yoga, Pilates, and Qi Gong activate all the muscles, tendons, ligaments, organs, and circulation (blood and plasma) in and around the pelvis. When your pelvis is open and balanced, the plasma flows easily, which allows it to cleanse your tissues and boost your immune system. A stagnant, misaligned pelvis will multiply (and in some cases cause) your prostate problems.

## Diet

A plant-based, whole food diet like the Paleo Diet is vital to a healthy body and mind. The Paleo Diet is based on how humans ate in their native state 15,000 years ago — before the agricultural revolution shifted us from hunter/gathers to grain eaters. The Paleo Diet is comprised of approximately 65-80 percent vegetables (which tend to alkalize your body) and low-glycemic fruits (berries), and the rest is lean animal protein and healthy fat. We can't say enough about selecting animal products that are free of all the chemicals, antibiotics, and other junk associated with conventional agriculture. We highly recommend that all your meat be grass fed, hormone-free, antibiotic free — preferably wild (fish) or organic if you can afford it. Also, we strongly recommend that prostate cancer patients avoid eating soy in any form: soy milk, tofu, tempeh, edamame, miso, and so on. The "estrogenic" (estrogen-like) compounds in soy can tip your testosterone/estrogen balance in the wrong direction, which can have dire consequences for the health of your prostate.

## Digestive Enzymes

If you haven't already, try taking digestive enzymes such as Bromelain (from pineapples). Pancreatic enzymes also help with digestion. Once these enzymes are done breaking down the protein in your lunch or dinner, they go to work on the cancer in your body, which is why it is best to take enzymes a couple of hours before or after meals.

## Community Heals

Connecting with your community (family, friends, co-workers, neighbors, and people who share your interests and values) is critical when it comes to feeling vibrant and alive. If you tend towards isolation (TV, books, video games, Facebook, and so on), reach out to real live human beings and invite them to join you for a

- cup of coffee or tea
- movie
- trip to a local museum
- sports event
- cultural event
- concert

Disease festers in isolation. Whatever you do, do it with a friend. Being part of something outside yourself promotes friendship and a feeling of belonging. Community heals.

## Help Others

Nothing snaps you out of a funk faster than helping people who are less fortunate than you. Volunteering is a great way to feel better about yourself by doing something for others. Do you enjoy spending time with seniors, children, veterans, people with disabilities, or dogs and cats? Do you have a skill or talent that you could offer a local nonprofit or religious organization (carpentry, accounting, plumbing, taxes, organizing, marketing, greeting people, you name it)? Just a couple of hours a week of helping other people will take the emphasis off your own worries and concerns, reduce your stress level, and improve your immune function.

## Environmental Estrogens

Avoid estrogenic compounds in food (soy), water (most plastic water bottles leach estrogen-like chemicals into the water), and personal products (lotions and shampoos). Maintaining a healthy testosterone/estrogen balance is crucial to a man's health, especially as he ages. Environmental estrogen exposure has been linked to a host of prostate issues in men (and breast cancer in women).

## Limit Alcohol Consumption

In 1988, the World Health Organization classified alcohol as a Group 1 carcinogen. Regular heavy alcohol consumption increases the risk for seven different types of cancer, including breast, prostate, colon, oral, and liver. We strongly recommend that you limit alcohol consumption to one drink per day. Better yet, stop drinking alcohol, at least during this healing crisis.

## Stop Smoking

Cigarette smoking is harmful for every body — the smoker, the people near the smoker, even the smoker's yet to be conceived offspring. Smoking doubles the risk of death from all causes between the ages of 35-69. Smoking while you drink is a lethal combination that amplifies the worst aspects of both habits.

## Biofeedback/Stress Reduction

Stress is associated with every major illness, including cancer. Lowering your stress level is perhaps the most important thing you can do to avoid prostate cancer and other diseases. It's easier than you think. There are several excellent books, audio programs, and DVDs available about stress reduction and biofeedback. We recommend you visit Amazon, Sounds True, or iTunes to see which programs work best for you.

## Meditation

The antidote to stress is meditation. The healing power of meditation is greatly underplayed in Western cultures. One of the best stories about how meditation heals is that of Australian author, Ian Gawler, who healed himself of bone cancer through meditation. All it takes is 20 minutes twice a day.

## Resolve Past Traumas

The connection between unresolved emotional issues and illness is well documented. For example, feelings of helplessness generate an inflammatory response that facilitates the growth and spread of cancerous tumors. If you know you're dragging around some demons from your past, there are many different kinds of therapy that can help.

## Have Fun

Last but not least, have fun. Life is short — even if you live to be 100.

If you delay happiness by saying, "I'll let myself be happy when ... I am healed from prostate cancer, get a new job, buy a new house, the kids move out ... you might be waiting for a long time.

Instead of waiting, we recommend that you give yourself a little dose of happiness every day.

Take 20 minutes out of every day to:

- Finish reading that novel you started last year (or start a new one)
- Play with your kids, grandkids, friends' kids ... any kids
- Practice playing a musical instrument
- Study a second language
- Paint
- Write
- Dance
- Sing (in the shower, your car, join a choir)
- Do whatever gives you the greatest sense of joy

**Remember:** It doesn't have to be the same thing every day. You'll be surprised what an impact these simple practices can have on your level of happiness, your overall health, and the health of your prostate.

# GLOSSARY

**4Kscore Test** - The 4Kscore Test is a blood test that ranks a man's risk for having aggressive prostate cancer.

**AUA Score** - A questionnaire that helps men quantify their urinary symptoms and their treatment(s). Also known as the International Prostate Symptom Score (IPSS).

**Benign Prostatic Hyperplasia (BPH)** - BPH is an enlarged prostate gland. If an enlarged prostate pinches off the urethra, it can cause urinary problems.

**Bio-individuality** - The concept that each person's biochemical make-up is unique (non-identical), even with identical twins. This includes biochemical process from nutritional requirements to the proteins that DNA instructs individual cells to make.

**Bladder** - A mucular organ that stores the urine produced by the kidneys before it is excreted.

**Bone Scan** - A type of X-ray that is used to determine if prostate cancer has spread to the bones.

**Brainspotting** - A somatic therapy for reducing anxiety, fear, and Post Traumatic Stress Disorder (PTSD)

**CAT Scan (**Computerized Axial Tomography Scan) - A painless form of X-rays that generates cross-sectional views of a patient's body.

**ConfirmMDx -** a biopsy based test that helps doctors rule out the need for a repeat biopsy or indicate the presence of "hidden cancer" that a previous biopsy missed.

**Cortisol -** A steroid hormone produced by the adrenal gland in response to stress or low blood sugar. Cortisol is also called "hydrocortisone" when used as a medication.

**DHEA** - An adrenal gland hormone that is a precursor of both male and female sex hormones.

**DHT** - This powerful male sex hormone is the most important male hormone inside the prostate, where DHT has a 5-10 times greater affinity for male sex hormone receptors than testosterone.

**Digital Rectal Exam (DRE)** - A procedure where a doctor inserts a gloved finger (digit) into the rectum in order to examine the prostate through the thin muscular wall of the rectum.

**DNA (deoxyribonucleic acid)** - The building blocks of life on Earth. Long strands of DNA, called "genes," determine everything from skin color to the likelihood of developing prostate cancer.

**EMDR** - Eye Movement Desensitization and Reprocessing is a psychotherapy technique for treating disturbing memories and PTSD.

**Emotional Freedom Technique (Tapping)** - A form of somatic therapy that integrates acupuncture, neuro-linguistic programming, and other treatments to release negative emotions and unwanted habits.

**Epigenetic Testing** - Tests that use tissue samples from a prostate biopsy look for biomarkers that indicate the presence (or absence) of prostate cancer.

**Erectile Dysfunction (ED)** - The inability to have or maintain an erection.

**Extracapsular Extension** - Prostate cancer that extends into or beyond the capsule (membrane) of the prostate.

**False Negative** - A negative result for a test, like a prostate biopsy, that failed to detect the presence cancer.

**Genetic Testing** - Tests that look for certain genetic markers in cancer cells taken from tissue samples, like a prostate biopsy. These markers indicate how aggressive the cancer is.

**Gene** - A portion of a DNA molecule that controls the development of one or more physical traits (heredity) or physiological responses (the likelihood of developing one or more traits).

**Gleason Score** - A method that pathologists use to determine how aggressive a certain sample of prostate cancer is. A Gleason score includes two numbers, which are added together to produce a sum. For example, 3 + 4 = 7.

**GMO (Genetically Modified Organism)** - Any living organism, typically crops and vegetables, that are modified for enhanced to modify certain traits, like crop yield.

**Hormones** -  A substance created by a gland, which circulates in the blood and stimulates the cells of different organs, glands, or tissues.

**Imaging**- X-rays, MRI, CAT scans, ultrasound, and other similar diagnostic tests.

**Insulin** - The hormone that moves sugar from the blood into the cells of the body where it can be metabolized as fuel or stored for future use.

**Lab Tests** - Blood, urine, and tissue sample tests used to determine the presence (or absence) of prostate cancer.

**Lumbosacral** - The lowest part of the back where the end of the lumbar spine meets the sacrum.

**Lymph Node** - A network of small pockets along the lymphatic system where lymph (also called "plasma" or "serum") is filtered and lymphocytes (white blood cells) are made.

**Magnetic Resonance Imaging (MRI)** - a type of imaging that uses magnetic fields and radio waves to create detailed images of the organs and tissues.

**Methylation** - A higher than normal concentration of methyl groups ($CH_3$) in a tissue sample, which indicates the presence of prostate cancer.

**MRI Fusion Prostate Biopsy** - A type of prostate biopsy that overlays an MRI image of the prostate on top of a standard ultrasound image, allowing for pinpoint accuracy and the ability to sample the same spot in the prostate multiple times.

**Mutation** - Any alteration in DNA structure or sequence that may be transmitted to future generations.

**Needle Cores** - The tissue samples collected during a prostate biopsy.

**Neuromodulation Technique** - The alteration of nerve activity through the delivery of electrical stimulation or chemical agents to targeted sites of the body.

**PCA3** - A urine test for a particular gene that is only found in prostate cancer cells. The PCA3 test is not affected by prostate size (BPH), PSA, or prostatitis.

**Pelvic Floor** - An interwoven web of muscles and connective tissues that form a hammock that supports the intestines, urinary tract, and other internal organs.

**PIN** - a pre-cancerous condition that causes the prostate's epithelial cells (cells that line the small sacs inside the prostate) to undergo microscopic changes.

**PNI** - Cancer that has spread into the space that surrounds a nerve.

**Prostate Biopsy** - An in-office procedure that looks for prostate cancer by taking 12-24 small tissue samples, which are then analyzed under a microscope.

**Prostate Cancer** - A disease of the prostate gland in which cells develop abnormally. These abnormal cells can form tumors, grow at an uncontrollable rate, and spread throughout the body.

**Prostate Zones** - The prostate is divided into 3 zones: Central, Peripheral, and Transitional.

**Prostatitis** - An inflammation of the prostate.

**PSA (Prostate Specific Antigen)** - A protein produced by the prostate that helps transport and nourish sperm after ejaculation. A certain amount of PSA leaks into the blood stream and is detectable by a PSA blood test.

**PSA Density** - A measurement of PSA that factors in the size of a man's prostate. (Bigger prostates leak more PSA into the blood stream.)

**PSA Free** - PSA that is NOT attached (bound) to any proteins. A higher concentration of Free PSA indicates a lower likelihood of prostate cancer.

**PSA Testing** - A blood test that detects the concentration of PSA.

**PSA Total** - A measurement of PSA Free + PSA bound to other proteins.

**PSA Velocity** - The rate of rise (or fall) of any PSA number over time.

**Rectum** - The final straight portion of the intestines that ends at the anus.

**Sacroiliac** - The two hinge joints that occur between the major bones of the pelvis: the sacrum and the ilium.

**SelectMDx** - A non-invasive urine-based molecular test that helps identify men with a higher risk of developing aggressive prostate cancer.

**Seminal Vesicle** - A pair of two small glands that connect to the top of the prostate and produce about 70 percent of the fluid in semen (seminal fluid).

**Seminal Vesicle Fluid** - The fluid produced by the seminal vesicles during ejaculation.

**Seminal Vesicle Involvement** - Prostate cancer that has spread to the seminal vesicles.

**Standard American Diet** - A style of eating characterized by a high intake of sugar, processed foods, red meat, processed meat, high-fat dairy products, refined grains, simple carbohydrates — and an absence of fresh fruits and vegetables.

**TRUS (standard) Biopsy** - A standard ultrasound-guided prostate biopsy. Also called a "Random" biopsy because of this procedure's lack of accuracy.

**TURP** - A type of surgery (rotor-rooter) to relieve the urinary symptoms caused by "BPH" (see above).

**Ultrasound** - The most common type of imaging used during a prostate biopsy.

**Urethra** - The tube by which urine flows from the bladder to the end of the penis.

**Urinary Frequency** - The feeling of having to urinate frequently.

**Urinary Retention** - Being unable to completely empty the bladder.

**Urinary Sphincter** - Another name for the "Pelvic Floor" (see above).

**Urinary Stricture** - Scar tissue that forms in the urethra.

**Urinary Urgency** - The feeling of having to urinate "right now"!

**Western Diet** - See "Standard American Diet"

# INDEX

# REFERENCES

## Introduction

1   Paquette EL, Sun L, Paquette LR, Connelly R, Mcleod DG, Moul JW. Improved prostate cancer-specific survival and other disease parameters: impact of prostate-specific antigen testing. *Urology*. 2002;60(5):756-759. *http://www. ncbi.nlm.nih.gov/pubmed/12429290*. Accessed September 10, 2016.

2   Pogliano D, Strum S. *A Primer on Prostate Cancer. The Empowered Patient's Guide*. second. Life extensions foundation; 2005.

3   Beliveau, R, Gingras, D. *Foods to Fight Cancer*. London: DK; 2007.

## Chapter 1

1   Tran E, Ahmadzadeh M, Lu Y-C, et al. Immunogenicity of somatic mutations in human gastrointestinal cancers. *Science*. 2015;350(6266):1387-1390. doi:10.1126/science.aad1253.

2   American Cancer Society. Cancer Facts & Figures 2010. Atlanta: American Cancer Society; 2010. *http://www.cancer.org/acs/groups/content/@nho/ documents/document/acspc-024113.pdf*.

3   National Cancer Institute. SEER Stat Fact Sheets: Prostate. Bethesda, MD: National Cancer Institute; 2011. *http://seer.cancer.gov/statfacts/html/prost. html*.

## Chapter 2

1   Bans L. Prostate Solutions of Arizona Takes Aim at Prostate Cancer Awareness. *Phoenix Ed*. 2006;6(3).

2   McDonald ML, Parsons JK. 4-Kallikrein Test and Kallikrein Markers in Prostate Cancer Screening. *Urol Clin North Am*. 2016;43(1):39-46. doi:10.1016/j. ucl.2015.08.004.

3   Vedder MM, de Bekker-Grob EW, Lilja HG, et al. The added value of percentage of free to total prostate-specific antigen, PCA3, and a kallikrein panel to the ERSPC risk calculator for prostate cancer in prescreened men. *Eur Urol*. 2014;66(6):1109-1115. doi:10.1016/j.eururo.2014.08.011.

## Chapter 3

1   Reiter RE. Risk stratification of prostate cancer 2016. *Scand J Clin Lab Invest Suppl*. 2016;245:S54-9. doi:10.1080/00365513.2016.1208453.

2   Moschini M, Spahn M, Mattei A, Cheville J, Karnes RJ. Incorporation of tissue-based genomic biomarkers into localized prostate cancer clinics. *BMC Med*. 2016;14:67. doi:10.1186/s12916-016-0613-7.

3   Falzarano SM, Ferro M, Bollito E, Klein EA, Carrieri G, Magi-Galluzzi C. Novel biomarkers and genomic tests in prostate cancer: a critical analysis. *Minerva Urol Nefrol*. 2015;67(3):211-231. *http://www.ncbi.nlm.nih.gov/ pubmed/26054411*. Accessed September 12, 2016.

4   Boström PJ, Bjartell AS, Catto JWF, et al. Genomic Predictors of Outcome in Prostate Cancer. *Eur Urol.* 2015;68(6):1033-1044. doi:10.1016/j.eururo.2015.04.008.

5   Sartori DA, Chan DW. Biomarkers in prostate cancer: what's new? *Curr Opin Oncol.* 2014;26(3):259-264. doi:10.1097/CCO.0000000000000065.

## Chapter 4

## Chapter 5

1   Makarov D V, Trock BJ, Humphreys EB, et al. Updated nomogram to predict pathologic stage of prostate cancer given prostate-specific antigen level, clinical stage, and biopsy Gleason score (Partin tables) based on cases from 2000 to 2005. *Urology.* 2007;69(6):1095-1101. doi:10.1016/j.urology.2007.03.042.

2   Eifler JB, Feng Z, Lin BM, et al. An updated prostate cancer staging nomogram (Partin tables) based on cases from 2006 to 2011. *BJU Int.* 2013;111(1):22-29. doi:10.1111/j.1464-410X.2012.11324.x.

## Chapter 6

1   Habibian DJ, Katz AE. Emerging minimally invasive procedures for focal treatment of organ-confined prostate cancer. *Int J Hyperthermia.* 2016;32(7):795-800. doi:10.1080/02656736.2016.1195925.

2   Jereczek-Fossa BA, Ciardo D, Petralia G, et al. Primary focal prostate radiotherapy: Do all patients really need whole-prostate irradiation? *Crit Rev Oncol Hematol.* 2016;105:100-111. doi:10.1016/j.critrevonc.2016.06.010.

3   Marra G, Gontero P, Valerio M. Changing the prostate cancer management pathway: why Focal Therapy is a step forward. *Arch españoles Urol.* 2016;69(6):271-280. *http://www.ncbi.nlm.nih.gov/pubmed/27416630.* Accessed September 13, 2016.

4   Wildeboer RR, Panfilova AP, Mischi M, Wijkstra H. Imaging modalities in Focal Therapy: Multiparametric Ultrasound. *Arch españoles Urol.* 2016;69(6):281-290. *http://www.ncbi.nlm.nih.gov/pubmed/27416631.* Accessed September 13, 2016.

5   Sivaraman A. High intensity focused ultrasound for Focal Therapy of prostate cancer. Arch españoles Urol. 2016;69(6):311-316. *http://www.ncbi.nlm.nih.gov/pubmed/27416634.* Accessed September 13, 2016.

6   Tay KJ, Polascik TJ. Focal Cryotherapy for Localized Prostate Cancer. *Arch españoles Urol.* 2016;69(6):317-326. *http://www.ncbi.nlm.nih.gov/pubmed/27416635.* Accessed September 13, 2016.

## Chapter 7

1   Morgentaler A, Benesh JA, Denes BS, Kan-Dobrosky N, Harb D, Miller MG. Factors influencing prostate-specific antigen response among men treated with testosterone therapy for 6 months. J *Sex Med*. 2014;11(11):2818-2825. doi:10.1111/jsm.12657.

2   Morgentaler A, Zitzmann M, Traish AM, et al. Fundamental Concepts Regarding Testosterone Deficiency and Treatment: International Expert Consensus Resolutions. *Mayo Clin Proc*. 2016;91(7):881-896. doi:10.1016/j.mayocp.2016.04.007.

3   Davidson E, Morgentaler A. Testosterone Therapy and Prostate Cancer. *Urol Clin North Am*. 2016;43(2):209-216. doi:10.1016/j.ucl.2016.01.007.

## Chapter 8

1   Yao S-L, Lu-Yao G. Population-Based Study of Relationships Between Hospital Volume of Prostatectomies, Patient Outcomes, and Length of Hospital Stay. *JNCI J Natl Cancer Inst*. 1999;91(22):1950-1956. doi:10.1093/jnci/91.22.1950.

2   Stephenson RA, Stanford JL. Population-based prostate cancer trends in the United States: patterns of change in the era of prostate-specific antigen. *World J Urol*. 1997;15(6):331-335. *http://www.ncbi.nlm.nih.gov/pubmed/9436281*. Accessed June 13, 2013.

3   Chou R, Dana T, Bougatsos C, et al. Treatments for Localized Prostate Cancer: Systematic Review to Update the 2002 U.S. Preventive Services Task Force Recommendation. *Evid Synth Number*. 2011;91. *www.ohsu.edu/epc*. Accessed September 13, 2016.

4   Lilleby W, Fosså SD, Waehre HR, Olsen DR. Long-term morbidity and quality of life in patients with localized prostate cancer undergoing definitive radiotherapy or radical prostatectomy. *Int J Radiat Oncol Biol Phys*. 1999;43(4):735-743. *http://www.ncbi.nlm.nih.gov/pubmed/10098428*. Accessed August 28, 2016.

5   Talcott JA, Manola J, Clark JA, et al. Time course and predictors of symptoms after primary prostate cancer therapy. *J Clin Oncol*. 2003;21(21):3979-3986. doi:10.1200/JCO.2003.01.199.

6   Resnick MJ, Koyama T, Fan K-H, et al. Long-Term Functional Outcomes after Treatment for Localized Prostate Cancer. *N Engl J Med*. 2013;368(5):436-445. doi:10.1056/NEJMoa1209978.

7   Frank SJ, Pisters LL, Davis J, Lee AK, Bassett R, Kuban DA. An assessment of quality of life following radical prostatectomy, high dose external beam radiation therapy and brachytherapy iodine implantation as monotherapies for localized prostate cancer. *J Urol*. 2007;177(6):2151-6; discussion 2156. doi:10.1016/j.juro.2007.01.134.

8   Bostwick DG, Waters DJ, Farley ER, et al. Group consensus reports from the Consensus Conference on Focal Treatment of Prostatic Carcinoma, Celebration, Florida, February 24, 2006. *Urology.* 2007;70(6 Suppl):42-44. doi:10.1016/j.urology.2007.07.037.

9   Donnelly BJ, Saliken JC, Brasher PMA, et al. A randomized trial of external beam radiotherapy versus cryoablation in patients with localized prostate cancer. *Cancer.* 2010;116(2):323-330. doi:10.1002/cncr.24779.

10  Bahn DK, Silverman P, Lee F, Badalament R, Bahn ED, Rewcastle JC. Focal prostate cryoablation: initial results show cancer control and potency preservation. *J Endourol.* 2006;20(9):688-692. doi:10.1089/end.2006.20.688.

11  Robinson JW, Donnelly BJ, Siever JE, et al. A randomized trial of external beam radiotherapy versus cryoablation in patients with localized prostate cancer: quality of life outcomes. *Cancer.* 2009;115(20):4695-4704. doi:10.1002/cncr.24523.

12  Compliance With NCCN Guidelines for Prostate Cancer- SEER Database Review.

13  Loeb S, Carter HB, Berndt SI, Ricker W, Schaeffer EM. Complications After Prostate Biopsy: Data From SEER-Medicare. *J Urol.* 2011;186(5):1830-1834. doi:10.1016/j.juro.2011.06.057.

14  Wilt TJ, Brawer MK, Jones KM, et al. Radical prostatectomy versus observation for localized prostate cancer. *N Engl J Med.* 2012;367(3):203-213. doi:10.1056/NEJMoa1113162.

15  Bill-Axelson A, Holmberg L, Filén F, et al. Radical prostatectomy versus watchful waiting in localized prostate cancer: the Scandinavian prostate cancer group-4 randomized trial. *J Natl Cancer Inst.* 2008;100(16):1144-1154. doi:10.1093/jnci/djn255.

16  Johansson E, Steineck G, Holmberg L, et al. Long-term quality-of-life outcomes after radical prostatectomy or watchful waiting: the Scandinavian Prostate Cancer Group-4 randomised trial. *Lancet Oncol.* 2011;12(9):891-899. doi:10.1016/S1470-2045(11)70162-0.

## Chapter 9

## Chapter 10

1   Lustig, R. Fat Chance: *Beating the Odds Against Sugar, Processed Food, Obesity, and Disease.* New York: Hudson Street Press; 2013.

2   Taubes, G. Why *We Get Fat: And What To Do About It.* New York: Anchor Books; 2011.

3   Christofferson, T. *Tripping Over the Truth: The Return of the Metabolic Theory of Cancer Illuminates a New and Hopeful Path to a Cure.* North Charleston: CreateSpace Independent Publishing Platform; 2014.

4   Perlmutter, D. Grain Brain: *The Surprising Truth about Wheat, Carbs and Sugar — Your Brain's Silent Killers.* New York: Little, Brown and Company; 2013.

## Digging Deeper

1 Schröder FH, Hugosson J, Roobol MJ, et al. Screening and pros-
tate-cancer mortality in a randomized European study. *N Engl J Med.*
2009;360(13):1320-1328. doi:10.1056/NEJMoa0810084.

2 Sellers TA, Potter JD, Rich SS, et al. Familial Clustering of Breast and
Prostate Cancers and Risk of Postmenopausal Breast Cancer. *JNCI J Natl
Cancer Inst.* 1994;86(24):1860-1865. doi:10.1093/jnci/86.24.1860.

3 Odedina FT, Akinremi TO, Chinegwundoh F, et al. Prostate cancer disparities in Black men of African descent: a comparative literature review of
prostate cancer burden among Black men in the United States, Caribbean,
United Kingdom, and West Africa. *Infect Agent Cancer.* 2009;4(Suppl 1):S2.
doi:10.1186/1750-9378-4-S1-S2.

4 Albain KS, Unger JM, Crowley JJ, Coltman CA, Hershman DL. Racial
disparities in cancer survival among randomized clinical trials patients of
the Southwest Oncology Group. *J Natl Cancer Inst.* 2009;101(14):984-992.
doi:10.1093/jnci/djp175.

5 Loeb S, Vellekoop A, Ahmed HU, et al. Systematic review of complications of prostate biopsy. *Eur Urol.* 2013;64(6):876-892. doi:10.1016/j.euru-
ro.2013.05.049.

6 Rosario DJ, Lane JA, Metcalfe C, et al. Short term outcomes of prostate
biopsy in men tested for cancer by prostate specific antigen: prospective
evaluation within ProtecT study. *BMJ.* 2012;344:d7894. *http://www.ncbi.
nlm.nih.gov/pubmed/22232535.* Accessed August 31, 2016.

7 Manoharan M, Ayyathurai R, Nieder AM, Soloway MS. Hemospermia
following transrectal ultrasound-guided prostate biopsy: a prospective
study. *Prostate Cancer Prostatic Dis.* 2007;10(3):283-287. doi:10.1038/
sj.pcan.4500955.

8 Chowdhury R, Abbas A, Idriz S, Hoy A, Rutherford EE, Smart JM. Should
warfarin or aspirin be stopped prior to prostate biopsy? An analysis of
bleeding complications related to increasing sample number regimes. *Clin
Radiol.* 2012;67(12):e64-70. doi:10.1016/j.crad.2012.08.005.

9 Helfand BT, Glaser AP, Rimar K, et al. Prostate cancer diagnosis is associated with an increased risk of erectile dysfunction after prostate biopsy. *BJU
Int.* 2013;111(1):38-43. doi:10.1111/j.1464-410X.2012.11268.x.

10 Nam RK, Saskin R, Lee Y, et al. Increasing hospital admission rates for urological complications after transrectal ultrasound guided prostate biopsy. *J
Urol.* 2013;189(1 Suppl):S12-7-8. doi:10.1016/j.juro.2012.11.015.

11 Zani EL, Clark OAC, Rodrigues Netto N. Antibiotic prophylaxis for transrectal prostate biopsy. *Cochrane database Syst Rev.* 2011;(5):CD006576.
doi:10.1002/14651858.CD006576.pub2.

12 Feliciano J, Teper E, Ferrandino M, et al. The incidence of fluoroquinolone resistant infections after prostate biopsy--are fluoroquinolones still effective prophylaxis? *J Urol.* 2008;179(3):952-5; discussion 955. doi:10.1016/j.juro.2007.10.071.

13 Carignan A, Roussy J-F, Lapointe V, Valiquette L, Sabbagh R, Pépin J. Increasing risk of infectious complications after transrectal ultrasound-guided prostate biopsies: time to reassess antimicrobial prophylaxis? *Eur Urol.* 2012;62(3):453-459. doi:10.1016/j.eururo.2012.04.044.

14 Taylor AK, Zembower TR, Nadler RB, et al. Targeted antimicrobial prophylaxis using rectal swab cultures in men undergoing transrectal ultrasound guided prostate biopsy is associated with reduced incidence of postoperative infectious complications and cost of care. *J Urol.* 2012;187(4):1275-1279. doi:10.1016/j.juro.2011.11.115.

15 Park DS, Hwang JH, Choi DK, et al. Control of infective complications of transrectal prostate biopsy. *Surg Infect (Larchmt).* 2014;15(4):431-436. doi:10.1089/sur.2013.138.

16 Sarkar S, Das S. A Review of Imaging Methods for Prostate Cancer Detection. *Biomed Eng Comput Biol.* 2016;7(Suppl 1):1-15. doi:10.4137/BECB.S34255.

17 Jiang X, Zhang J, Tang J, et al. Magnetic resonance imaging - ultrasound fusion targeted biopsy outperforms standard approaches in detecting prostate cancer: A meta-analysis. *Mol Clin Oncol.* 2016;5(2):301-309. doi:10.3892/mco.2016.906.

18 Alcover J, Filella X. Identification of Candidates for Active Surveillance: Should We Change the Current Paradigm? *Clin Genitourin Cancer.* 2015;13(6):499-504. doi:10.1016/j.clgc.2015.06.001.

19 Newcomb LF, Brooks JD, Carroll PR, et al. Canary Prostate Active Surveillance Study: design of a multi-institutional active surveillance cohort and biorepository. *Urology.* 2010;75(2):407-413. doi:10.1016/j.urology.2009.05.050.

20 Reichard CA, Stephenson AJ, Klein EA. Applying precision medicine to the active surveillance of prostate cancer. *Cancer.* 2015;121(19):3403-3411. doi:10.1002/cncr.29496.

21 Magnan S, Zarychanski R, Pilote L, et al. Intermittent vs Continuous Androgen Deprivation Therapy for Prostate Cancer. *JAMA Oncol.* 2015;1(9):1261. doi:10.1001/jamaoncol.2015.2895.

22 Fang F, Keating NL, Mucci LA, et al. Immediate Risk of Suicide and Cardiovascular Death After a Prostate Cancer Diagnosis: Cohort Study in the United States. Journal of the National Cancer Institute 2010;102:307-14. PMID: 20124521.

3 Llorente MD, Burke M, Gregory GR, et al. Prostate cancer: a significant risk factor for late-life suicide. Am J Geriatr Psychiatry 2005; 13:195–201.

4 *The Complete Skinny on Obesity.* La Jolla: University of California Television; 2014.

5 Mercola J. *mercola.com.* Take Control of Your Health. 2016. Available at *http://www.mercola.com/.* Accessed January 7, 2016.

# ABOUT THE AUTHORS

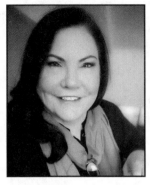

**EMILIA A. RIPOLL, MD** - Dr. Ripoll has been practicing urology and urologic oncology in the Denver metro area for more than 25 years.

Born in Barcelona, Spain and educated in the United States, Dr. Ripoll graduated from the University of Colorado School of Medicine with honors, did her residency and post-doctorate fellowship at Baylor College of Medicine, and received her medical acupuncture training at UCLA.

As an American Urological Association Foundation Scholar, Dr. Ripoll researched genetic predisposition and the role of proto-oncogenes in the development of prostate cancer.

For more information about Emilia A. Ripoll, visit *emiliaripollmd.com*

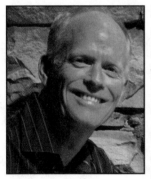

**MARK B. SAUNDERS** is a writer, editor, and 10-year cancer survivor. As an active surveillance prostate cancer patient, Mark did not receive traditional treatment like surgery or some form of radiation. Instead, he dramatically overhauled his lifestyle — and his cancer went away — and hasn't come back since.

As a prostate cancer survivor, Mark has dedicated his life to sharing what he has learned about health and wellness. A journey that he calls, "Inside out, round-about, and back again."

For more information about Mark B. Saunders, visit *markbsaunders.com*

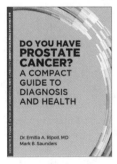

Dr. Emilia A. Ripoll and Mark B. Saunders are also the authors of ***Do You Have Prostate Cancer? A Compact Guide to Diagnosis and Health***. This book is for men who have had some unusual prostate test results but have not received a prostate cancer diagnosis. For more information, visit *health-otb.com*

**NOTES:**

**NOTES:**

**TES:**

**NOTES:**